# The Geripause

MEDICAL MANAGEMENT
DURING THE LATE MENOPAUSE

# The Geripause

## MEDICAL MANAGEMENT DURING THE LATE MENOPAUSE

**BERNARD A. ESKIN,** MD
*Drexel University College of Medicine, Philadelphia, PA*

AND

**BRUCE R. TROEN,** MD
*University of Miami School of Medicine, Miami, FL*

## The Parthenon Publishing Group
### International Publishers in Medicine, Science & Technology

A CRC PRESS COMPANY
BOCA RATON    LONDON    NEW YORK    WASHINGTON, D.C.

**Library of Congress Cataloging-in-Publication Data**
The geripause : medical management during the late
menopause/B.A. Eskin and B.R. Troen
   p. ; cm.
  Includes bibliographical references and index.
  ISBN 1-84214-037-X (alk. paper)
  1. Menopause. 2. Aged women–Health and hygiene.
I. Eskin, Bernard A. II. Troen, B. R. (Bruce R.)
[DNLM: 1. Aged, 80 and over. 2. Postmenopause.
WP 580 G369 2002]
RG186 .G477 2002
618.97′0082–dc21
                      2002192652

**British Library Cataloguing in Publication Data**

Eskin, Bernard A.
  The geripause : medical management during the late
menopause
  1.Middle aged women – Health and hygiene
I. Title  II.Troen, B. R.
613′.0434

ISBN 184214037X

Published in the USA by
The Parthenon Publishing Group
345 Park Avenue South, 10th Floor
New York, NY 10010, USA

Published in the UK and Europe by
The Parthenon Publishing Group
23–25 Blades Court, Deodar Road
London SW15 2NU, UK

Copyright © 2003 The Parthenon Publishing Group

Typeset by Siva Math Setters, Chennai, India

Printed and bound by Bookcraft (Bath) Ltd.,
Midsomer Norton, UK

# Contents

# List of Contributors

**Neil Alexander**, MD
Division of Geriatric Medicine
University of Michigan
1500 East Medical Center Drive
Ann Arbor, MI 48109-0926
USA

**Hugh R.K. Barber**, MD
Cornell University College of Medicine
Lenox Hill Hospital
100 East 77th Street
New York, NY 10021-1883
USA

**Tamara G. Bavendam**, MD
Centers for Women's Health
MCP-Hahnemann University
Philadelphia, PA 19129
USA

**Alan P. Berg**, PhD, MD
Home Visit Doctor
1 Penn Boulevard
Philadelphia, PA 19144
USA

**Brian M. Berger**, MD
Beth Israel Medical Center
Harvard Medical School
and
Boston IVF
The South Shore Center
2300 Crown Colony Drive
Quincy, MA 02169
USA

**Melissa M. Bottrell**, MPH, PHD
Division of Nursing
New York University
6th Floor, 246 Greene St
New York, NY 10003
USA

**Christine Cassel**, MD
School of Medicine
Oregon Health and Science University
3181 SW Sam Jackson Park Road
Portland, OR 97239
USA

**William P. Castelli**, MD
Boston University School of Medicine
and
Framingham Cardiovascular Institute
Metrowest Medical Center
115 Lincoln Street
Framingham, MA 01702
USA

**Karen L. Dahlman**, PhD
Department of Psychiatry
The Mount Sinai School of Medicine
Box 1230
One Gustave L. Levy Place
New York, NY 10029
USA

**Nina S. Davis**, MD, FACS
Centers for Women's Health
MCP-Hahnemann University
Philadelphia, PA 19129
USA

**Helen K. Edelberg**, MD, MPH
Brookdale Department of Geriatrics and
  Adult Development
The Mount Sinai School of Medicine
Box 1070
One Gustave L. Levy Place
New York, NY 10029-6574
USA

**Bernard A. Eskin, MS, MD**
Department of Obstetrics
   and Gynecology
Center for Menopause and Geripause
Drexel University College of Medicine
3300 Henry Avenue
Philadelphia, PA 19129
USA

**Karen E. Hall, MD, PhD**
Division of Geriatric Medicine
Department of Internal Medicine
University of Michigan
2215 Fuller Road
Ann Arbor, MI 48105-2399
USA

**Angela M. Inzerillo, MD**
Division of Endocrinology, Diabetes
   and Bone Disease
Departments of Medicine and Geriatric
   and Adult Development
The Mount Sinai School of Medicine
Box 1055
One Gustave L. Levy Place
New York, NY 10029
USA

**Rosanne M. Leipzig, MD, PhD**
Brookdale Department of Geriatrics
   and Adult Development
The Mount Sinai School of Medicine
Box 1070
One Gustave L. Levy Place
New York, NY 10029
USA

**Richard C. Mohs, PhD**
Department of Psychiatry
The Mount Sinai School of Medicine
Box 1230
One Gustave L. Levy Place
New York, NY 10029
USA

**Isaac Schiff, MD**
Harvard Medical School
and
Women's Care Division
Massachusetts General Hospital
Boston, MA
USA

**Margaret C. Sewell, PhD**
Department of Psychiatry
The Mount Sinai School of Medicine
Box 1230
One Gustave L. Levy Place
New York, NY 10029
USA

**Frederick T. Sherman, MD, MSc**
Brookdale Department of Geriatrics
   and Adult Development
The Mount Sinai School of Medicine
70 East 96th Street 7A
New York, NY 10128-0749
USA

**Bruce R. Troen, MD**
Division of Gerontology and Geriatric
   Medicine
Department of Medicine
University of Miami School of Medicine
Miami Veterans Affairs Geriatric Research
   Education and Clinical Center
11 GRC
1201 NW 16 Street
Miami, FL  33125
USA

**Mone Zaidi, MD, PhD**
Division of Endocrinology,
   Diabetes and Bone Disease
Departments of Medicine and
   Geriatric and Adult Development
The Mount Sinai School of Medicine
Box 1055
One Gustave L. Levy Place
New York, NY 10029
USA

# Foreword

*Geripause* is the felicitous term coined by Bernard Eskin to describe a newly defined phase in the feminine life cycle. Geripause is seen to begin just after menopause, with its loss of reproductive capability, and covers the time of anatomic and hormonal changes due to aging that set in during these postmenopausal years. The present text is unique in that it makes every effort to treat reproductive loss and physiologic aging as separately evolving entities. It should prove invaluable to all physicians who care for women in their later years. Authors Eskin and Bruce Troen, a gynecologist/ endocrinologist and a gerontologist, respectively, have also included in their book authoritative chapters written by researchers in diverse fields of expertise, which provide both basic and clinical information concerning the medical, endocrine, psychologic, and sociologic aspects of aging.

The book is divided into three sections. In the first, *The Effects of Age*, the demographics of aging are seen to project an evident increase in the postmenopausal population, because of the rise in human survival. This section assesses and responds to the growing demands of a knowledgeable and interested aging population. The unique aspects of caring for the geriatric patient – such as the inevitable physiological deceleration, patient attitude, and physician strategies – are discussed, and examples furnished. The observations made will certainly provide the concerned physician with a new outlook on patient expectations. Several chapters describe conditions that relate mainly to aging while simultaneously evaluating the loss of reproductive status and estrogen deficiency. Both conditions show major effects on the endocrinology, pharmacology, cognition, sexuality, and gynecology of the mature woman. The clinical conditions are described and potential preventive and therapeutic approaches are addressed. It's unfortunately the case that the physiology/pathology of the mature woman has been studied only in recent decades, so that much of the information we now possess remains controversial. The clinical data that have been obtained from trials are described and discussed. On the basis of this knowledge, practical approaches are outlined to assist in diagnosis and treatment of various conditions.

In the second section, *Care of the Older Patient*, the general gerontologic concepts that apply to all patients are discussed. In women, however, menopause brings on a complex of deficiencies from reproductive loss, particularly a severe reduction in estrogen and other related hormones. The geripausal woman thus faces additional problems both from residual menopausal symptoms and aging itself. In menopausal women, therapies to deal with sex hormone loss are also a consideration. This section presents an update of available treatments with hormones and with alternative medications. The geriatric factors dealt with include the neuromuscular, cardiovascular, skeletal, urologic, and gastroenterologic – all of them with specific reference to the geripausal woman. Both medical and surgical approaches to particular postmenopausal and geripausal conditions are informatively discussed.

In the third section, *Conclusions and Commentary*, end-of-life care is given the serious attention it deserves. Ethical aspects are reviewed in light of medical treatments available. The question of whether these therapies provide a better quality of daily life is sensitively discussed. The authors further discuss the period they refer to as late geripause, the terminal phase of a woman's life. The emotional and social support provided at the time of death also comprises an essential component of basic medical care. Thus the authors define desirable clinical care in elderly women and balance the discussion by opposing the benefits of treatment with the risks and burdens involved.

By singling it out and by actually naming it, authors Eskin and Troen have focused attention on an important period in a woman's life that may have been lost in the medical shuffle. No longer. With this book, which brings together as it does our present knowledge of the postmenopausal and geripausal states, serious interest in the health and well-being of elderly women is sure to grow and, with the growth of that interest, an assured improvement in the quality and style of the life of these women is sure to follow. *The Geripause: Medical Management During the Late Menopuase* is an important and most welcome contribution to the literature.

Isaac Schiff, MD
Joe Vincent Megis Professor
Harvard Medical School
and
Chief, Vincent Memorial Obstetrics
and Gynecology Service
Massachusetts General Hospital

# Preface

Our society is undergoing a profound transformation. The latter part of the twentieth century and the first half of the twenty-first century will bear witness to a remarkable increase in the percentage of older people. While seen at all ages over 65, this phenomenon is particularly striking for those over the age of 85. Undoubtedly this demographic shift will exert significant changes upon our culture, not least of which will be our approach to maintaining the health of our population. We strongly believe that many, if not most, health care providers will need to enhance their knowledge and skills to help care for both those who are aging successfully and are relatively healthy, and those that are beset with the burden of multiple illnesses. Towards this end, we have sought to provide a primer describing the age-related changes and diseases associated with the later stages in life that we have identified as the geripause. In *The Geripause: Medical Management During the Late Menopause*, we have chosen to focus on the aging woman. However, many of the basic principles in this book are applicable to men. We hope that our book will not only be a resource to the practitioner, but that it will enhance the awareness of the geripause, act as a starting point for future and ongoing learning by health care providers, and ultimately help to improve the quality of life of our older patients.

*Bernard A. Eskin*, MD
*Bruce R. Troen*, MD

# Acknowledgements

We are grateful to Parthenon/CRC Press Publisher David Bloomer and United States Editor Nat Russo for their interest and assistance in introducing this new life phase of women's health. "Thank you" to our Editor Stephen Nicholls for his precise monitoring and expedition of this textbook. We extend our appreciation to all of our contributors, and the assistance of Dr. Morton Schiff. We are particularly appreciative to Lynn Eskin for her work in collating and preparing the chapters for the editorial staff at Parthenon.

I personally thank my wife, Lynn, for her patience and understanding of the time spent on this new book venture (BAE).

I appreciate greatly the support, patience, and understanding that my wife, Suzanne, has given me for the time that I have been devoting to my professional activities and the development of this book (BRT).

# Part I
# The Effects of Age

# 1

# Geripause

*Bruce R. Troen*

## Introduction

A demographic revolution is occurring that will change the landscape of medical care. The growth in numbers of people aged 65 and older is greater than that of the general population, and the most rapid increase is occurring in the group aged 85 and above. This pattern will be maintained and even accelerate in the next 35 years. Therefore, not only are there more elderly, but also there are more of the oldest old. The ramifications of such a population shift are profound and will force us to reassess our notions of 'old age' and the approach to delivering medical care to these patients. This will be especially important for women, who are a significant majority of those 65 and older. Until recently, the phases of maturity for a woman were composed of childbearing age (premenopausal), followed by the menopause (or a perimenopausal period) and ending in a postmenopausal state. It is now clear that the term postmenopausal insufficiently describes the years after menopause. Instead, the post-menopausal period is more the penultimate stage of life and is increasingly often the prelude to a prolonged epoch for many women – the geripause. In order to provide the best possible care, we must approach the geripausal/geriatric patient in a manner that recognizes that the patient's physiology and response to stress and illness are markedly different from those at earlier times in life.

## Demography

The average/median life span (also known as life expectancy) is represented by the age at which 50% of a given population survive, and the maximum life span potential (MLSP) represents the longest-lived member(s) of the population or species. The average life span of humans has increased dramatically over time, yet the MLSP has remained approximately constant and is usually stated to be 90–100 years (Figure 1)[1]. For 99% of our existence as a species, the average life expectancy for humans was very short compared to the present. During the Bronze Age (circa 3000 BC), the average life expectancy was 18 years, owing to disease and accidents. Average life expectancy in 275 BC was still only 26 years. By 1900 improved sanitation helped to improve the average life expectancy at birth for humans to 47 years, but infectious disease was still a major killer. From 1995, better diet, health care and reduced infant mortality has resulted in an average life expectancy of 76 years[2]. The increase in the average life expectancy has resulted in a compression of morbidity and mortality (a rectangularization of the survival curve) towards the end of the lifespan (Figure 1). Evidence for the continuation of this trend is the increase in life expectancy at the age of 65 by 3.3 years since 1960[3]. In 1997, people reaching the age of 65 had an average life expectancy of 17.6 more years (19 for females and 15.8 for males). From 1991, 85 year olds have had an average life expectancy of more than 5 years[3]. Life expectancy at birth has also continued to increase (Table 1). The longest-lived human for whom documentation exists was Jeanne Calment, who died at the age of 122 in August 1997. The longest-lived male was Christian

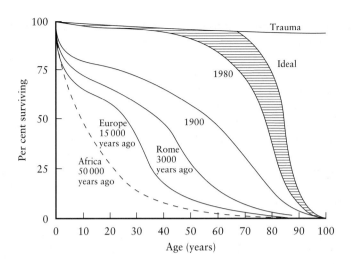

**Figure 1** Per cent survival curve for humans at different times in history with varying environments, nutrition and medical care. The 50% survival values have improved, but maximum life span potential has remained the same (adapted from reference 1).

**Table 1** Life expectancy at birth by race and sex: USA, 1940–96 (data from reference 42)

| | All races | | | Caucasian | | | All other | | | | | |
| | | | | | | | Total | | | African-American | | |
| Year | Both sexes | Male | Female | Both sexes | Male | Female | Both sexes | Male | Female | Both sexes | Male | Female |
|---|---|---|---|---|---|---|---|---|---|---|---|---|
| 1996 | 76.1 | 73.1 | 79.1 | 76.8 | 73.9 | 79.7 | 72.6 | 68.9 | 76.1 | 70.2 | 66.1 | 74.2 |
| 1990 | 75.4 | 71.8 | 78.8 | 76.1 | 72.7 | 79.4 | 71.2 | 67.0 | 75.2 | 69.1 | 64.5 | 73.6 |
| 1980 | 73.7 | 70.0 | 77.4 | 74.4 | 70.7 | 78.1 | 69.5 | 65.3 | 73.6 | 68.1 | 63.8 | 72.5 |
| 1970 | 70.8 | 67.1 | 74.7 | 71.7 | 68.0 | 75.6 | 65.3 | 61.3 | 69.4 | 64.1 | 60.0 | 68.3 |
| 1960 | 69.7 | 66.6 | 73.1 | 70.6 | 67.4 | 74.1 | 63.6 | 61.1 | 66.3 | — | — | — |
| 1950 | 68.2 | 65.6 | 71.1 | 69.1 | 66.5 | 72.2 | 60.8 | 59.1 | 62.9 | — | — | — |
| 1940 | 62.9 | 60.8 | 65.2 | 64.2 | 62.1 | 66.6 | 53.1 | 51.5 | 54.9 | — | — | — |

—, Data not available

Mortensen, who died in 1998 at the age of 115. As causes of early mortality have been eliminated through public health measures and improved medical care, more individuals have approached the maximum life span. Between 1960 and 1994, the population of those aged 85 and over grew by 274%, whereas the elderly population in general rose by 100% and the entire US population grew by only 45%[3]. The number of people aged 100 years and over has doubled since 1980. Life expectancy at birth varies depending upon gender and race; in 1996 it was almost 80 years for Caucasian females, 74 years for African-American females, 73 years for Caucasian males and 66 years for African-American males (Table 1). Continued increases in life expectancy in the 21st century, the greater life expectancy for women, and the tendency for women to marry men older than they, lead to the projection that 70% of 'baby boom' women will outlive their husbands and can expect to be widows for 15 or more years.

In 2000, those 65 and older numbered 35 million and accounted for 12.4% of the US population[4]. During the next 35 years, the number of people aged 65 and older will more than double, and the number aged 85 and older will triple[4]. Women account for a significant majority of the elderly population. In 1997, there were 20.1 million women and 14 million men aged 65 and over. This imbalance increases with age: almost 60% of those aged 65–69 are women, over 70% of those aged 85 and over are women and approximately 80% of centenarians are women[3]. The older population will continue to grow significantly in the coming decades (Figure 2). Growth slowed during the 1990s because of the relatively small number born during the Great Depression of the 1930s. By 2010, the first group of 'baby boomers' will reach the age of 65. Consequently the older population will mushroom between the years 2010 and 2030, when the 'baby boom' generation reaches age 65 and beyond[5]. Between now and 2030, the number of people 65 and older will double and account for 20% of the population. By 2050 almost 25% of the elderly will be 85 and older. One can appreciate further the increasing longevity of those who reach the age of 65 by considering the following: 14% of 65 year olds in 1960 were expected to reach the age of 90; 26% of 65 year olds in 2000 will be expected to reach the age of 90; and 42% of 65 year olds in 2050 will probably live to the age of 90[3].

## Normal aging

There is evidence supporting at least five common characteristics of aging (Table 2):

(1) *Increased mortality with age after maturation.* In the early 19th century, Gompertz first described the exponential increase in mortality with aging due to various causes, a phenomenon that still persists today[6]. In 1995, the death rate for all causes between the ages of 25 and 44 was 189.5/100 000 and for the ages of 65 and over was 5069/100 000: a > 25-fold increase[7].

(2) *Changes in biochemical composition in tissues with age.* There are notable age-related decreases in lean body mass and total bone mass in humans[8,9]. Although subcutaneous fat is either unchanged or declining, total fat remains the same[8]. Consequently, the percentage of adipose tissue increases with age. At the cellular level, many markers of aging have been described in various tissues from different organisms[10]. Two of the first to be described were increases in lipofuscin (age pigment)[11] and increased cross-linking in extracellular matrix molecules such as collagen[12,13]. Additional examples include age-related changes in both the rates of transcription of specific genes and the rate of protein synthesis' and numerous age-related alterations in post-translational protein modifications, such as glycation and oxidation[14,15].

(3) *Progressive decrease in physiological capacity with age.* Many physiological changes have been documented in both cross-sectional and longitudinal studies[16–18]. Declines in various organ systems include: cardiac output and heart rate in response to stress, peripheral blood vessel compliance, bone mineral density, cartilaginous resiliency, creatinine clearance, renal blood flow, maximum urine osmolality, forced vital capacity and expiratory volume, maximal oxygen uptake, intestinal motility, visual accommodation and acuity, color sensitivity, depth perception, high-frequency perception, speech discrimination, T-cell immune response, total sleep time and time in rapid eye movement (REM) sleep, and psychomotor performance. These decreases occur linearly from about the age of 30. However, the rate of physiological decline is quite heterogeneous from organ to organ and individual to individual[19,20]. As described in detail elsewhere in this book, women experience a dramatic decline in estrogen at the time of the menopause. Growing evidence suggests that testosterone,

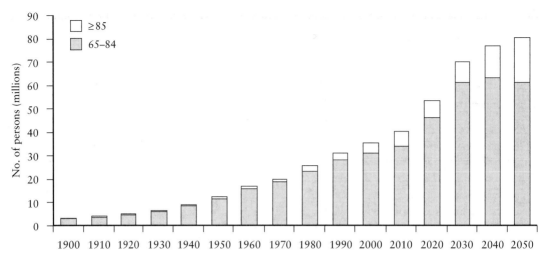

**Figure 2** Number of persons aged ≥ 65: 1900–2050 (data from reference 3)

**Table 2** Characteristics of aging

Increased mortality with age after maturation
Changes in biochemical composition in tissues with age
Progressive decrease in physiological capacity with age
Reduced ability to respond adaptively to environmental stimuli with age
Increased susceptibility and vulnerability to disease with age

dehydroepiandrosterone, and growth hormone levels also decline with age[21].

(4) *Reduced ability to respond adaptively to environmental stimuli with age.* A fundamental feature of senescence is the diminished ability to maintain homeostasis[22]. This is manifest, not primarily by changes in resting or basal parameters, but in the altered response to an external stimulus such as exercise or fasting. The loss of 'reserve' can result in blunted maximum responses as well as in delays in reaching peak levels and in returning to basal levels. For example, the response of heart rate and cardiac output to exercise and sympathetic nervous system stimulation are significantly reduced in the elderly[23].

(5) *Increased susceptibility and vulnerability to disease with age.* The incidence and mortality rates for many diseases increase with age and parallel the exponential increase in mortality with age[24]. For the five leading causes of death for people over 65, the relative increase in death rates compared with people aged 25–44 is: heart disease, 92-fold; cancer, 43-fold; stroke, > 100-fold; chronic lung disease, > 100-fold; and pneumonia and influenza, 89-fold[7]. The basis for these dramatic rises in mortality is incompletely understood, but presumably involves changes in the function of many types of cell that lead to tissue/organ dysfunction and systemic illness.

## Health status

Increasing age is accompanied by poorer health, as manifested by higher disease rates

**Table 3** Leading causes of death in people 65 years and over in the USA in 1996 (adapted from reference 41)

| Cause | All people | | Men | | Women | |
|---|---|---|---|---|---|---|
| | % | Rate | % | Rate | % | Rate |
| Cardiovascular | 35.7 | 1808 | 35.2 | 1983 | 36.2 | 1686 |
| Cancer | 22.3 | 1131 | 25.6 | 1442 | 19.6 | 915 |
| Cerebrovascular | 8.2 | 415 | 6.6 | 374 | 9.5 | 443 |
| Chronic obstructive pulmonary disease and allied conditions | 5.3 | 270 | 6.0 | 338 | 4.8 | 223 |
| Pneumonia and influenza | 4.4 | 221 | 4.2 | 236 | 4.5 | 212 |
| Diabetes | 2.7 | 137 | 2.5 | 139 | 2.9 | 136 |
| Accidents and adverse effects | 1.8 | 91 | 1.9 | 110 | 1.7 | 78 |
| Alzheimer's disease | 1.3 | 62 | 0.9 | 49 | 1.5 | 71 |
| Renal | 1.2 | 62 | 1.2 | 70 | 1.2 | 56 |
| Septicemia | 1.0 | 51 | 0.9 | 50 | 1.1 | 52 |

Rate, per 100 000 population

and increasing levels of frailty and disability. More than a quarter of those over 65 categorize their own health as fair or poor[25]. The leading causes of death in the elderly are listed in Table 3. Cardiovascular disease caused the most deaths in this age group in 1996. Cancer was responsible for the second highest number of deaths. Given the growth of the elderly population, the number of incident cancers is projected to more than double in the first part of the 21st century[26]. Most people over 65 report at least one chronic ailment, including (in descending prevalence) arthritis, hypertension, heart disease, diminished hearing, cataracts, orthopedic impairment, sinusitis, and diabetes (see Table 3). Cerebrovascular disease rates quadruple, heart disease rates triple, and arthritis and hypertension rates double between the perimenopausal era (45–64 years) and the geripause (≥ 65 years). Women suffer from higher rates of arthritis and hypertension, whereas men have higher rates of heart disease and hearing impairment. Several conditions that do not explicitly appear in Table 3 merit mention. There are more than 1.3 million osteoporotic fractures a year in the USA, including 500 000 in the spine, 250 000 in the hip and 240 000 in the wrist[27]. This results in significant morbidity (manifest often as decreased mobility) and economic cost. Up to 50% of women above the age of 50 are osteopenic and 18% are osteoporotic[28]. One-third of all women and one-sixth of all men who reach the age of 90 suffer a hip fracture; 26% of hospital discharges for hip fracture in 1994 were for men[28]. Urinary incontinence affects 15–30% of community dwelling elderly and up to 50% of those in long-term care facilities[29]. Perimenopausal women experience more stress incontinence, whereas urge and mixed incontinence predominate in the elderly[30]. Incontinence is associated with isolation, depression and the risk of institutionalization. Dementia is one of the most common causes of disability in the elderly. More than 25% of those aged 85, and more than 50% of those aged 95 and over suffer dementia[31]. Alzheimer's disease accounts for two-thirds or more of dementia, with a prevalence in the community dwellers of 10% of those over 65 years and 47% of those older than 85[32]. Because women have a longer life expectancy, they experience a higher rate of dementia. It is interesting to note that out-patient screening for breast and cervical cancer is decreased in women with a higher number of chronic conditions[33].

Frailty in the elderly has a distinct phenotype that includes unexplained weight loss,

**Table 4** Chronic conditions (per 1000 persons) by age (years) in the USA in 1996 (data from reference 25)

|  | All 45–64 | All ≥ 65 | Male ≥ 65 | Female ≥ 65 |
|---|---|---|---|---|
| Arthritis | 233 | 490 | 405 | 550 |
| Hypertension | 223 | 403 | 349 | 442 |
| Heart disease | 121 | 308 | 367 | 224 |
| Hearing impairment | 145 | 284 | 362 | 268 |
| Deformity/orthopedic impairment | 176 | 178 | 166 | 187 |
| Chronic sinusitis | 179 | 153 | 135 | 167 |
| Diabetes mellitus | 64 | 126 | 124 | 128 |
| Cerebrovascular disease | 15 | 71 | 80 | 65 |

**Table 5** Disability prevalence with age (data from reference 42)

| Age (years) | Any disability | Severe disability | Difficulty with ≥ 1 ADL | Difficulty with ≥ 1 IADL | Needs personal assistance with ≥ 1 ADL or IADL |
|---|---|---|---|---|---|
| 45–54 | 24.5 | 11.5 | 3.1 | 4.5 | 3.3 |
| 55–64 | 36.3 | 21.9 | 6.0 | 8.1 | 6.1 |
| 65–79 | 47.3 | 27.8 | 10.5 | 15.3 | 11.5 |
| ≥ 80 | 71.5 | 53.5 | 27.5 | 40.4 | 34.1 |

ADL, activities of daily living; IADL, instrumental activities of daily living

exhaustion, weak grip, slow walking speed and low energy[34]. Of those 65 years and older living alone, 7% had at least three criteria for frailty, while 46% had none. Women, African-Americans, people 75 years and older, the less educated and the poor are more likely to be frail. The most common co-existing illnesses in the frail include arthritis, hypertension and diabetes. Over a period of 3 years, frail elderly suffered more falls, worsening mobility and disability, hospitalization and, most importantly, death. After 7 years, 43% of those who were frail died, compared to 12% of those who had no initial indicators of frailty. Increasing numbers of studies now show that frail elders are more likely to suffer prolonged or repeated hospitalizations and undergo protracted or limited recovery[35]. Triggers for such events often include multiple co-morbid conditions and possibly a fall and/or fracture. The loss of homeostatic reserve (including increased reaction time, decreased strength, decreased vision) and the presence of osteoporosis and/or polypharmacy probably play important roles in worsening the outcomes of

acute illness in the frail elderly. Fortunately, knowledge of the phenotype of frailty will hopefully permit the development of better assessment tools and interventions to enhance the health of frail elders.

Many of the elderly suffer from multiple chronic, conditions, and these restrict the activities of older people (Table 4). Over 50% of those 65 and over reported at least one disability, with a third experiencing severe disabilities. Women spend approximately twice as many years disabled prior to death as their male counterparts[36]. With increasing age, disabilities and difficulties performing activities of daily living (ADL) and instrumental activities of daily living (IADL) become more prevalent (Table 5). ADL include bathing, dressing, eating, and ambulation[37]. IADL include meal preparation, shopping, managing money, using the telephone, doing housework and laundry, having the ability to travel, and taking medication[38]. It is important to note, however, that over 70% of people aged 65 and over report their health status as good, very good, or excellent, despite the prevalence of chronic conditions in this group[25]. Furthermore, despite the prevalence of chronic conditions and increasing disability, more than 90% of the elderly live in the community and 75% of those 85 and older still live at home.

## Conclusion

As described above, the number of people 65 years and older will continue to increase dramatically well into the 21st century. The physiology of the elderly and their response to pathology markedly differ from those of younger individuals, including women who are premenopausal and perimenopausal. Furthermore, the most explosive growth will occur in the group of people 85 years and older. We are beginning to learn that these 'old' old may represent a distinct subgroup in the elderly population. Indeed, in the not too distant future, we may use the term 'elderly' to refer to those 85 and over. Despite the prevalence of chronic illness and the rapid age-related increase in mortality in those 65 and over, there is some

evidence to suggest that future cohorts may be healthier. Manton and co-workers reported that age-related disability declined between 1982 and 1994[39]. In addition, since 1953, Americans have engaged in healthier behaviors: per capita tobacco consumption has declined by 40%, butter consumption is down one-third, use of whole milk and cream is down one-fourth, and the use of saturated animal fats in cooking is down by 40%[40]. It is possible that such behaviors, often associated with the 'baby boomers' as they have matured, may reduce future rates of chronic disease. These changes, along with advances in health care, may continue to fuel the increase in life expectancy that has been driving the rectangularization of the survivorship curve. It is unknown what impact there will be on health-care utilization. At the very least, it has become clear that the demographic shift towards a progressively aged and aging population will necessitate that providers pay more and more attention to maintaining and enhancing the health of the elderly.

# References

1. Cutler RG. Evolutionary perspective of human longevity. In Hazzard WR, Andres R, Bierman EL, et al., eds. *Principles of Geriatric Medicine and Gerontology*. New York: McGraw-Hill, 1985:16
2. Monthly Vital Statistics Report. National Center for Health Statistics, Hattysville, MD, 1997;45 No. 11(S)2
3. Hobbs FB, Damon BL. *65+ in the United States*. U.S. Bureau of the Census. Current Population Reports, Special Studies, P23-90. Washington, DC, 1996
4. Administration on Aging. *A Profile of Older Americans: 2001*. US Department of Health and Human Services. Washington, DC, 2001
5. Day JC. *Population Projections of the United States by age, sex, race, and Hispanic Origin: 1995 to 2050*. Current Population Reports, Series P25-1130. Washington, DC, 1996
6. Gompertz B. On the nature of the function expressive of the law of human mortality and on a new mode of determining life contingencies. *Philos Trans R Soc Lond* 1825;115:513
7. Rosenberg HM, Ventura SJ, Maurer JD, et al. Births and deaths: United States, 1995. *Monthly Vital Stat Rep* 1996;45:31–3
8. Shock NW, Greulich RC, Andres R, et al. *Normal Human Aging: The Baltimore Longitudinal Study of Aging*. Washington, DC: US Department of Health and Human Services, 1984
9. Riggs BL, Melton LD. Involutional osteoporosis. *N Engl J Med* 1986;314:1676–86
10. Florini JR. Composition and function of cells and tissues. In Florini JR, ed. *Handbook of Biolochemistry in Aging*. Boca Raton: CRC Press, 1981
11. Strehler BL. *Time, Cells, and Aging*. New York: Academic Press, 1977
12. Bjorksten J. Cross linkage and the aging process. In Rothstein M, ed. *Theoretical Aspects of Aging*. New York: Academic Press, 1974:43
13. Kohn RR. Aging of animals: possible mechanisms. *Principles of Mammalian Aging*. Englewood Cliffs, NJ: Prentice-Hall, 1978

14. Finch CE. Introduction: Definitions and concepts. Longevity, Senescence, and the Genome. Chicago: University of Chicago Press, 1990

15. Levine RL, Stadtman ER. Protein modifications with aging. In Schneider EL, Rowe JW, eds. *Handbook of the Biology of Aging*. San Diego: Academic Press, 1996:184–97

16. Shock NW. Longitudinal studies of aging in humans. In Finch CE, Schneider EL, eds. *Handbook of the Biology of Aging*. New York: Van Nostrand Reinhold, 1985:721

17. Kane RL, Ouslander JG, Abrass IB. *Clinical Implications of the Aging Process. Essentials of Clinical Geriatrics*. New York: McGraw-Hill Health Professions Division, 1999:3–18

18. Taffet GE. Age-related physiologic changes. In Cobbs EL, Duthie EH, Murphy JB, eds. *Geriatric Review Syllabus*. Dubuque, IA: Kendall/Hunt Publishing, 1999:10–23

19. Lakatta EG. Changes in cardiovascular function with aging. *Eur Heart J* 1990;11(Suppl. C): 22–9

20. Lindeman RD, Tobin J, Shock NW. Longitudinal studies on the rate of decline in renal function with age. *J Am Geriatr Soc* 1985;33:278–85

21. Roshan S, Nader S, Orlander P. Ageing and hormones. *Eur J Clin Invest* 1999;29:210–13

22. Adelman RC, Britton GW, Rotenberg S, *et al.* Endocrine regulation of gene activity in aging animals of different genotypes. In Bergsma D, Harrison DE, eds. *Genetic Effects on Aging*. New York: Alan R Liss, 1978:355

23. Lakatta EG. Cardiovascular aging research: the next horizons. *J Am Geriatr Soc* 1999;47: 613–25

24. Brody JA, Brock DB. Epidemiological and statistical characteristics of the United States elderly population. In Finch CE, Schneider EL, eds. *Handbook of the Biology of Aging*. New York: Van Nostrand Reinhold, 1985:3

25. Benson V, Marano MA. *Current Estimates from the National Health Interview Survey, 1995*. National Center for Health Statistics, Vital Health and Statistics, Hattysville, MD. 1998;10

26. Polednak AP. Projected numbers of cancers diagnosed in the US elderly population, 1990 through 2030. *Am J Public Health* 1994; 84:1313–16

27. Christiansen C. Consensus development conference: diagnosis, prophylaxis, and treatment of osteoporosis. *Am J Med* 1993;94:646–50

28. Looker AC, Orwoll ES, Johnston CC Jr, *et al.* Prevalence of low femoral bone density in older U.S. adults from NHANES III [see comments]. *J Bone Miner Res* 1997;12:1761–8

29. Resnick NM. Urinary incontinence. *Lancet* 1995;346:94–9

30. Thom D. Variation in estimates of urinary incontinence prevalence in the community: effects of differences in definition, population characteristics, and study type. *J Am Geriatr Soc* 1998;46:473–80

31. Ebly EM, Parhad IM, Hogan DB, Fung TS. Prevalence and types of dementia in the very old: results from the Canadian Study of Health and Aging [see comments]. *Neurology* 1994; 44:1593–600

32. Evans DA, Funkenstein HH, Albert MS, *et al.* Prevalence of Alzheimer's disease in a community population of older persons. Higher than previously reported. *J Am Med Assoc* 1989; 262:2551–6

33. Kiefe CI, Funkhouser E, Fouad MN, May DS. Chronic disease as a barrier to breast and cervical cancer screening. *J Gen Intern Med* 1998;13:357–65

34. Fried LP, Tangen CM, Walston J, *et al.* Frailty in older adults: evidence for a phenotype. *J Gerontol A Biol Sci Med Sci* 2001;56: M146–56

35. Perry HM 3rd. The endocrinology of aging. *Clin Chem* 1999;45:1369–76

36. La Croix AZ, Newton KM, Leveille SG, Wallace J. Healthy aging. A women's issue. *West J Med* 1997;167:220–32

37. Katz S, Downs TD, Cash HR, Grotz RC. Progress in development of the index of ADL. *Gerontologist* 1970;10:20–30

38. Lawton MP, Brody EM. Assessment of older people: self-maintaining and instrumental activities of daily living. *Gerontologist* 1969;9: 179–86

39. Manton KG, Stallard E, Corder LS. The dynamics of dimensions of age-related disability 1982 to 1994 in the U.S. elderly population. *J Gerontol A Biol Sci Med Sci* 1998;53: B59–70

40. Longino CF. Myths of an aging America. *American Demographics* 1994;16:36–42

41. Peters KD, Kochanek KD, Murphy SL. *Deaths: Final Data for 1996. National Vital Statistics Reports*, vol. 47. Hyattsville, MD: National Center for Health Statistics, 1998

42. McNeil JM. Americans with disabilities: 1994-95. US Bureau of the Census. Current Population Reports, P70-61. US Department of Commerce, Washington, DC, 1997

# 2

# Diversity of health-related attitudes and strategies of older patients

*Alan P. Berg*

## Introduction

This chapter is one geriatrician's attempt to make explicit some of the subjective lives of older people facing illness. There are two key sections. The first focuses on attitudes, the biases of individuals and how these influence health-related behaviors and responses to illness. The second focuses broadly on some strategies that individuals might employ to provide relief from an illness and promote their health. Inevitably, we will look beyond the individual to the social and demographic contexts within which decision-making occurs.

A variety of attitudes and strategies are documented, testimony to the fact that each of us lives a singular life, each life trajectory and pattern of aging unique. For each person, life is perceived somewhat differently from that of all others, even when compared to members of the same household. Moreover, for any one person, perceptions about health evolve over the years. This chapter attempts to elaborate on such diversity.

Inadvertent wisdom from a 97-year-old patient:

'Doctor, I don't understand what is happening.'
'Please tell me more, Mrs Klein'
'Well, for one thing, I've never been this old before.'

## Illness, health and health care

Illness and health are common words with well understood, but often ill-defined meanings.

Before using these terms, some definitions might be useful[1]. Illness will refer to individual suffering, whereas disease will refer to medically definable pathology. A person may be ill without disease, or diseased without being ill. Medicine deals well with diseases.

'Health' may be harder to define so directly, because the term is used in so many ways, ranging from 'full functioning of all internal organs' to the utopian statement of the World Health Organization that health is 'a state of complete physical, mental, and social well-being and not merely the absence of disease or infirmity'. Nevertheless, there is broad agreement that health is good in itself, as well as a means or precondition for normal functioning. Good health implies functioning as a whole, in harmony with self and surroundings.

Factors that threaten health may include such pathogens as infections, cancer, vascular disease or trauma, all falling within the realm of medical care as usually conceived. Additional 'pathogens' might include poverty, lack of education, environmental toxins or war, all things beyond the realm of medical intervention. A person may carry a disease but function in a healthy manner. Consider this scenario: a 78-year-old woman slowly walks a mile every morning and feels healthy, whereas her doctor, documenting electrocardiogram changes at moderate levels of exertion, might conclude otherwise.

Post-Flexnerian American medicine and the stunning technical successes of recent decades often partially blind us to the fact that illness and health belong to individuals, the proper focus of care. Even with evidence-based medicine, and a focus on results and on the bottom line in much of health care, it is challenging but wise to understand the patient's concepts and responses to her own illness and health[2,3].

## Attitudes

Every geriatrician has encountered a variety of attitudes towards health and an equal diversity of personal responses to being ill. To be ill is to encounter some personal limitation, and to be challenged both physically and in existential, moral and symbolic spheres, the latter often missing from the 'H and P' (history and physical examination). While we speak of the patient, much of what is said here also applies directly to carers. Following are some scenarios illustrating responses to being ill.

For some people, being ill is a nuisance. Changes in self-perception and adjustments in lifestyle are needed. The limitations illness imposes are perceived as relatively minor. Something previously taken for granted reaches consciousness. For example, movement is less spontaneous or less comfortable. Standing balance now requires both eyes open and extra attention. Walking is more tiring. Foods once tolerated cause symptoms. Easily remembered phone numbers require a Rolodex. Nevertheless, life goes on pretty much as usual. The relation between present and future remains uncompromised and social relationships continue. There is no pressing need for urgent advance planning. The glitch (illness) will be mended, or mend itself in due time, even if medications or treatments are needed.

For some people, illness is destiny. Something has happened to make 'me' different from who I was. Health is compromised. There is loss of the usual energy, resilience, comfort, outlook. In a way, this is how it is supposed to be. For some, getting older and having disease go hand in hand; that is the expectation. As proof, one has only to look at older family members and reports on the obituary page. Expectations are

for further sickness as time goes on. One may not like it, but that's the way it is.

For some people, illness has to be dealt with, but not at the expense of work, family, religion, or recreation. Illness denied is illness tamed.

For some people, illness is an 'excuse' not to cope actively. I'm sick – leave me alone. How can I work, or care for my appearance or my family because I'm hurting?

Beneath such scenarios lie some of the personal threats of being ill, now sketched out.

The patient may feel alone, isolated, even stigmatized into avoiding social contact.

The patient may well become more dependent, less potent, and autonomous; there is loss of wholeness, of abilities, possible worries about loss of income or ability to pay for care, more need for care and loving (TLC) from family, community or hired helpers.

The patient may face loss of the familiar, and perceive deficits in self-knowledge, along with an urgent need to acquire missing information and insights.

The patient may become overwhelmed, become perplexed with all that needs to be done, begin to doubt the integrity of her or his own body, experience shrinking of future expectations and focus almost exclusively on the present, or on death.

The patient might feel a need to change some aspect of lifestyle, as this holds the promise to cure or correct the present problem. However, now there is less freedom to act. Adopting better health habits offers possible redemption.

The patient may realize that something she/he did caused all this, and she/he is afraid. There is the possible threat of a much shorter life. Then, there is the additional fear that, by emphasizing illness, the doctor will make things feel worse.

One should not conclude that all attitudes are fixed for life. In fact, attitudes can and do mutate with age[4,5].

## Strategies

All strategies for dealing with illness or for fostering health are successful to some extent when measured against the underlying assumptions of the patient. Not all strategies objectively improve health, well-being or functional status, or necessarily lessen morbidity or mortality.

People cope with illness in a multitude of ways. Which mechanisms are 'chosen' will hinge partly on the specific medical problem and its severity, as well as the kinds of personal issues (see above) unleashed by illness. The approach will be illustrative of the personal adjustments set in motion, with the primary goal of making the clinician aware of some of the complexities of real-life decision making. Some of the strategies are simple and practical, others quite sophisticated; some address immediate needs and others deep personal issues. One common strategy will be for the patient to choose a geriatrician who can appreciate their problems at many levels, counsel and be able to discuss without fear or anger many of the difficult issues facing the older patient.

Illness may reduce independence in activities of daily living, forcing a reduction in daily scope or increased dependence on others. Such becomes painfully obvious in a person who has had a stroke or major heart attack. Nevertheless, some temporary loss of independence may occur with almost any illness. When the patient lives among supportive people, and is willing to relinquish some independence, a long-term change in lifestyle may not be necessary. However, families may be small, involved in work or raising children, be themselves ill or non-supportive, or may live far away. Strategies may range from buying or renting a mechanical aid (cane, bedside commode), moving the patient's bed from a second-floor bedroom to a first-floor dining room, rearranging the schedule of a family member, finding outside help, or engaging a nursing agency.

Loss of potency or wholeness rudely strikes many ill people, even if only for a short while. Strategies range from pulling back, restricting activities and contacts, to seeking help actively as quickly as possible, to address both the particulars of the medical problems underlying the loss of wholeness and the secondary trauma of lost potency and wholeness. This is an area where counselling can help, to better understand the possibilities and time lines to healing, or help in dealing with long-term infirmity. It is also an area often inadequately discussed by both patients and their physicians.

Illness can be expensive. It strains resources in many ways, from loss of earning capacity for those still working, to increases in all sorts of expenses for almost everyone. Costs for prescriptions can increase, sometimes markedly. Family coffers can be strained when a relative has to leave work to care for an older relative, or when someone has to be hired. In this context, help available through the area offices on aging or from visiting nursing agencies may be too little, and terminate too soon. When long-term infirmity is anticipated, many people are forced to cut back on expenses, refinance their home (or take a reverse mortgage), spend down personal savings and/or consider transfer to an institution.

We are creatures of habit and inertia. Illness may force deviation from familiar routines and habits. If the old ways are quickly regained, the effects may be minimal, but for some, illness begets first distrust of the self, then distrust of the stability of the world. Strategies for dealing with loss of trust include overcoming the current illness as soon as possible, noting, improvements in functioning over time, and seeking the company of others.

All the following call for ongoing help and counseling: being overwhelmed; facing uncertainty and doubts about one's own integrity and the integrity of the world; feeling out of control of one's future; fearing the unknown; having the perception that one's options and time left are decreased; and fearing death.

So where do medical doctors and medical professionals fit in? In some ways, doctors lead, staying at the front and center of the patient's view. Not unexpectedly, people choose their doctors, expecting many differing kinds of support. Here are some of these: a provider of bad news; an ear to listen to woes and difficulties; a shoulder to lean on; a source of knowledge, who is able to tie together loose ends coherently; an expert, yet one who can communicate difficult matters simply; a mechanic, with the skill to make specific things better; a mender, to help rebalance things gone awry; a mediator of conflicts; a priest or shaman; a source of hope or at least a road to hope; and a source of inspiration.

Regardless of the specific role(s) played, the doctor is expected to 'educate' his patients following values and lines of thought brought to consciousness through his medical education, and hopefully reflecting the local society. Fortunately, within a society, there is a high level of agreement between the premises and conclusions of patients and their physicians[6], although substantial differences between the priorities of patient and physician have been documented[7].

We turn now from illness strategies to strategies for improving health. There are fascinating contrasts between dealing with illness and striving to improve health. Strategies for addressing illness attempt to alleviate pain, suffering and limitations. They must focus on the present, possibly to the exclusion of future living. Often they are rooted in the crisis of forced change. They may supplement purely medical interventions, and often require these to be effective. Strategies for improving health focus more on the future, are relatively free of crisis and may or may not include medical components, often being effective on their own. In practice, approaches to illness and to health can co-exist, complementing each other.

Examples of goals for bettering health and a few of the strategies[8] employed to foster these goals are listed below. Any one person will probably utilize only one or a few of these[9].

(1) *Increasing vitality*. Strategies might include improving nutrition quality; working towards a more ideal weight[10]; changing attitudes towards food; eating and nutrition, dieting where necessary; and working on changing body image and ideals. A key component will be integrating regular and health-appropriate exercise into one's life[11].

(2) *Increasing resistance to disease*. Strategies might include smoking cessation, some of the 'herbal remedies' (proven or not)[12] as well as choosing from among any one of numerous 'alternative' therapies, some of which are slowly being integrated into Western medicine.

(3) *Increasing one's ease of life, improving ability to relax*. Strategies might include centering; meditating, stretching and relaxing; learning to handle stress without strain; getting rid of unnecessary clutter and simplifying one's obligations; and letting go where desirable and possible.

(4) *Increasing or maintaining independence as much as possible*. Strategies might include optimizing resources for retirement, although this is not always easy[13]; fulfilling a lifelong dream, such as a vacation, or a trip to a homeland; learning to cut expenses where necessary; moving into a smaller residence or apartment (for some); adapting the current home for improved access and ease; or moving into a relative's home, a retirement community, or assisted living or nursing facility, as appropriate[14,15].

(5) *Optimizing medical resources including doctors and social services*. Strategies might include lifelong learning, learning as much as possible about one's own health problems; and becoming one's own 'local world's authority' and taking charge where possible.

(6) *Enhancing hope and faith*. Strategies might include joining groups, cultivating a sense of belonging and appreciation, even with changing roles and limitations; having the support or trust of family and community; partnering with others, as opportunities and desires allow; and joining support groups[16].

## Beyond the individual patient: a digression or a necessity?

Unique to each of us is a personal history, of both events and of past decisions. Our attitudes and strategies derive from this personal history, and incorporate those of our families, group values and our society's institutions, expectations and taboos.

At a personal level, it matters how perceptions of illness and compromise were taught to us, and at what age we first encountered illness in others and in ourselves. At what age did health concepts develop? Was there a gradual shift in priorities or was there a crisis? Have we led a lifetime aware that 'aging' begins in childhood and we can choose health, or has health been a non-issue? If sick, where are we on the road from shock to acceptance or hope? Do we have incontinence, which compromises the freedom of our social interactions (unless something is done); diabetes, where daily care and prudence do not greatly limit our interactions and functioning; or progressive and untreatable cancer, where our options are greatly limited? Are we becoming demented in such a way as to function fairly well, perhaps not as badly as others say we do?[17]

At the family level, what values have we lived by? What precepts from childhood continue to hold our attention and guide our teaching of self and others? How did our parents and elders cope with their illnesses and their deaths? What kinds of decisions can and should I make in caring for my own sick spouse or other relative? Am I ready to re-prioritize my life?

At the community level, what medical and social services are available, paid for and sanctioned? What medical models and treatments are awarded and which are shunned? Who bears the costs for various interventions? If I get very sick, will my health insurance plan be there in full? Will I be able to stay in my own home with the expectation of receiving help there? Can I afford long-term care insurance?

At the societal level, what does it mean to be old? What did it mean when we were younger? At the turn of the 20th century, far fewer people reached their eighties and nineties than do now. Then, to be 50 or 60 was 'old'. Now, the reality in First World countries is different, with substantial numbers of people leading active, able lives well into their ninth decade[18,19]. Key attitudes of many of today's older seniors were formed at a time when 'old' commonly meant something very different from what it does today[20]. How are we, as a society, going to adapt to the demographics and economics of a stable or slowly declining population, and the potential of its many older citizens to remain healthy and productive for long years?[21-23]

At the cultural level, considerable differences in assumptions, world view and outlook exist between people from various cultures and sub-cultures[24-26]. The most effective practices are those culturally familiar to the patient. Likewise, the most effective doctors are those who employ culturally familiar outlooks and treatments.

'Happiness is good health and a bad memory'

Ingrid Bergman

# References

1. Mordacci R, Sobel R. Health: a comprehensive concept. *Hastings Center Rep* 1998;28:34–7

2. Nordenfelt L. On chronic illness and quality of life: a conceptual framework. *Health Care Anal* 1995;3:277–81

3. Adelman RD, Greene MG, Ory MG. Communication between older patients and their physicians. *Clin Geriatr Med* 2000;16:1–24

4. Krosnick JA, Alwin DF. Aging and susceptibility to attitude change. *J Pers Soc Psychol* 1989;57:416–25

5. Tyler TR, Schuller RA. Aging and attitude change. *J Pers Soc Psychol* 1991;61:689–97

6. Hurwicz ML. Physicians' norms and health care decisions of elderly Medicare recipients. *Med Anthropol Q* 1995;9:211–35

7. Root MJ. Communication barriers between older women and physicians. *Public Health Rep* 1987;Suppl:152–5

8. Gilbert SB. Health promotion for older Americans. *Health Values* 1986;10:38–46

9. Berman RL, Iris MA. Approaches to self-care in late life. *Qual Health Res* 1998;8:224–36

10. Fallaz AF, Bernstein M, Van Nes MC, *et al.* Weight loss preoccupation in aging women: a review. *J Nutr Health Aging* 1999;3:177–81

11. Spencer G. The role of exercise in successful ageing. *Prof Nurse* 1999;15:105–8

12. Butler RN, Fossel M, Pan CX, *et al.* Anti-aging medicine. What makes it different from geriatrics? [Comment]. *Geriatrics* 2000;55:36, 39–43

13. Levy SM. The adjustment of the older woman: effects of chronic ill health and attitudes toward retirement. *Int J Aging Hum Dev* 1980; 12:93–110

14. Kraus AS, Spasoff RA, Beattie EJ, *et al.* Elderly applicants to long-term care institutions. I. Their characteristics, health problems and state of mind. *J Am Geriatr Soc* 1976;24:117–25

15. Brown JB, McWilliam CL, Mai V. Barriers and facilitators to seniors' independence. Perceptions of seniors, caregivers, and health care providers. *Can Fam Physician* 1997;43:469–75

16. Powell DA, Milligan WL, Furchtgott E. Interaction of physio-medical and psychosocial variables in age-related functional impairments. *Int J Aging Hum Dev* 1984;19:235–52

17. Weinberger M, Samsa GP, Schmader K, *et al.* Comparing proxy and patients' perceptions of patients' functional status: results from an out-patient geriatric clinic. *J Am Geriatr Soc* 1992; 40:585–8

18. Kerschner H, Pegues JA. Productive aging: a quality of life agenda. *J Am Diet Assoc* 1998; 98:1445–8

19. O'Reilly P, Caro FG. Productive aging: an overview of the literature. *J Aging Soc Policy* 1994;6:39–71

20. Weg RB. The image and reality of 'old': time for a change. *J Am Optom Assoc* 1982;53: 21–9

21. Somers AR. Aging in the 21st century: projections, personal preferences, public policies – a consumer view. *Health Policy* 1988;9:49–58

22. Berg RJ. Development as if all generations mattered. Presented at the 29th *Annual Educational Conference of the Senior Services of Washington*, September 2000

23. Dychtwald K. 'Age power': how the new-old will transform medicine in the 21st century. Interview by AV Luddington. *Geriatrics* 1999; 54:22–7

24. Goodwin JS, Black SA, Satish S. Aging versus disease: the opinions of older black, Hispanic, and non-Hispanic white Americans about the causes and treatment of common medical conditions. *J Am Geriatr Soc* 1999;47:973–9

25. Ontiveros JA, Black SA, Jakobi PL, *et al.* Ethnic variations in attitudes toward hypertension in adults ages 75 and older. *Prev Med* 1999;29: 443–9

26. Sommer B, Avis N, Meyer P, *et al.* Attitudes toward menopause and aging across ethnic/racial groups. *Psychosom Med* 1999;61:868–75

# 3

# Endocrinology of postmenopause and geripause

*Bernard A. Eskin*

## Introduction

Most theories of aging describe intracellular changes that are appropriate throughout the body. Actually, most scientific matter on aging characterizes only those tissues we associate with clinical senescence, i.e. skin, neurological and vascular tissues, muscle and bone. In these specific areas, anatomical and physiological modifications have been presented and hypothetical models established.

However, the endocrine system is unique in that, besides apparent losses of tissue growth and metabolism, secretory activity may in some cases be inhibited, modified or even completely reversed by the aging process. Essential hormones generally required for normal physiological functioning of other parts of the body may be lost[1]. Particularly applicable is a reduction in muscle strength, which leads to frailty[2,3].

A series of histological modifications, which are not unique, occurs in the endocrine glands due to aging[1]. Connective tissue increases in the gland capsule and connective tissue elements replace secretory cells. In the endocrine cell, mitotic rate decreases and fragmentation of mitochondria and nuclear damage often appear. Thus, alterations in the endocrine tissues with aging relate to both secretory and target organ functions[4]. The changes are: (1) primary loss of functional tissue by hypoplastic or atrophic changes in secreting cells; (2) decrease in secretory rate as a result of these cellular changes; (3) decrease of metabolic clearance of hormones produced; and (4) decrease in end-organ response to the hormones.

## Objectives

This chapter discusses the endocrine changes that occur in the menopause as it progresses to the postmenopause and further, into the geripausal years. At present, the research and therapies for these women are restricted because of the relative recency of recognition of this phase of a woman's life. Most of the changes are gradual, except for those related to ovarian demise. Clinically, the most evident and important modifications are hormonal, but age-related factors are present and often difficult to factor out. Those hormones considered most evident and present are: gonadal hormones; thyroid hormones; pancreatic hormones in diabetes mellitus; adrenal hormones; and the neurological and secretory hormonal controls in the brain. Our discussion entails those that are considered most affected by the postmenopause and geripause. Most evident are the gonadal and thyroid hormones; however, some information has become available concerning other postmenopausal endocrinopathies, which are described briefly. Perhaps future research will uncover other useful relationships for endocrine entities in the maintenance of good health status during these periods.

## Gonadal hormones

The most dramatic and rapidly occurring change in women around the age of 50 is menopause[5]. Estradiol cyclicity during the reproductive years is replaced by a very low estradiol level, which then gradually declines.

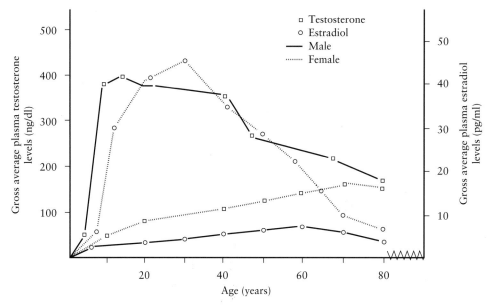

**Figure 1**    Plasma levels of estradiol and testosterone in human females and males according to age

While the prevailing theory was that menopause resulted from an exhaustion of ovarian follicles, ultrasound and stimulatory therapy have disproved that. Age-related changes in the central nervous system (CNS) and hypothalamic–pituitary–ovarian axis may initiate the menopausal transition. Obviously, both the ovary and the brain are key pacemakers in instituting and maintaining the ensuing changes of the postmenopause and geripause[6]. Changes in the activity of the hypothalamic–pituitary–testis axis in males are more subtle and range over a longer time.

In most women, this period of decline in estrogens is accompanied by vasomotor reactions, atrophism of the perineum, uterus, Fallopian tubes and breasts, depressed mood, and changes in skin and body composition (increase in body fat and decrease in muscle mass). In the subsequent years, loss of estrogens is followed by a loss of bone mass, cognitive impairment and probably a higher incidence of cardiovascular disease[7]. The average age of menopause remains 51.4 years and is largely determined by genetic factors. As life expectancy increases, the time a woman spends after menopause constitutes more than one-third of her life[8].

## Endogenous sex hormones

In Figure 1, the apparent average changes in testosterone and estrogen in human females and males are graphically presented. The rapid fall of estrogen at menopause is followed by the lesser decline throughout late postmenopause and into geripause. During the late menopause and geripause, testosterone appears enhanced, perhaps by the decreased availability of the aromatase enzymes. Eventually, after the menopause, estrogen is below the threshold needed to maintain an active endometrium (Figure 1).

Using average 30-day estrogen levels, Figure 2 shows a curve plotted representing the life span[9]. During the transition, these serum estrogens show a gradual decrease. The premenopause has occasional estrogen increases that are due to feedback-activated elevations of follicle stimulating hormone (FSH) stimulating small increments in ovarian release. These cause periods of mild increases

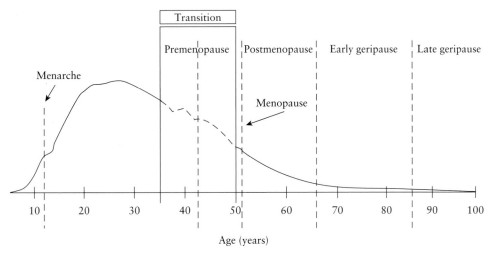

**Figure 2** Lifetime estrogen levels of women. Reproduced from Eskin BA. Epilogue. In: Eskin BA, ed. *The Menopause Comprehensive Management*, 4th edn. Carnforth, UK: Parthenon Publishing, 2000:299–302

**Table 1** Normal serum estrogen values obtained in a general laboratory* in women during the indicated ages

| Age (years) | Normal estrogen (pg/ml) |
| --- | --- |
| 35–45 | 20–300 |
| 45–55 | 0–200 |
| 55–65[†] | < 20 |
| > 65[†] | < 10 |

*Clinical Laboratories, Inc.; [†]after natural menopause

in estrogen until menopause occurs. In the postmenopause (from 1 year after the last uterine bleeding is observed) a sustained decrease in estrogen can be measured. By early geripause estrogen levels are less than 10 pg/ml[10]. As seen in Table 1, the level of estrogen during reproductive cycles is extremely variable and is dependent on ovulatory activity. However, by postmenopause the level becomes stable and shows the inability to further stimulate reproduction.

## Gonadotropins

The hypothalamic–pituitary–orarian axis is no longer functioning reproductively in the postmenopause. Gonadotropin release from the secretory cells of the anterior pituitary is excessively high, and minimal storage occurs. This phenomenon is probably caused by depletion of estrogen feedback and reduced availability of the gonadotropin receptors. This also is definitive evidence of negative responses from the ovaries. In the late postmenopausal period and entering the geripause, studies in our laboratory and others have shown that a fall in FSH is seen to occur at 64–66 years of age[10]. Luteinizing hormone (LH), which has also steadily risen, begins its decline shortly after that of FSH. There are no studies that have indicated what triggers these decreases in gonadotropins. However, it may be surmised that some of the features unique to the geripause may be a result of the dissipation of FSH and LH release.

There are no direct data that show monamine stimulatory changes in the hypothalamus, but, since vasomotor thermal changes such as hot flushes occur, a reduction in activity may be the cause. In addition, hot flushes may decrease or clear during late postmenopause or early geripause. Newer diagnostic means for both neuroanatomical and neuroresponsive measurement in the geripause may be useful in this determination.

## Clinical manifestations

Critical changes that occur with menopause may involve: enhanced vasomotor reactions; atrophy of vulva, vagina, uterus and breast; mild to moderate depression; and changes in skin/hair composition. These problems are evident and increase from the beginning of menopause (cessation of bleeding) through the postmenopause, but by the onset of the geripause they are modified.

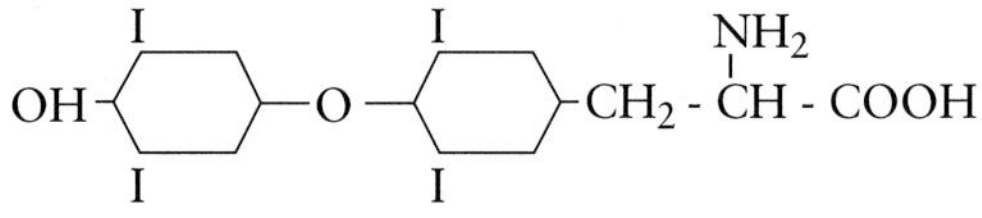

## Thyroid hormones

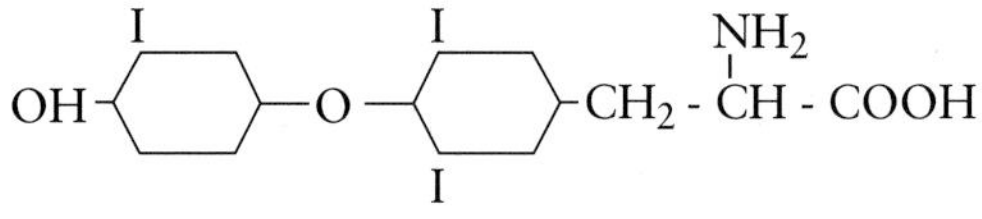

Age-related thyroid dysfunction is common in the postmenopause and geripause[11]. Overall, there is a lower plasma thyroxine ($T_4$) level with an anticipated increase in thyrotropin stimulating hormone (TSH) concentration in 5–10% of elderly women[11]. These changes are the result of the autoimmunity that commonly transpires in women in the course of disease states on the thyroid as they age[12,13]. The aging process shows a measurable decrease in pituitary TSH release[10], but is mostly characterized by a decreased peripheral degradation of $T_4$. The gradual age-dependent decline in serum tri-iodothyronine ($T_3$) concentration is the direct result of this breakdown, while $T_4$ levels seem to have minimal change[14]. This modest decrease in plasma $T_3$ concentration occurs largely within the normal range of a healthy elderly population. As described below, this has not been convincingly related to functional changes during aging[11].

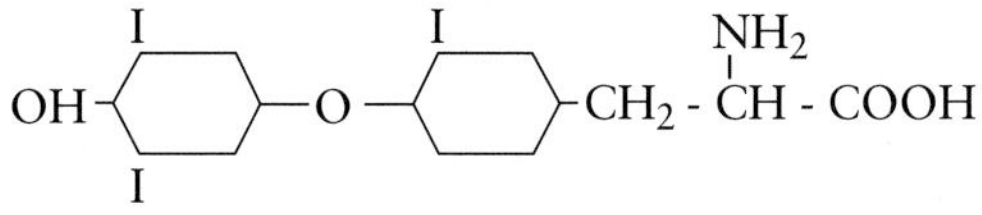

The thyroid gland in adult women normally weighs about 12–20 g and is responsible for extraordinary metabolic activity. The thyroid is essential to women's health, with diagnoses of abnormal states occurring five times more often than in men. During the menopause, the thyroid gland ages and, while relieved from the modifications caused by sex hormone and reproductive cyclicity, it exhibits the influences of anatomical transformations and physiological conversions of aging.

In general, thyroid disorders increase with aging. Thyroid endocrinopathies may be subtle,

Figure 3 Thyroid hormones

non-specific and confusing, with function tests that can be misleading. These irregularities may be attributed to normal aging or acute and chronic diseases seen in the post-menopausal–geripausal individual[15]. Emphasis is directed towards the perimenopausal and geripausal woman and, where evident, differences that may exist from menstruating women.

The thyroid gland secretes the thyronines: $T_4$, $T_3$ and reverse $T_3$ ($rT_3$), which appear to be synthesized from simple substrates of tyrosine and iodine (Figure 3). All of these exist in plasma. $T_4$ is highest in concentration and appears to be the only one that arises solely from the thyroid gland. Under normal conditions, $T_3$ is secreted to a slight extent from the thyroid, but most $T_3$ is obtained from peripheral metabolism. Present in infants and aging patients, $rT_3$ and secondary thyronines are derived from peripheral conversion of $T_4$[16]. This hormone becomes apparent during the postmenopause and continues to increase during geripause.

The formation of tyrosines, monoiodotyrosine (MIT) and di-iodotyrosine (DIT), occurs in approximately equal amounts. Since non-iodinated thyronine has not been demonstrated, the intracellular thyroproteins $T_4$ and $T_3$ must arise from iodotyrosines. $T_4$ would arise from doubling of two DIT molecules, while $T_3$ would be the result of DIT and MIT moieties. This is the 'coupling reaction'.

The thyroid hormones $T_4$ and $T_3$, as well as other iodinated tyrosyls, are transported in the blood bound firmly although reversibly to the serum proteins: thyroid binding globulin (TBG), thyroid binding prealbumin (TBPA) and albumin. The biological activities – transport through the body as well as degradation of the thyroid hormones – are influenced by the binding affinities of these proteins to the hormones. However, clinical responses are dependent on the quantity of the free thyroid hormones available.

$T_4$ is the primary secretory thyronine from the thyroid gland, and is derived only by direct secretion from the thyroid gland. $T_3$ and $rT_3$ are present in greater quantities in the blood than can be assigned to thyroid gland secretion only. Peripheral synthesis from $T_4$ has become apparent quantitatively. Under these circumstances, the formation of $T_3$ occurs in peripheral locations in such diverse places as nervous tissues (including the CNS), liver, kidney and generalized fat.

Reverse $T_3$, found in greater amounts in postmenopausal and geripausal patients, appears to be biologically inactive[16]. Reverse $T_3$ may be involved in receptor response in some tissues; thus, when $rT_3$ is formed, the parent $T_4$ shares the receptor pool. This reduction in the thyroid hormone response decreases thyroid hormone overactivity and may prevent hyperthyroid disease in the tissues, most commonly in the geripausal patient.

## Endocrinology of thyroid activity

Regulatory mechanisms that are affected during menopause are known to exist for thyroid gland activity and menopause. These are the hypothalamic–pituitary–thyroid axis, peripheral synthesis and cellular regulation.

### Hypothalamic–pituitary–thyroid axis

Iodine transport, hormone synthesis and hormone secretion in the thyroid gland are

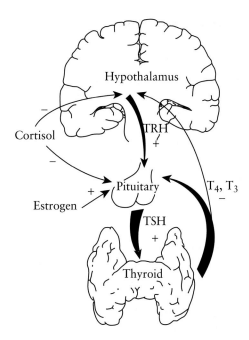

**Figure 4** Endocrine control of thyroid hormone secretion. TRH, thyroid releasing hormone; TSH, thyroid stimulating hormone; $T_4$, thyroxine; $T_3$, tri-iodothyronine

controlled by TSH from the anterior pituitary. Furthermore, it appears that TSH influences both thyroid structure and thyroid function, and is involved in the amount and effectiveness of the vascularity, the changes in the epithelial cells, especially their height, and the total amount of stored colloid that occurs in the thyroid gland. It has been known for many years that TSH is able to control peripherally the intrathyroidal metabolic processes which include glucose oxidation, phospholipid synthesis and RNA synthesis. The release of TSH from the pituitary is caused by the feedback on the pituitary by the free (unbound) forms of both $T_4$ and $T_3$ (Figure 4). The specific effect of $rT_3$ remains moot.

Unlike several other endocrine pituitary control systems, the pituitary secretion (TSH) has the primary control of thyroid metabolism. While the hypothalamus secretes thyrotropin releasing hormone (TRH), it does not appear to be the major regulator of the thyroid through feedback control. The hypothalamus has a modulating influence on the pituitary and resulting TSH secretion. Since there are other factors evident that control pituitary secretions, the final result is often unpredictable (Figure 4). It appears that TRH acts to stimulate first the release and later the synthesis of TSH, while thyroid hormones act to inhibit these functions. Thyroid hormones seem to mediate the feedback regulation of TSH secretion, while TRH determines its set point. Receptor systems for both $T_4$ and $T_3$ are present in the pituitary, although binding affinity varies. Some mechanisms that regulate TSH secretion have been seen to affect TRH receptors, which are located on pituitary thyrotropin surfaces. These are modified also by both thyroid and steroid hormones (Figure 4). Small doses of thyroid hormone reduce the clinical effectiveness of exogenous TRH on pituitary secretion of TSH. Iodides cause the reverse.

## Peripheral synthesis and cellular regulation

It has become apparent that extrathyroidal metabolism maintains the level and type of thyroid hormone available. Peripheral metabolism consists of first, synthesis of thyroid hormones and second, peripheral action at the target cells.

## Clinical aspects of the thyroid

Abnormalities of thyroid function may generate universal abnormal metabolic and hormonal states. Probably owing to the repetitive perturbations or reproductive hormone cyclicity and irregularities of menstruation prior to the menopause, thyroid disturbances occur more commonly in women. In the menopause, the thyroid is associated with a number of morphological and functional changes, such as decreased serum $T_3$ and mean TSH concentrations, which are to some extent independent of intercurrent non-thyroidal illnesses[17]. The result is an endocrine pattern in the thyroid that is unpredictable[1]. There are specific changes found in menopausal women that are responsible for the increasing morbidity seen (Table 2). Thyroid diseases in women occur

**Table 2** Postmenopausal thyroid physiology

*Decreased*
Renal iodide clearance
Thyroid iodide clearance
Total $T_4$ production
Serum TBG concentration
$T_3$ concentration
TSH response to TRH
Diurnal variation of TSH

*Increased*
$T_4$ degradation
Reverse $T_3$ concentration

*Same*
Serum $T_4$ concentration

$T_4$, thyroxine; TBG, thyroid binding globulin; $T_3$, tri-iodothyronine; TSH, thyrotropin stimulating hormone; TRH, thyrotropin releasing hormone

often later in life. Evaluation of function and clinical examination of the thyroid are *a priori* requirements of the complete evaluation in the menopause and geripause. The clinical symptoms manifested are more subtle, because it is anticipated that an aging patient will show energy loss, lethargy, sexual dysfunction, mild depression and other non-definitive incapacitations brought on by the consequences of aging.

Hypothyroidism, hyperthyroidism, as well as thyroid malignancies are more common in the postmenopause. While men also have an increased risk for thyroid disease as they age, the resulting numbers characteristically still favor older women in a ratio of at least 5 : 1. Since this chapter refers to endocrine changes seen with aging, reference only to functional diseases will be made – hypothyroidism and hyperthyroidism. Characteristic pathologies in benign and malignant neoplasms will be left to other textbooks.

## Menopausal screening for thyroid disease

In light of the high occurrence rate, it is advisable to screen postmenopausal women, generally at 50 and 55 years of age. Obviously, tests should be done if functional thyroid disease is suspected at any time, particularly in the geripause. A number of pathophysiological changes occur in thyroid metabolism at the time of the menopause. Many times these conditions will appear although no immediate medical abnormality or concern is visible (Table 2). Some geriatricians practice preventive medicine by conducting studies in all patients, men and women, at 65 years of age. It is necessary to recognize that thyroid function tests for screening are not always accurate when acute psychiatric or medical illnesses are present, because of interference with laboratory procedures, particularly by the medications[2].

Patients with symptoms of failure to thrive, depression and disability benefit from physical examination and screening for thyroid disease. Subtle evidence of early thyroid problems can be easily treated as needed. The quality of life is greatly improved, and conditions such as elevated cholesterol, apathy and anxiety can be relieved. The screening test most easily performed and providing the most accurate results is the high-sensitivity test for TSH.

## Hypothyroidism

Hypothyroidism is a condition caused by thyroid failure, where there is an inadequate supply of thyroid hormone available as required by the individual's peripheral tissues. The range of the thyroid dificiency is extensive; often it is present only subclinically[4]. Myxedema is the term applied to the most severe expression of hypothyroidism, and often follows total or subtotal thyroidectomy or radioactive iodine treatment for hyperthyroidism. When it occurs spontaneously it is considered to be iodiopathic myxedema or Gull's disease. Both Gull's and Hashimoto's thyroiditis are the end results of an autoimmune process. Other causes for hypothyroidism include drug induction, goiters (idio pathic as iodine deficient) or reduced stimulation from hypothalamic or pituitary abnormalities.

## Prevalence

The prevalence of hypothyroidism has been reported to increase with age, and in up to 10%

**Table 3** Hypothyroidism in the postmenopause

*Primary causes*
Drugs
   iodine-containing drugs: amiodarone, iodinated glycerol
   antithyroid drugs: propylthiouracil, methimazole lithium
Chronic autoimmune thyroiditis
Radiation
   [131]I-therapy for hyperthyroidism
   radiation therapy for head and neck cancer
Surgical thyroidectomy

*Secondary causes*
Hypothalamic tumors or granuloma
Radiation
Pituitary tumors
Pituitary surgery

of postmenopausal women[18]. Thirty per cent of these cases are of iatrogenic origin and require careful analysis for cause (Table 3). The onset of this disease is subtle and since myxedema is rare, hospital care is seldom required. In menopausal women, the pathogenesis is almost entirely on the basis of chronic autoimmune thyroiditis or Hashimoto's disease. Often, a pre-existing viral infection may destroy thyroid cells during which time a temporary hyperthyroidism occurs. Soon, however, the destroyed area becomes ineffective and hypothyroidism occurs. Several causes have been described by thyroidologists to characterize the disease, as seen in Table 3. Chronic autoimmune thyroiditis is characterized by a focal or diffuse lymphocytic infiltration of thyroid parenchyma, damaged or atrophic follicles and the presence of autoantibodies in the serum. In postmenopausal and geripausal women the increase in thyroid autoimmunity is due to the severe estrogen loss[19].

## Diagnosis

Prominent clinical features include a puffy face, a pleasant personality, non-pitting myxedema, marked cold intolerance, and coarse, dry skin and hair[20]. Clinical features of hypothyroidism in the menopause are listed in Table 4. Enlargement of the heart shadow

**Table 4** Clinical features of hypothyroidism in postmenopausal women

*Cutaneous*
Dry skin
Hair loss
Edema of face and eyelids

*Cardiovascular*
Bradycardia
Pericardial effusion
Congestive heart failure

*Neurological*
Parasthesia (carpal tunnel syndrome)
Ataxia
Dementia

*Psychiatric and behavioral*
Depression
Apathy or withdrawal
Psychosis
Cognitive dysfunction

*Metabolic*
Weight gain
Hypercholesterolemia
Hyperglyceridemia
Peripheral edema

*Musculoskeletal*
Myopathy
Arthritis/arthralgia

is frequently due to a pericardial effusion. Cardiac output is decreased and the body is less sensitive to catecholamines. Adrenal function is decreased with urinary 17-ketosteroid/hydroxycorticoid excretion reduced and serum cortisol and corticoid serum levels lowered, particularly in the morning. Certain signs are readily seen, such as reflex relaxation time, which is markedly prolonged, decreased metabolic rate and increases in blood cholesterol and other lipid fractions.

The postmenopausal signs and symptoms of hypothyroidism tend to be non-specific because of the insidious onset of the disease and its long progression[21]. The diagnosis of primary hypothyroidism is confirmed by finding an elevation of serum TSH accompanied by a reduced free $T_4$ level while total $T_4$ is adequate[2]. The hypothalamic–pituitary axis is so sensitive that it is often possible to detect TSH elevation indicating thyroid damage before the patient notices symptoms. The condition is termed subclinical hypothyroidism.

## Therapy

Therapy of primary hypothyroidism should be instituted with levothyroxine at a dose that takes into account the age of the patient, the severity and duration of the hypothyroidism and the presence of co-existing medical conditions, particularly symptomatic coronary artery disease. Partial substitution of $T_3$ for $T_4$ has been suggested as improving mood and neuropsychological function in older women. This finding suggests a specific effect of $T_3$[22].

An important consideration is whether therapy should be instituted slowly at a lower dose and increased after treatment observation. In the premenopausal patient, with no complicating illnesses, a starting levothyroxine replacement dose of 0.6–0.7 µg/lb ideal body weight (1.6–1.8 µg/kg) can be given immediately. However, lower doses should be always instituted in postmenopausal or geripausal patients and those with illnesses that may compromise the capacity of the cardiorespiratory system to respond to an increased metabolic demand[23].

## Hyperthyroidism

The clinical syndrome of hyperthyroidism is usually caused by Graves' disease or diffuse toxic goiter. Thyroiditis as a cause for hyperthyroidism is much less common in menopausal than in premenopausal women[24]. Thyrotoxicosis (symptomatic hyperthyroidism) may also be produced by toxic multinodular goiter, toxic adenomas, excessive thyroid hormone ingestion, early viral diseases, and several rare syndromes. In older patients, toxic multinodular goiter is more common, reaching as many as one-half of the patients, especially in geographic areas of iodine deficiency.

Graves' disease, a disease of autoimmunity, which shows hyperfunctioning of the thyroid gland, has a strong hereditary tendency. When

**Table 5** Clinical features of hyperthyroidism in the postmenopause

*Cardiovascular*
Palpitation
Chronic or intermittent atrial fibrillation
Congestive heart failure

*Psychiatric and behavioral*
Depression
Apathy
Lethargy
Irritability

*Gastrointestinal*
Decreased appetite
Weight loss
Nausea
Constipation

*Musculoskeletal*
Proximal muscle weakness
Muscle atrophy

fully expressed, Graves' disease includes thyrotoxicosis, goiter, exophthalmos and pretibial myxedema, but it has been shown to be present with one or more of these features (Table 5). Inheritance of specific HLA antigens has been shown to predispose to Graves' disease. Psychic trauma, sympathetic nervous system activation, strenuous weight reduction and iodide administration have also been associated with the initiation of hyperthyroidism.

An immune response is characterized by the presence of abnormal antibodies directed against specific thyroid tissue antigens that particularly bind with the thyrotropin receptor. These antibodies act as either agonists or antagonists, thus stimulating or blocking TSH, usually resulting in suppression of TRH stimulation. Antibodies of this type can be measured in 80–100% of untreated patients with Graves' disease. The serum factor TSAb (long-acting thyroid stimulators, LATS) is measurable and most commonly involved. Serum TSH is typically suppressed and may be near zero. When $T_3$ is administered, the thyroid gland is not suppressed, while small levels of $T_4$ may reduce the thyroid outflow. The pituitary response to TRH is also suppressed. The gland is unusually responsive to iodide, which both blocks further hormone synthesis and inhibits release of hormone from the gland.

## Prevalence

In studies, the incidence of Graves' disease ranges from 3.4 to 6.8% of postmenopausal women. Approximately 10–17% of all hyperthyroid patients are over the age of 60 years. As previously stated, the frequency in women is always greater than in men.

Thyrotoxicosis itself is associated with pathological changes including damage to muscles and mild damage to the liver. Graves' disease is associated with thyroid hyperplasia with lymphoid infiltration, generalized lymphoid hyperplasia, and the specific changes in infiltrative ophthalmopathy and pretibial myxedema.

## Diagnosis

In the postmenopause, the classic features of thyrotoxicosis are described as nervousness, diminished sleep, tremulousness, tachycardia, increased appetite, weight loss and increased perspiration[25]. Graves' disease shows specific symptoms and signs that are associated with goiter, occasionally with exophthalmos and rarely with pretibial myxedema. Physical findings include fine skin and hair, tremulousness, a hyperactive heart, 'Plummer's nails', muscle weakness, accelerated reflex relaxation, occasional splenomegaly and often peripheral edema. Plummer's nails (thinning of the nails and marked posterior eversion of the hyponychium) are more common in the late postmenopause and geripause. Thyroid changes seen in menopausal Graves' disease are given in Table 4. Skin changes appear to be autoimmune vitiligo or hives. The extent and degree of hyperthyroid bone diseases, particularly osteoporosis, surpass the effects of postmenopause on the bone mass and can often be more extensive[26].

Absence of some of the typical manifestations of hyperthyroidism in the menopause and geripause was called 'apathetic hyperthyroidism' because there was only slight evidence of hypermetabolism. In the older patient, the diagnosis of hyperthyroidism is often overlooked because of apathy, and the dominant clinical findings may be weight loss, and cardiac or gastrointestinal manifestations. The prevalence of subclinical hyperthyroidism is higher than that of subclinical hypothyroidism in older women and it might involve non-autoimmune factors[27].

Hyperthyroidism typically begins gradually in premenopausal women and steadily worsens if not treated by the postmenopause. Muscle weakness in frequent, myasthenia may co-exist, and hypokalemic periodic paralysis may be induced by thyrotoxicosis. While hypercalciuria is frequent, kidney stones rarely occur. Complications of thyrotoxicosis are congestive heart failure, mitral valve prolapse, atrial tachycardia and cardiac fibrillation. Other medical conditions may include normocytic anemia, diarrhea without malabsorption, minimal liver damage and hyperbilirubinemia.

The laboratory tests that are most effective for evaluating the status of thyroid function are the sensitive TSH assay and any technique measuring free $T_3$. As an initial single test, a highly sensitive TSH assay is most cost-effective and direct. Although the results may range slightly, depending on the kit or technique employed, sensitive TSH tests should yield 0–0.1 µIU/ml in thyrotoxicosis. In menopausal women a range of 0.1–0.25 is sometimes seen, especially with the toxic form of multinodular goiters, which are more common at this age.

A variety of free thyroxine techniques have become available and are often suitable as a single testing system as well. However, if clinical judgement places considerable doubt on a normal result, an additional test may be employed: serum $T_3$ level determined by radioimmunoassay. It is almost always elevated in thyrotoxicosis. Interpretations can be made without correcting for protein binding. The serum $T_4$ level is elevated in 86% of menopausal hyperthyroid patients, providing a reasonably sensitive alternative for hyperthyroidism. However, there are hyperthyroxinemic patients without hyperthyroidism, indicating a low specificity of the serum total $T_4$ assay.

## Treatment

The choice of treatment of all forms of thyrotoxicosis requires full patient participation. As indicated, thyrotoxicosis in untreated cases leads to cardiovascular damage, bone loss and fractures, or inanition, and can be fatal. The long-term history also includes spontaneous remission in some cases, and eventual spontaneous development of hypothyroidism if autoimmune thyroiditis co-exists and destroys the thyroid gland.

Primary treatment of Graves' disease follows three pathways: blocking of thyroid hormone synthesis in the thyroid by the use of antithyroid drugs; complete destruction of the thyroid tissues by radioactive iodine; and partial or complete surgical ablation of the thyroid.

(1) Women in the menopause often do very well on antithyroid medications given for 6 months to 1 year and then discontinued and observed[28]. This may require longer periods of time or repetitive therapy after an unsuccessful trial. The spontaneous successes from medical therapy are satisfying, since both radiation and surgery may induce damage to the thyroids, parathyroids or recurrent nerves. However, side-effects and complications of the medications for the individual must be weighed in each case.

(2) Radioactive ablation, which is commonly used in postmenopausal and geripausal women, may cause some damage to the peripheral tissues and commonly results in hypothyroidism with a need for thyroid replacement treatment. A population-based study (in 1999) showed a decrease in overall cancer incidence and mortality in those treated for hyperthyroidism with radioiodine[29]. The absolute risk of cancers of the small bowel and thyroid remained low, but an increased relative risk was considered a problem requiring long-term vigilance. However, the simplicity of the treatment is useful, since in many cases the older patient cannot tolerate long-term medical therapy or surgery.

(3) Surgery, the usual therapy until 1950, is minimally used for hyperthyroidism. It is generally resorted to when the patient chooses not to have radioactive treatment and medical treatment has been unsuccessful.

## Diabetes

The subject of diabetes mellitus can be only briefly mentioned here. Although it is an important endocrinopathy, particularly in the geripause, the complexity of the pancreatic hormone and carbohydrate metabolism deserves a dedicated book. Most women in the postmenopause, not already diagnosed with insulin-dependent diabetes mellitus (IDDM; DM1), will fall into the second category of non-insulin-dependent diabetes mellitus (NIDDM; DM2), which commonly occurs after 40 years of age. Although estrogen may already be decreasing, this decisive division is not gender-affected[30].

Approximately 40% of individuals 65–74 years of age and 50% of individuals older than 80 years have impaired glucose tolerance or a form of diabetes mellitus, and nearly half of elderly diabetics are undiagnosed[31,32]. These persons are at risk of developing secondary, mainly macrovascular, complications at an accelerated rate[33]. Pancreatic, insulin receptor, and post-receptor changes associated with aging are critical components of the endocrinology of aging. Apart from decreased (relative) insulin secretion by the beta cells, peripheral insulin resistance related to poor diet, physical inactivity, increased abdominal fat mass and decreased lean body mass contribute to the deterioration of glucose metabolism[33].

Therapy may be more difficult for IDDM patients and re-evaluation is usually required for these women entering the menopause. Most of the new cases will be considered as NIDDM, because the onset of disease was much later in life. Dietary management, exercise, oral hypoglycemic agents and insulin are the four components of treatment of these patients, although the medical care is costly and intensive[34]. These changes in insulin sensitivity

that occur in the aging population are of clinical importance and are recognized and seriously treated as diseases.

## Adrenal hormones

Aging of the adrenal gland has been shown to occur primarily in the cortex. The secretory aspects most affected by postmenopause are related to 'sex hormones' and their precursors. A deficiency of aromatizing enzyme has been suggested, but not proven, which accounts for a modest reduction in estrogen (as estrone) and similarly, the adrenal as a source for androgens is slightly decreased. This occurs even though gonadotropins increase and cross-stimulation by LH has been described.

Age-related changes in the circulating levels of the most representative adrenal androgen, dehydroepiandrosterone (DHEA) and its sulfate (DHEAS), show a gradual decline presenting a change in steroidogenesis[35–37]. Adrenal secretion of DHEA diminishes progressively over the last decades of life, whereas adrenocorticotropin (ACTH) secretion, which is physiologically linked to plasma cortisol levels, remains largely unchanged[38]. The decline in DHEA(S) levels in the postmenopausal woman contrasts with plasma cortisol levels, which remain at the premenopausal levels. Both DHEA and DHEAS seem to be caused by a selective decrease in the number of functional zone reticularis cells in the adrenal cortex rather than through deregulation by the hypothalamus[36]. Recent studies have shown that levels of these δ5-steroids at age 70 and 80 years are only 20–30% of those obtained between age 20 and 30[37–39]. There may be anatomical changes in the adrenal medulla that may also modulate this steroidogenesis[40].

Interestingly, stimulation of the adrenal cortex with exogenous or endogenous ACTH consistently results in decreased DHEA responses in older individuals as compared to premenopausal controls[41,42]. Corticosteroid production except for androgens remains adequate during normal physiological aging, although it is possibly up-regulated for glucosteroids and down-regulated for mineralocorticoids[43].

Clinically, these changes are not evident and usually a need for replacement has not been suggested. One condition that has shown relative risk evidence when there are enhanced levels of cortisol with decreased levels of DHEA is Alzheimer's disease. Several important clinical trials have been undertaken to evaluate theory. Enhancement of the immune system and of the growth hormone axis with replacement of DHEA has been described in preliminary studies[44,45].

Basically, adrenal activity with aging has been insufficiently studied in postmenopausal and geripausal women. This complex area needs further clarification.

## Growth hormone

The growth hormone (GH)–insulin-like growth factor I (IGF-I) axis gradually declines in activity during aging[46,47]. Mean pulse amplitude, duration and fraction of GH secreted, but not pulse frequency, have been seen to decrease gradually during aging. Similarly, there is a progressive fall in circulating IGF-I levels in both sexes[47]. GH is secreted by the pituitary, but is stimulated primarily by hypothalamic hormone. Pituitary somatotropes, regardless of age, can be restored to premenopausal secretory capacity when treated with GH-releasing pulsatile peptides.

The hormone secretions that might be reduced because of an aging brain seem to be difficult at this time to implicate. The central pacemaker of aging has been considered to be the hypothalamus[37]. Although studies using the hypothalamic peptide GH show an effect on pituitary release, this is not universal and not understood. Gonadotropin releasing hormone (GnRH) responses indicate that the thermal change that occurs in menopause may at least partially be due to hypothalamic dysfunction because of the proximity of GnRH secretion to the thermal control area[48]. Use of GnRH therapy is independent of the total function of the hypophysial–pituitary–ovarian axis and appears to restore some gonadotropin effects, but fails with complete ovarian failure.

While aging is involved in the endocrine problems seen in the postmenopause and geripause, there are some problems in the endocrine system that are directly influenced by menopause.

The most impressive endocrine conditions caused by ovarian failure are in the thyroid gland. Normal function is essential for cyclicity and reproduction. It is apparent that thyroid disease occurs in women eight times more frequently than in men of the same age. Following this interaction is essential for good quality of life in the mature woman. Diabetes and pancreatic hormone changes seem to have some correlation with ovarian function. This is evidenced in premenopausal variables such as polycystic ovarian disease and diabetic mothers. The ovarian demise is responsible for many further problems that occur, particularly in steroidogenesis in the adrenal and ovary.

Endocrine changes in the postmenopause/geripause are evident and are steadily modified with aging as the hormonal systems adjust. Much more basic information is needed before clinical recognition and replacement therapies can be applied. The ovarian demise is responsible for many further problems that occur, particularly in steroidogenesis.

# References

1. Hershman JM, Pekary AE, Berg L, *et al*. Serum thyrotropin and thyroid hormone levels in elderly and middle-aged euthyroid persons. *J Am Geriatr Soc* 1993;41:823–8
2. Brent GA, Hershman JM. Effects of nonthyroidal illness on thyroid function tests. In Van Middlesworth L, ed. *The Thyroid Gland*. Chicago: Year Book Medical Publishers, 1986:83–102
3. Fox B. Venous infarction of the adrenal glands. *J Pathol* 1976;57:211–21
4. Figg J, Lennung M, Goodman AD, *et al*. The clinical evaluation of patients with subclinical hyperthyroidism and free triiodothyronine toxicosis. *Am J Med* 1994;96:229–34
5. Guyton AC, ed. *Textbook of Medical Physiology*, 8th edn. Philadelphia: Saunders, 1991:899–914

6. Wise PM, Krajnak KM, Kashon ML. Menopause: the aging of multiple pacemakers. *Science* 1996;273:67–70

7. Lindsay R, Bush TL, Grady D, *et al.* Therapeutic convroversy: estrogen replacement in menopause. *J Clin Endocrinol Metab* 1996;81:3829–38

8. Jones EC. The postreproductive phase in mammals. *Front Horm Res* 1975;3:1–19

9. Eskin BA. Epilogue. In Eskin BA, ed. *The Menopause: Comprehensive Management*, 4th edn. Carnforth, UK: Parthenon Publishing, 2000;299–302

10. Eskin BA, Trivedi RA, Weideman C, Walker RF. Positive feedback disturbances and infertility in women over 30. *Am J Gynecol Health* 1988;2:110–17

11. Mariotti S, Franceschi C, Cossarizza A, Pinchera A. The aging thyroid. *Endocr Rev* 1995;16:686–715

12. Hijmans W, Radl J, Bottazzo GF, Daniach D. Autoantibodies in highly aged humans. *Mech Ageing Dev* 1984;26:83–9

13. Mariotti S, *et al.* Thyroid and other organ-specific autoantibodies in healthy centurions. *Lancet* 1992;339:1506–8

14. Rubenstein HA, Butler, Werner SC. Progressive decrease in serum triiodothyronine concentrations with human aging. *J Clin Endocrinol Metab* 1973;37:247–53

15. Wong TK, Hershman JM. Changes in thyroid function in nonthyroid illness. *Trends Endocrinol Metab* 1992;3:8–18

16. Nishikawa M, Inada M, Naito K, *et al.* Age related changes of serum 3,3′-diiodothyronine, 3′,5′-diiodothyronine, and 3,5-diiodothyronine concentrations in man. *J Clin Endocrinol Metab* 1981;52:517–22

17. Chrovato L, Minotti S, Pinchera A. Thyroid diseases in the elderly. *Baillière's Clin Endocrinol Metab* 1997;11:251–70

18. Faughnan M, LePage R, Fugere P, *et al.* Screening for thyroid disease at the menopausal clinic. *Clin Invest Med* 1995;18:11–18

19. Lotz H, Salabe GB. Lipoprotein(a) increase associated with thyroid autoimmunity *Eur J Endocrinol* 1997;136:87–91

20. Doucet J, Travalle C, Chassagne P, *et al.* Does age play a role in clinical presentation of hypothyroidism? *J Am Geriatr Soc* 1994;42: 984–6

21. Bemben DA, Hamm RM, Morgan L, *et al.* Thyroid disease in the elderly: I. Prevalence of undiagnosed hypothyroidism. *J Fam Pract* 1994;38:577–82

22. Buneorcius R, Kazanavicius G, Zalinkaviciars R, Prange AJ. Effects of $T_4$ as compared with $T_4$ and $T_3$ in patients with hypothyroidism. *N Engl J Med* 1999;340:424–9

23. Biondi B, Fazio S, Carella C, *et al.* Cardiac effects of long term thyrotropin-suppressive therapy with levothyroxine. *J Clin Endocrinol Metab* 1993;77:334–8

24. Davis PJ, Davis FB. Hyperthyroidism in patients over the age of 60 years. *Medicine* 1974;53:161–81

25. Trivalle C, Doucet J, Chassagne P, *et al.* Differences in the signs and symptoms of hyperthyroidism in older and younger patients. *J Am Geriatr Soc* 1996;44:50–3

26. Jodar E, Munoz-Torres M, Escobar-Jimenez F, *et al.* Bone loss in hyperthyroid patients and in former hyperthroid patients controlled on medical therapy: influence of aetiology and menopause. *Clin Endocrinol* 1997;47:279–85

27. Chuang CC, Wang ST, Wang PW, Yu ML. Prevalence study of thyroid dysfunction in the elderly of Taiwan. *Gerontology* 1998;44:162–7

28. Yamada T, Aizawa T, Koizumi Y, *et al.* Age-related therapeutic response to antithyroid drugs in patients with hyperthyroid Graves' disease. *J Am Geriatr Soc* 1994;42:513–16

29. Franklyn JA, Maisoneuve P, Sheppard M, *et al.* Cancer incidence and mortality after radioiodine treatment for hyperthyroidism: a population-based cohort study. *Lancet* 1999;353: 2111–15

30. Lamberts SWJ, van den Beld HW, van der Lely A-J. The endocrinology of aging. *Science* 1997; 278:419–24

31. Minaker KL. Peripheral insulin sensitivity in healthy young and old adults. *Am J Clin Nutr* 1990;52:524–8

32. Harris MI, Klein R, Welborn TA, Knuiman MW. Onset of NIDDM occurs at least 4–7 years before clinical diagnosis. *Diabetes Care* 1992; 15:815–19

33. Davidson MB. The effect of aging on carbohydrate metabolism. *Metabolism* 1979;28: 688–705

34. Fink RI, Kolterman OG, Olefsky JM. The physiological significance of the glucose intolerance of aging. *J Gerontol* 1984;39:273–8

35. Ravaglia G, *et al.* The relationship of DHEAS to endocrine-metabolic parameters and functional status in the oldest-old. *J Clin Endocrinal Metab* 1996;81:1173–8

36. Hernert J. The age of DHEA. *Lancet* 1995;345: 1193

37. Labrie F, Belanger A, Simard J, *et al.* DHEA and peripheral androgen and estrogen formation – interacinology. *Ann NY Acad Sci* 1995; 774:16–28

38. Kroboth PD, Salek FS, Pittenger AL, *et al.* DHEA and DHEA-S: a review. *J Clin Pharmacol* 1999;39:327–48

39. Angeli A, Masera RG, Magri F, Ferrari E. The adrenal cortex in physiological and pathological

aging: issues of clinical relevance. *J Clin Endocrinol Invest* 1999;22(Suppl 10):13–18

40. Troiano L, Pini G, Petruzzi E, *et al*. Evaluation of adrenal function in aging. *J Endocrinol Invest* 1999;22(Suppl 10):74–5

41. Tsagarakis S, Grossman A. The hypothalamic–pituitary–adrenal axis in senescence. In JE Morley, SG Korenman, eds. *Endocrinology and Metabolism in the Elderly*. Oxford: Blackwell Scientific Publications, 1992:70–8

42. Rasmuson S, Nasman B, Eriksson S, *et al*. Adrenal responsivity in normal aging and mild to moderate Alzheimer's disease. *Biol Psychiatry* 1998;43:410–7

43. Parker CR. Adrenal fuction in aging. *Curr Opin Endocrinol Diabetes* 1999;3:210–15

44. Irwin M, Hauger R, Brown M. Central corticotropin-releasing hormone activates the sympathetic nervous system and reduces immune function: increased responsivity of the aged rat. *Endocrinology* 1992;131:1047–53

45. Berr C, Lafont S, Debuire B, *et al*. Relationships of dehydroepiandrosterone sulfate in the elderly with functional, psychological and mental status, and short-term mortality. A French community-based study. *Proc Natl Acad Sci USA* 1996;93:13410–15

46. Rudman D, Rao UMP. Growth hormone effects in aging. In Morley JE, Korenman SG, eds. *Endocrinology and Metabolism in the Elderly*. Oxford: Blackwell Scientific, 1992: 50–68

47. Corpas E, Harman M, Blackman MR. Serum IGF-binding protein-3 is related to IGF-I, but not to spontaneous GH release. *Horm Metab Res* 1992;13:543–5

48. Perry HM 3rd. The endocrinology of aging. *Clin Chem* 1999;45:1369–76

# 4

# Pharmacology

*Helen K. Edelberg and Rosanne M. Leipzig*

## Introduction

Americans spend $92 billion a year on out-patient medications[1]. Nearly 2.5 billion prescriptions were dispensed at US pharmacies in 1998; 25–30% of these medications were consumed by the 13% of the population aged 65 years and older[2,3]. On average, community-dwelling older adults take three over-the-counter preparations and between four and five prescription medications each day[4,5]. The numbers are higher for older adults who receive residential long-term care at home or in a nursing home[2,6]. The use of non-prescription medications has not been shown to increase with age; however, with the recent trend toward switching the availability of prescription to non-prescription medications, this needs to be reinvestigated. The most commonly prescribed prescription drugs are cardiovascular, analgesic, central nervous system (CNS) and endocrine agents; the most common non-prescription drugs are analgesic and gastrointestinal, including nutritional supplements.

## Normal aging

### Changes in dose response with aging

Aging-related changes in dose response may be due to changes in pharmacokinetic (i.e. what the body does to the drug) or pharmacodynamic (i.e. what the drug does to the body) parameters (Figure 1). Although a number of studies have examined the pharmacokinetics of certain medications in essentially healthy 60–75 year olds, little is known about patients

over the age of 75 years or those with multiple medical conditions. Pharmacodynamic studies are more difficult to perform, since they require that the intensity of effect be quantifiable and measured at several points in time.

### Aging-related changes in pharmacokinetics

#### Absorption

Although there are many aging-related physiological changes in the gastrointestinal tract and in splanchnic blood flow, alterations in absorption contribute the least to aging-related changes in dose response. A recent cross-sectional study of community-dwelling older adults demonstrated that the vast majority are able to acidify gastric contents, challenging the previously held assumption that aging-related achlorhydria impedes drug absorption[7]. Although absorption tends to be complete in older adults, it may proceed at a slightly slower rate, resulting in a mild lowering of the peak concentration and/or an increase in the time to onset of drug effect. This is clinically significant mainly for symptom-relieving drugs, such as analgesics or anxiolytics, where the time to onset or peak concentration can influence whether the patient considers the medication to be effective. As shown in Table 1, lifestyle, co-morbidity and the use of other medications affect absorption more than does age alone.

The fraction of an oral drug that reaches the systemic circulation, known as the drug's

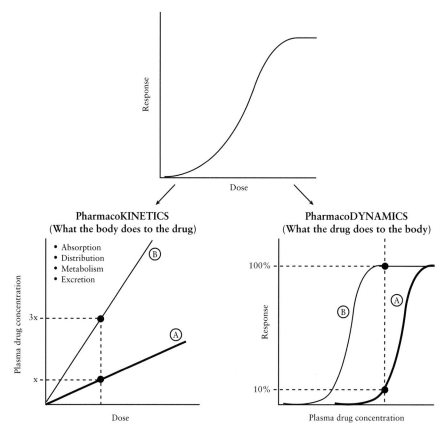

**Figure 1** Variability in dose response. In each lower graph, A and B represent two possible dose–concentration relationships (left graph) or concentration–response relationships (right graph). When age-related pharmacokinetic or pharmaco-dynamic changes occur, the relationship usually shifts from A to B. See text for more complete descriptions. Adapted from Leipzig RM. Avoiding adverse drug effects in elderly patients. *Cleve Clin J Med* 1998;65:47–8

bioavailability, is a function of absorption and first-pass metabolism – the metabolism that occurs prior to the drug's entry into the circulation. If the amount of first-pass metabolism decreases, the bioavailability and therefore the systemic concentration of the drug will be higher than expected, potentially leading to a concentration-related enhanced response or an adverse drug effect. Drugs with high first-pass metabolism can be identified by the large difference between the parenteral (intravenous) and oral dose. The bioavailability of most drugs is unchanged with aging; however labetolol, levodopa, lidocaine, nifedipine, omeprazole and ondansetron have been shown to have increased bioavailability in older adults.

## Distribution: weight and body composition

Body weight correlates with the size of the spaces into which drug distributes, e.g. body water and muscle mass, as well as with the function and blood flow of organs, including those involved in drug clearance. In general, adult weight begins to decline in the seventh or eighth decade; many frail older adults weigh significantly less than the average 70-kg adult. Dosage adjustment by weight has not been tested as a mechanism for reducing adverse events (ADEs); nevertheless, an increasing number of drug dosage recommendations adjust dose by weight as a means of improving

**Table 1** Examples of pharmacokinetic variability. Adapted with permission from Leipzig RM. Pharmacology and appropriate prescribing. In: Cobbs EL, Duthie EH, Murphy JB, eds. *Geriatric Review Syllabus: A Core Curriculum in Geriatric Medicine.* Dubuque, USA: Kendall-Hunt Publishing Company, 1999:30–35

| | Life style | | Drugs | Disease | |
| --- | --- | --- | --- | --- | --- |
| | *Agent* | *Effect* | *Drugs* | *Disease* | *Effect* |
| *Absorption/bioavailability* | | | | | |
| ↑ Nifedipine, omeprazole | grapefruit juice | ↑ CCB | cimetidine, ranitidine: ↑ alcohol famotidine: no effect on alcohol | gastroparesis | ↓ time to onset and peak concentration of slow-release drugs |
| | milk | ↓ norfloxicillin, ciprofloxicillin | Maalox: ↓ time to onset of effect of diazepam, chlordiazepoxide | cirrhosis | ↑ propranolol |
| ↑ Alcohol | food | ↓ alendronate | metaclopramide: ↑ lithium iron: ↓ thyroid hormone | diarrhea | ↓ bioavailability slow-release drugs |
| *Distribution* | | | | | |
| ↑ Loading-dose digoxin, lithium | obesity | ↓ loading-dose aminoglycoside | quinidine: displaces digoxin from binding protein; may cause digoxin toxicity | ascites | ↑ loading-dose aminoglycosides |
| *Hepatic metabolism* | | | | | |
| ↓ Clearance: felodipine, ketoprofen, paroxetine | smoking | ↓ clearance theophylline | see Table 2 | CHF | ↓ clearance: lisinopril, furosemide, lidocaine, prazosin |
| | chronic alcohol | see Table 2 | | acute hepatitis | ↓ clearance: amlodipine, amiloride, diazepam, propranolol |
| | | | | cirrhosis | ↓ clearance: fluoxetine, paroxetine, glyburide, nifedipine, isosorbide dinitrate |
| | | | | other genetics | poor metabolizers: ↑ drug concentration |
| *Renal excretion* | | | | | |
| ↓ Excretion of digoxin, amantadine, enalapril, famotidine | | | HCTZ: ↓ excretion lithium | renal disease | see Table 3 |

CCB, calcium channel blockers; CHF, congestive heart failure; HCTZ, hydrochlorothiazide the risk/benefit ratio in frail older adults[8]. Examples include weight-adjusted dosing of low-molecular-weight and unfractionated heparin for treatment of deep vein thrombosis (DVT), and non-steroidal anti-inflammatory drugs (NSAIDs) and narcotics for pain in cancer patients.

Aging is associated with a decrease in total body water and lean body mass and an increase in body fat. In older adults the loading dose or initial dose needed to produce a target plasma concentration should be reduced for drugs that are mainly water soluble, such as lithium, aminoglycosides and alcohol, or for those that bind to skeletal muscle, such as digoxin. In theory, fat-soluble drugs require a greater initial dose in older adults, but for pharmacodynamic reasons many of these drugs, such as diazepam, thiopental and trazodone, are actually given in lower doses.

## Protein binding

With normal aging there is minimal change in the concentrations of the major drug-binding proteins, albumin and $\alpha_1$-acid glycoprotein[9]. Although changes in the concentration and binding ability of these proteins can occur with disease, these changes usually have little clinical significance, since the proportions of bound and free drug rapidly re-equilibrate. These changes may affect the interpretation of plasma drug concentration levels.

## Hepatic metabolism

Age, genotype, lifestyle habits, cardiac output, disease and interactions with other medications result in marked interindividual variability in hepatic drug metabolism (Table 1), at times resulting in as much as a 100-fold difference in plasma drug levels for the same dose of oral medication. Drugs can be biotransformed in the liver by oxidative metabolism through the cytochrome P450 system, or by acetylation or conjugation (Table 2). For some drugs, such as warfarin, diazepam, naproxen and phenytoin, the aging-related decline in clearance may be due to a reduction in liver mass, resulting in decreased hepatic metabolic capacity[10]. There

is inconclusive evidence for an aging-related decline in the activity of biotransforming enzymes. Propranolol, morphine, verapamil and desipramine are examples of drugs whose rate of metabolism is limited by the amount of drug delivered to the liver. For these drugs, decreased clearance is probably due to the 40–50% aging-related decline in hepatic blood flow. Unfortunately, there is no convenient clinical method to measure changes in hepatic drug metabolism comparable to creatinine clearance for changes in renal drug excretion. The rates of acetylation and conjugation do not decline in any clinically meaningful way with aging, but drugs that are conjugated, such as temazepam, may need to be given to older adults in lower doses for pharmacodynamic reasons.

## Renal excretion

In approximately two-thirds of adults the glomerular filtration rate (GFR) decreases with aging. Renal mass and blood flow also decrease[11]. The 24-hour creatinine clearance provides an accurate estimate of GFR in older adults; GFR can be used to estimate initial dosing regimens in drugs primarily eliminated by the kidney. The aging-related decrease in lean body mass reduces creatinine production, allowing a decrease in renal function to occur without elevating serum creatinine. Although several formulas have been developed to estimate creatinine clearance using the patient's age, actual or lean body weight or body mass index, serum creatinine, and sex, these have been demonstrated to have poor predictive accuracy[12,13]. Since the blood urea nitrogen (BUN) reflects serum urea, and much urea is derived from protein, the BUN in patients with malnutrition and renal insufficiency may remain within normal limits. Dosage adjustment is required for several commonly prescribed drugs when a patient's GFR is reduced to 10–50 ml/min, and is suggested for certain drugs when the GFR is 51–70 ml/min (Table 3). Some of the drugs listed in Table 3 are not primarily renally excreted, but should be used cautiously in patients with renal insufficiency. Examples include tetracycline, which may produce azotemia in patients with

**Table 2** Examples of hepatically metabolized drugs. Adapted with permission from: Bertz RJ, Granneman GR. Use of *in vitro* and *in vivo* data to estimate likelihood of metabolic pharmacokinetic interactions. *Clin Pharmacokinet* 1997;32:210–58

| Primary transformation | Drugs | Inducers | Inhibitors |
|---|---|---|---|
| *Cytochrome P450s* | | | |
| CYP1A | TCAs, neuroleptics, theophylline, caffeine, acetaminophen, tacrine | cigarette smoke, cruciferous vegetables, charcoal broiled beef | |
| CYP2C9 | diclofenac, ibuprofen, indomethacin, piroxicam, phenytoin, tolbutamide, s-warfarin | phenytoin | fluconazole, itraconazole, ketoconazole, methylphenidate, cimetidine |
| CYP2D6 | hydrocodone, oxycodone, codeine, tramadol, propafenone, most oxidized psychotropic drugs (e.g. TCAs, paroxetine, fluoxetine, classic neuroleptics, risperidone), metoprolol, timolol, propranolol | not inducible | propoxyphene, chloroquine, propafenone, quinidine, fluoxetine, paroxetine, perphenazine, thioridazine, methylphenidate, cimetidine |
| CYP2E1 | acetaminophen, ethanol, fluorinated volatile anesthetics (e.g. halothane) | alcohol | |
| CYP3A | fentanyl, methadone, erythromycin, clarithromycin, itraconazole, ketoconazole, amiodarone, lidocaine, quinidine, all calcium channel blockers, cisapride, sertraline, alprazolam, zolpidem, triazolam, astemizole, loratadine, terfenadine, cyclosporine, sex hormones, cortisol, acetaminophen, carbamazepine, nefazodone | barbiturates, glucocorticoids, carbamazepine, phenytoin | erythromycin, clarithromycin, diltiazem, nicardipine, itraconazole, verapamil, ketoconazole, fluoxetine, methylphenidate, cimetidine |
| *Acetylation* | isoniazid, hydralazine, procainamide, sulfonamides | | |
| *Conjugation* | | | |
| Glucuronidation | morphine, codeine, lorazepam | phenytoin, barbiturates carbamazepine, rifampin | valproate |
| Sulfation | acetaminophen, steroids, methyldopa | | |

TCA, tricyclic antidepressant

**Table 3** Drugs requiring dosage modification for diminished glomerular filtration rate (GFR). Adapted with permission from Leipzig RM. Avoiding adverse drug effects in elderly patients. *Cleve Clin J Med* 1998;65:470–8

|  | GFR | |
|---|---|---|
|  | *51–70 ml/min* | *10–50 ml/min* |
| *Antimicrobial drugs* | | |
| Acyclovir | | X |
| Amantadine | X | X |
| Aminoglycosides | X | X |
| Amphotericin | | X |
| Aztreonam | | X |
| Cephalosporins | X (some) | X (many) |
| Imipenem | | X |
| Penicillins | X (ticarcillin only) | X (most) |
| Quinolones | | X (most) |
| Sulbactans | | X |
| Sulfonamides | | X |
| Tetracycline | X | X |
| TMP/SMZ | | X |
| Vancomycin | X | X |
| *Antihypertensives/cardiovascular drugs* | | |
| ACE inhibitors | | X (most) |
| Atenolol | | X |
| Digoxin | | X |
| Methyldopa | | X |
| Nadolol | | X |
| Sotalol | | X |
| *Psychotropic drugs* | | |
| Lithium | | X |
| *Analgesics* | | |
| Acetaminophen | | X |
| Meperidine | | X |
| *Others* | | |
| Albuterol | | X |
| Glyburide | ? | X |
| $H_2$ blockers | X (cimetidine only) | X (most) |
| Insulin | | X |

TMP, trimethoprim; SMZ, sulfamethoxazole; ACE, angiotensin converting enzyme; X, requires modification

end-stage renal disease, acetaminophen, whose active metabolites may be nephrotoxic to impaired kidneys, and meperidine, procainamide and enalapril, all of which are hepatically metabolized to active metabolites that are renally excreted.

## Therapeutic drug monitoring

Variation in pharmacokinetics can be detected by measuring plasma drug concentrations. This is most useful for drugs with a low therapeutic index, substantial interindividual variability in dose response – when it is not possible to use a direct measure of the desired effect, as with anticonvulsants or oral anticoagulants – or when the patient is at high risk for an ADE or ineffective therapy. In general, drug levels should be drawn at the end of a dosing interval, after steady state has been achieved, to allow drug distribution to be complete and to accurately relate the results to the laboratory's 'therapeutic levels'. In older adults, toxicity may occur with a plasma level within therapeutic range.

Plasma drug levels may be misinterpreted when the concentration of binding proteins differs from normal. Albumin is the binding protein for acidic drugs such as phenytoin, warfarin and naproxen, and its concentration decreases with malnutrition, cirrhosis, burns, nephrotic syndrome, and end-stage renal disease. $\alpha_1$-acid glycoprotein, an acute-phase reactant whose concentration may increase during trauma, surgery, acute myocardial infarction, infections, inflammatory diseases, and cancer, among other disorders, binds mainly basic drugs (for example, tricyclic antidepressants, quinidine, and lidocaine). Plasma drug concentrations are reported as total drug, both free and protein-bound. Drug response is usually correlated with the unbound concentration. As a result, the phenytoin level in patients with hypoalbuminemia reflects a greater concentration of unbound drug than that level would reflect in normoalbuminemic individuals. A hypoalbuminemic patient with a 'low' phenytoin level may actually have a 'therapeutic' unbound phenytoin level, i.e. a level adequate to prevent seizures in most adults; the same patient with a 'therapeutic' level may have a higher than desired unbound phenytoin level. Similarly, lidocaine levels appear toxic in patients with an acute myocardial infarction (MI), since $\alpha_1$-acid glycoprotein levels and therefore total (bound and free) drug level increase during an MI. The concentration of free drug, however, is within normal limits. Binding protein concentrations as well as the patient's clinical state need to be considered in the interpretation of drug levels.

## Effect of pharmacokinetic changes on drug action

Most studies that find differences in aging-related pharmacokinetics detect either a prolongation of drug half-life (the time it takes for the plasma concentration to fall 50%) and/or a diminished clearance (the rate of drug elimination) in older adults. These changes produce either an increase in the amount of time it takes to reach steady state and/or an increase in the concentration of the drug at steady-state. It takes four half-lives to reach 94% of a drug's steady-state concentration. The steady-state concentration of diazepam, whose half-life is about

90 hours in older adults, may not be reached until 2 weeks after starting the medication or increasing the dose. Once the diazepam is stopped, it will take another 2 weeks for the drug to be completely eliminated from the patient's system. Steady-state drug concentrations increase with drug dosage, bioavailability and impairment in drug clearance. Decreasing the dose and/or increasing the dosing interval can counteract a decrease in drug clearance.

## Aging-related changes in pharmacodynamics

If aging-related pharmacokinetic differences are not evident, dosage recommendations may still need to be modified for older compared with younger adults. For example, fentanyl and alfentanil do not have aging-related changes in pharmacokinetic parameters; however, older adults need a lower plasma level than younger persons to produce the same degree of sedation as measured by electroencephalogram (EEG)[14]. This is a pharmacodynamic difference, as illustrated in Figure 1.

Pharmacodynamic differences, which can result in increased or decreased responsiveness to a drug, may be due to alterations in receptors or post-receptor events, tissues or end-organs, or compensatory or homeostatic mechanisms. The only known example of aging-related decreased sensitivity is the diminished heart rate response to a given plasma level of isoproterenol in older adults, and the greater plasma level of propranolol needed to block this effect[15]. These responses appear to be due to a decrease in the proportion of high-affinity β-adrenoreceptors and the subsequent decrease in the generation of cAMP. Pharmacodynamically increased drug sensitivity can lead to a greater therapeutic benefit or to an adverse effect. For example, older adults experience greater pain relief at a particular morphine plasma level, enhanced sedation and memory impairment at similar diazepam plasma concentrations, and greater cardiac and CNS toxicity at similar theophylline levels compared with younger adults[16,17].

Many aging-related changes contribute to a narrowing of homeostatic reserve in older adults, termed 'homeostenosis' by some. This

**Table 4** Principles of appropriate prescribing for elderly patients. Adapted with permission from Leipzig RM. Pharmacology and appropriate prescribing. In: Cobbs EL, Duthie EH, Murphy JB, eds. Geriatrics Review Syllabus: A Core Curriculum in Geriatric Medicine. Dubuque, USA: Kendall-Hunt Publishing Company, 1999:30–35

Obtain a complete medication history. Have patients bring all medications to the office visit for review including non-prescription medications, vitamins and products bought at health-food stores. Ask about allergies, adverse reactions, use of tobacco, alcohol, caffeine, recreational drugs and also about other providers.

Use no drug before its time. Avoid prescribing when no diagnosis has been established, when symptoms are minor or non-specific, or when the benefit of the medication is questionable.

Use no drug beyond its time. Review medication lists at each visit and update them. Discontinue any medications that are no longer indicated. Monitor the use of drugs as needed and over-the-counter drugs.

Know the drugs you use. Know the pharmacological profile of the medications you prescribe and the potential adverse effects and toxicities. Monitor patients closely for deterioration in functional and cognitive parameters that could be drug related.

Start low, go slow. Always use the minimum dosage necessary for efficacy. Use drug levels when available and appropriate.

Treat adequately. Use dosages sufficient to achieve the therapeutic goal, as tolerated. Do not withhold therapy for treatable diseases.

Encourage treatment adherence. Clearly communicate with patients about the therapeutic goals and methods to achieve them. Give legible written instructions. Consider complexity of dosing schedules, expense and potential adverse effects when choosing a medication.

Use new agents with particular caution. Most new compounds have not been thoroughly evaluated in the elderly age group, and the risk/benefit ratio is often unknown.

results in a decreased reserve capacity for offsetting drug effects. For example, dehydrated older adults often have impaired thirst, antidiuretic hormone (ADH) secretion and renal concentrating responses. This can impair the ability to respond to drug-induced volume loss (diuretics, lithium-induced nephrogenic diabetes insipidus) or vasodilatation (centrally acting sympatholytics, nifedipine, $\alpha_1$-adrenergic antagonists such as tricyclic antidepressants, low-potency neuroleptics or prazosin-like drugs), resulting in orthostatic hypotension. In younger adults, a compensatory increase in catecholamines results in an increase in heart rate and therefore stroke volume to counteract the drop in blood pressure. Older adults generate the adrenergic response, but heart rate often does not increase, owing to the decreased numbers of high-affinity β-receptors discussed above, resulting in falls, syncope, or near-syncope. Another example of homeostenosis occurs with the production of vasoconstrictive prostaglandins to maintain renal blood flow

when effective circulating volume is decreased due to congestive heart failure (CHF), nephrotic syndrome, ascites, dehydration or hemorrhage. NSAIDs interfere with this homeostatic mechanism by inhibiting the formation of these prostaglandins, resulting in deterioration of renal function.

## Prescribing for older adults

Appropriate medication use by older adults requires balancing the benefits of treatment with its risks and burdens. Once the prescriber and the patient decide that the expected benefits are sufficient to warrant treatment, individualization of therapy may enhance the likelihood of successful treatment while avoiding predictable adverse outcomes. Therapy can be individualized by considering the patient's potential for having: an altered dose response; an adverse drug reaction; an interaction between the drug and others being taken; and difficulty in adhering to the treatment regimen;

as well as the patient's age, co-morbidity and life style.

## Principles of appropriate prescribing

Appropriate prescribing requires the individualization of therapy – the agent, dose, formulation, regimen – and explicit criteria for monitoring benefits and adverse events. An expert panel has recently reviewed medications used in older adults and made suggestions for prescribing (included in Table 5)[18]. Table 6 reviews many of the principles of prescribing for all patients, but particularly older adults who often have a narrow benefit/risk ratio.

## Medication review

It is most important to recognize the pitfalls in cataloging and maintaining an up-to-date list of all the medications a patient takes. Multiple prescribers and pharmacies, the use of non-prescription medications and supplements, and the shift to telephone consultation to monitor certain conditions rather than face-to-face visits, may all interfere with accurate record-keeping. The use of generic medications can add to the confusion, since the pills often look different and may be labeled with different drug names. A recent study of community-dwelling older adults found significant disagreement between doctor and patient perceptions of prescribed drug regimens[19]. Explicitly asking patients to bring all medications to appointments and inquiring whether they have seen any other health-care providers in between visits can help with this problem.

A regular review of medications can also prompt the provider to reassess whether these medications should be continued, and if so, whether the dosing regimen is still proper. Patients may no longer require medications initially prescribed as 'life-long'. Studies have shown that up to 40% of older adults remained normotensive 11 months after discontinuation of chronic antihypertensive medications[20] and that digoxin termination was well tolerated by the vast majority of nursing home residents in sinus rhythm without left ventricular dysfunction[21]. When the reason for continuing a medication is unclear, a cautious taper can provide evidence for or against renewing its prescription.

The conditions that influence pharmacokinetics and pharmacodynamics are dynamic, not static, and need to be regularly revisited. These include the use of tobacco, alcohol and recreational drugs, as well as weight and diet. Drugs that have been chronically taken and well tolerated may precipitate new problems as patients age. These conditions may be subtle and the possibility that they are drug-induced, especially from a long-term medication, might not be considered. But the possibility that any new condition in an older person may be drug-induced must be considered.

In 1996, the Food and Drug Administration approved 53 new molecular entities. Although the majority of new drugs are similar in action to older drugs, some provide a previously unavailable mechanism of action that could add substantially to the therapeutic armamentarium. Examples include zafirlukast (Accolate®), a leukotriene receptor blocker for asthma, zileuton (Zyflo®), a lipoxygenase inhibitor for asthma, pentosan polysulfate (Elmiron®), the first oral therapy for interstitial cystitis, fosfomycin (Monurol®), a single-dose antibiotic for uncomplicated urinary tract infections and mirtazapine (Remeron®) an $\alpha_2$ and serotonin receptor blocker antidepressant. However, very few geriatric patients participated in the clinical trials. Non-pharmacological and established pharmacological therapies should be exhausted before cautiously introducing a new medication.

## Medication management skills

Although the vast majority (85%) of older adults are responsible for taking their own medications, as many as 40% fail to take prescribed medications properly[22,23]. Medication management requires not only a defined set of mental and physical skills but also higher-level cortical processing and integration. Health literacy is a constellation of skills needed for medication management, including ability to

**Table 5** Prescribing considerations in older adults (recommendations from reference 18)

| Drug class | Implicated drugs | ADEs | Drug/dosage considerations |
|---|---|---|---|
| *Analgesics* | | | |
| Opioids | all | sedation, delirium, respiratory depression | always use lowest effective dose |
| | meperidine (Demerol®) and propoxyphene (Darvon®) | twitching, seizures | propoxyphene and meperidine should generally be avoided in the elderly, especially if giving multiple doses propoxyphene offers few analgesic advantages over acetaminophen, yet has the side-effects of other opioid drugs*. Meperidine requires huge doses, owing to poor bioavailability |
| | pentazocine (Talwin®) | confusion and hallucinations | pentazocine is a mixed agonist/antagonist, and should be avoided in the elderly* |
| NSAIDs | all | renal insufficiency hyperkalemia gastritis/ulcer painless GI bleeding | patients with decreased effective circulating volume due to CHF, nephrotic syndrome, ascites, dehydration or hemorrhage are at greater risk of developing renal insufficiency GI bleeding is least common with low-dose ibuprofen, and most common with piroxicam and possibly ketoprofen proton pump inhibitors (e.g. omeprazole), misoprostol, and high-dose famotidine (40 mg po bid) decrease UGI ulcers/bleeding by 40%. Usual-dose $H_2$ blockers are not effective |
| | phenylbutazone (Butazolidin®) | hematological complications | avoid in elderly* |
| | indomethacin (Indocin®) | CNS effects | avoid in elderly* |
| *Anticoagulants/antiplatelet agents* | | | |
| | dipyridamole ticlopidine | orthostatic hypotension rare neutropenia and thrombocytopenia | only beneficial in patients with artificial heart valves* no better than aspirin at preventing clotting and considerably more toxic. Avoid in elderly* may be useful in aspirin-intolerant patients require lower doses than younger people |
| | warfarin | increased risk of bleeding | multiple drug interactions – consider monitoring when other drugs are added or deleted from regimen |

*(Continued)*

**Table 5** Continued

| Drug class | Implicated drugs | ADEs | Drug/dosage considerations | Drugs of choice |
|---|---|---|---|---|
| | | | Co-morbidities | low-dose thiazide diuretics |
| *Cardiovascular medications* | | | *none or osteoporosis* | |
| Antihypertensives | alpha blockers (prazosin, terazosin, doxazosin, etc.) potent vasodilators (nifedipine, hydralazine, etc.) diuretics | orthostatic hypotension | | |
| | centrally acting antihypertensives (methyldopa, clonidine) lipophilic beta blockers (propranolol, metoprolol) | dementia or depression | LV dysfunction, DM angina, diastolic dysfunction | ACE inhibitors CCBs (e.g. verapamil and diltiazem), beta blockers |
| | methyldopa (Aldomet®) reserpine (Serpasil® or Hydropres®) | bradycardia, depression depression, sedation, impotence, orthostatic hypotension | unnecessary risk. Avoid in elderly* | |
| Digoxin | | confusion, anorexia | indications: CHF not responsive to diuretics and ACE inhibition; rapid AF. Does not prevent rapid AF in patients with paroxysmal AF because of decreased renal clearance, doses in elderly should rarely exceed 0.125 mg unless treating atrial arrhythmias* | |
| Antiarrhythmics | disopyramide | CHF, anticholinergic effects (confusion, constipation, urinary retention, sedation) | most potent negative inotrope. Avoid in elderly* | |
| *Central nervous system medications* | ergot mesyloids (Hydergine®) | | not effective for treatment of dementia* | |
| *Endocrine/metabolic medications* | insulin | | dosage will need adjustment as creatinine clearance declines | |

(Continued)

**Table 5** Continued

| Drug class | Implicated drugs | ADEs | Drug/dosage considerations |
|---|---|---|---|
| Oral hypoglycemics | chlorpropamide (Diabinese®) glyburide (Micronase®) | SIADH, prolonged hypoglycemia hypoglycemia | avoid in the elderly* may have greater rate of hypoglycemia than other oral sulfonylureas |
| | Metformin (Glucophage®) | Lactic acidosis, anemia | Monitor renal function. Hold prior to iodinated contrast study or surgical procedures |
| Thyroid hormone | | | the replacement dose in older adults is often less than in younger adults |
| Iron supplements | | constipation | rarely need to be given in doses of > 325 mg daily. Higher doses do not increase absorption but may increase constipation* |
| *Gastrointestinal and genitourinary medications* | | | |
| Antispasmotics | dicyclomine (Bentyl®) hyoscyamine (Levsin®, Levsinex®) propantheline (Pro-Banthine®) belladonna alkaloids (e.g. Donnatal®) clidinium-chlordiazepoxide (Librax®) | highly anticholinergic (confusion, constipation, urinary retention, sedation) | uncertain efficacy with substantial chance of toxicity avoid long-term use in the elderly* |
| H$_2$ blockers | oxybutynin (Ditropan®) all | delirium | dose must be decreased for impaired creatinine clearance review indicator for treatment post-hospitalization |
| *Psychotropics* | | | |
| Antidepressants | tertiary TCAs [amitriptyline (elavil®, Triavil®, Limbitrol®); doxepin (Sinequan®); imipramine (Tofranil®), clomipramine (Anafranil®)] | Sedation, confusion, urinary retention, orthostatic hypotension, prolonged Qt$_c$ or heart block | Tertiary amine TCAs are more anticholinergic, antiadrenergic and antihistiminergic than secondary TCAs [(nortriptyline (Aventyl®, Pamelor®) and desipramine (Norpramin®)]. Amitriptyline and doxepin have very strong anticholinergic and sedating properties and should rarely be the antidepressant of choice for elderly patients* |

*(Continued)*

**Table 5** Continued

| Drug class | Implicated drugs | ADEs | Drug/dosage considerations |
|---|---|---|---|
| | | | when using a TCA, always initiate therapy with a low dose of a secondary agent and monitor blood levels (steady state in about 3 days), owing to interindividual differences in metabolism and potential drug interactions. |
| | | | *Co-morbidity* — *Drug recommendations* |
| | | | LV dysfunction — consider nortriptyline or bupropion |
| | | | hepatically metabolized medications — fluoxetine and paroxetine inhibit the metabolism of certain drugs (Table 2) |
| | | | type Ia antiarrhythmics — TCAs relatively contraindicated |
| Barbiturates | all | sedation, confusion, falls | barbiturates cause more side-effects than most other sedative or hypnotic drugs in the elderly and are highly addictive. They should not be started as new therapy in the elderly except when used to control seizures* |
| Benzodiazepines | all, especially long-acting: diazepam (Valium®), chlordiazepoxide (Librium®), flurazepam (Dalmane®), clonazepam (Klonopin®) | sedation, confusion, falls or fractures | medium- and short-acting benzodiazepines are preferred. Older adults have increased sensitivity to these, so the following maximum total daily doses are suggested: lorazepam (Ativan®) 3 mg; oxazepam (Serax®), 60 mg; alprazolam (Xanax®), 2 mg; temazepam (Restoril® 15 mg); triazolam (Halcion®), 0.25 mg; zolpidem (Ambien®), 5 mg* parenteral administration is more likely to cause apnea, hypotension, or cardiac arrest |
| | meprobamate (Miltown®, Equanil®) | | highly addictive and sedating. Should avoid use in elderly, taper gradually* |
| Neuroleptics | all | sedation, new delirium coincident with drug usage, orthostatic hypotension, severe extrapyramidal symptoms | low-potency neuroleptics (e.g. chlorpromazine (Thorazine®), thioridazine (Mellaril®) are very anticholinergic, antiadrenergic and sedating |

*(Continued)*

**Table 5** Continued

| Drug class | Implicated drugs | ADEs | Drug/dosage considerations |
|---|---|---|---|
| | | | high-potency neuroleptics [e.g. haloperidol (Haldol®), perphenazine (Stelazine®)] are potent $D_2$ receptor blockers causing EPS and Parkinson's disease choose drug based on patient profile effective doses are much smaller than those used in younger adults, e.g. 0.25–0.5 mg haloperidol; 25 mg chlorpromazine |
| *Symptomatic relief* | | | |
| Antiemetics | trimethobenzamide (Tigan®) | extrapyramidal effects | trimethobenzamide is one of the least effective antiemetic drugs. When possible, it should be avoided in the elderly* |
| H₁ blockers | examples include chlorpheniramine, diphenhydramine (Benadryl®), hydroxyzine (Vistaril®, Atarax®), cyproheptadine (Periactin®), promethazine (Phenergan®). | sedation, delirium, respiratory depression | many antihistamines are very anticholinergic. Many cough and cold preparations are available without antihistamines, and these are safer substitutes in the elderly* diphenhydramine (Benadryl®) should not be used as a hypnotic in the elderly. When used to treat or prevent allergic reactions it should be used in the smallest possible dose and monitored carefully* fexofenadine (Allegra®) and loratadine (Claritin®) do not cross the blood–brain barrier and so are less likely to cause these problems. Terfenadine (Seldane®) and astemizole (Hismanal®) may be associated with prolonged Qtc interval when taken with inhibitors of the CYP3A isozyme of cytochrome P450 (see Table 2) |
| Muscle relaxants | methocarbamol (Robaxin®) carisoprodol (Soma®) chlorzoxazone (Paraflex®) metaxalone (Skelaxin®) cyclobenzaprine (Flexeril®) | anticholinergic side-effects, sedation, weakness | effectiveness at doses tolerated by the elderly is questionable. Whenever possible, they should not be used in the elderly* instead, use local measures (heat, cold, massage) and, if necessary, short-acting benzodiazepine |

*From Beers' criteria, reference 18; GI, gastrointestinal; CHF, congestive heart failure; UGI, upper gastrointestinal; CNS, central nervous system; LV, left ventricular; DM, diabetes mellitus; ACE, angiotensin converting enzymes; CCB, calcium channel blocker; AF, atrial fibrillation; SIADH, syndrome of inappropriate antidiuretic hormone; TCA, tricyclic antidepressant; EF, ejection fraction; EPS, extrapyramidal symptoms; NSAIDs, non-steroidal anti-inflammatory drugs. Adapted with permission from Beers MH. Explicit criteria for determining potentially inappropriate medication use by the elderly. An update. *Arch Intern Med* 1997;157:1531–6

**Table 6** Effect of food on drug absorption

*Increased drug absorption*
Alprazolam, amiodarone, carbamazepine, clarithromycin, diazepam, diltiazem, felodipine, hydralazine, hydrochlorothiazide, labetalol, metoprolol, nifedipine, nitrofurantoin, oxybutynin, phenytoin, propranolol, spironolactone theophylline, ticlopidine, tramadol

*Decreased drug absorption*
Acetaminophen, alendronate, atenolol, captopril, ciprofloxacin, digoxin, doxazosin, levodopa/carbidopa, methyldopa, metformin, methotrexate, norfloxacin, pravastatin, sotalol, sulpiride, verapamil

perform basic reading and numerical tasks required to function in the health-care environment; this set of skills includes ability to read and interpret medical instructions as well as the ability to calculate medication dosage and timing[23]. In a survey of 3260 older Medicare enrollees, one-third of the English- and one-half of the Spanish-speaking respondents had inadequate or marginal health literacy.[24]

## Non-adherence

Studies reporting compliance rates in older adults have found that the adherence rate ranges from 26 to 59%[25]. Treatment adherence can be difficult to ascertain in older adults. Patients may be unwilling or unable to discuss reasons for non-adherence such as financial concerns, difficulty obtaining or taking medications, or lack of belief that the medications are necessary[26]. Motivation and functional impairments, for example ambulation, vision, and manual dexterity, can interfere with taking medication as prescribed[25,27]. One study found that poor recall of the medication regimen, seeing numerous physicians, being female, having a medium income, using many medications, and believing that medications are expensive were factors independently associated with an increased risk of hospitalization due to non-adherence[28]. Among people over age 65 who take prescription drugs, an average of 3.1% of household income is spent on out-of-pocket expenses for drugs. Among severely disabled elderly persons, out-patient prescription drug costs account for over half of out-of-pocket expenditures for health care. Significantly higher rates of non-adherence have also been found among elders who live alone or use more than one pharmacy. Medications that must be taken several times a day are harder to take according to schedule. Aids exist to improve adherence, such as daily dose reminder boxes, and to improve the administration of inhalers, eye drops and insulin[29].

Lack of understanding (non-comprehension) of the expected regimen and lack of instructions on how to integrate medications at hospital discharge into the pre-hospitalization regimen account for a large portion of the 'non-compliance' seen post-hospitalization. Intelligent non-compliance occurs when the patient has a new symptom temporally associated with the initiation of drug therapy and the physician states that the medication could not possibly be responsible. Patients may then stop the medication or change the dose without telling the physician. This could result in serious complications if the patient is hospitalized and the physician's medication list is implemented.

## Estimates of drug efficacy and harm in older adults

Effective therapies are underprescribed to older adults, including thrombolysis for acute myocardial infarction[30], opioids for cancer pain[31,32], anticoagulation to prevent stroke in chronic atrial fibrillation[33], and beta blockers[34] and aspirin post MI[35]. Although older adults are often at greater risk for ADEs than younger adults, they are frequently more likely to benefit from treatment[36]. For example, 72 hypertensive adults ≥ 60 years old would need to be treated for 5 years to prevent one death, whereas 167 younger adults would need to be treated to obtain the same result. The best evidence of a drug's efficacy and the best estimate of the degree of its efficacy come from randomized clinical trials. Published randomized controlled trials, however, probably underestimate the prevalence of ADEs and fail to identify certain ADEs that will occur in the frail or older-old, or in older adults whose illnesses or medications would have excluded them from the study. Some of these ADEs will be due to age- and disease-related pharmacokinetic changes, and some due to drug interactions. Premarketing pharmacokinetic studies in older adults and drug interaction screening with both those drugs most commonly taken in patients with the condition being treated, as well as drugs that are likely to affect metabolism, are becoming more frequent. These are often noted in the prescribing information, and treatment can be modified accordingly.

There will always be unexpected ADEs that are detected post-marketing, since most clinical trials are relatively small and most ADEs are rare; large numbers of people need to be exposed to the drug before an association between the adverse event and the drug can be made. However, some ADEs may be common in older adults but not detected for the reasons noted above, for example interference with compensatory mechanisms that are less critical in healthier or younger adults, non-specific complaints often mimicking syndromes associated with aging, or pharmacodynamic effects due to aging- or disease-related changes in end-organs. Delirium, depression and oversedation are examples of ADEs that have been identified post-marketing in older adults.

## Medication errors and adverse drug events

Aging-related metabolic changes, polypharmacy, the complexity of medical regimens and individual-specific physiological and functional characteristics predispose older adults to ADEs[1,4,36,37]. Most medication errors and ADEs are unreported and undocumented[38–41]. According to a 1993 estimate published in the recent Institute of Medicine report, there are 7000 deaths/year due to medication errors[1]. Between 1983 and 1993 there was an 8.5-fold increase in the number of out-patient deaths due to medication errors; this number is expected to increase as new medications are introduced for a wider range of indications and as the US population ages[1,42]. Medication errors and ADEs

are associated with increased utilization of health-care resources – doctor visits, emergency room visits and acute hospitalizations[21,43,44]. In 1994 the cost of ambulatory drug-related morbidity and mortality was $76.6 billion. For every dollar spent on out-patient medications, another dollar is spent to treat new health problems related to that medication[1].

It is estimated that 5–15% of acute geriatric medical admissions are due to ADEs, defined as injuries resulting from medical interventions related to drugs. These adverse events may differ from those typically seen in younger patients and may be misinterpreted by physicians, patients and family members because: they resemble disorders thought to increase in prevalence in the elderly, e.g. falls, anorexia, fatigue, cognitive impairment, urinary incontinence and constipation; or they differ from the ADEs uncovered during clinical trials with younger, healthier subjects. A lowered index of suspicion can result in misdiagnosis and the prescription of additional medications, further increasing the chances of ADEs. For example, pharmacoepidemiological studies have identified temporal associations between the prescribing of beta blockers and antidepressants, as well as neuroleptics and anti-Parkinsonian agents. These data suggest that drug-induced depression and Parkinsonism are being under-recognized and pharmacologically treated rather than identified as ADEs, resulting in dosage reduction or a change in medication.

Although elderly patients experience more ADEs than younger patients, age alone has generally not been shown to be an independent risk factor. Pharmacokinetic changes affecting drug concentration and the increased use of medications with a low therapeutic index account for some potentially avoidable ADEs in elders. In several studies, the percentage of patients experiencing an ADE increases substantially with the number of drugs taken. It is not known whether this is due to drug–drug interactions or to the severity of illness, enhanced end-organ dysfunction, or impaired compensatory mechanisms associated with the prescription of multiple medications.

ADEs can be predictable or idiosyncratic; most are predictable. In predictable ADEs, almost every person given a sufficient quantity of drug will develop the ADE. The dose precipitating the ADE can vary substantially, however. Within an individual the ADE is usually dose-dependent, that is, the ADE does not occur with lower doses of drug. Examples include alcohol and intoxication as well as opioids and obtundation. In contrast, only certain people will develop an idiosyncratic ADE regardless of the quantity of drug given. Examples include renal insufficiency with angiotensin converting enzyme (ACE) inhibitors and gastrointestinal bleeding with NSAIDs. Susceptibility to an ADE may be due to genetic factors – such as inherited variant pathways of drug metabolism or increased susceptibility to a drug's effect, for example glucose-6-phosphate dehydrogenase deficiency – or to acquired conditions such as ACE inhibitor renal insufficiency due to hypovolemia, severe CHF, diabetes mellitus and hyponatremia, or acetaminophen hepatotoxicity in alcoholics or severely malnourished individuals. Previous ADEs can often suggest a predilection to future ADEs; examples include drug-induced confusion, unexpected high plasma concentrations of a drug – suggesting that the patient is a poor or slow metabolizer – or therapeutic failure due to low concentrations in a rapid metabolizer.

A recent case series of self-reported ADEs in older out-patients taking five medications or more found 95% to be predictable. Predictable ADEs are generally preventable, especially if new medications are started at a low dose and dosage increases made only after a steady-state has been reached. This is often feasible when treating chronic non-life-threatening conditions. Even some idiosyncratic reactions can probably be prevented once the risk factors are identified. Age ≥ 80 years, digoxin dose ≥ 0.25 mg, concurrent use of amiodarone, propafenone, verapamil or quinidine, and serum creatinine ≥ 1.36 mg/dl were found to be independent risk factors for digoxin toxicity in one study of hospitalized Italian patients. A prescriber attuned to the principles of geriatric pharmacology would have quickly recognized the need to adjust dosage because of renal impairment and to check for potential drug interactions. In this way, a predictable ADE

might have been prevented. Two recent studies of hospital in-patients of all ages found that 19–28% of in-patient ADEs were preventable.

## Drug interactions

Drug interactions can result in the attenuation of a therapeutic effect or the precipitation of an adverse event. They can be either pharmacokinetic or pharmacodynamic in nature; examples of pharmacokinetic interactions are shown in Tables 1 and 2. Drug interactions can occur with diseases, foodstuffs, or other medications.

*Drug–disease interactions*  When disease affects organs of drug metabolism or elimination such as the liver or the kidney, or the delivery of drugs to those organs, as in CHF or cirrhosis, pharmacokinetic drug–disease interactions can occur. The therapeutic effects of prodrugs such as codeine, enalapril and prednisone are diminished when hepatic metabolism is impaired, resulting in impaired production of their biologically active forms – morphine, enalaprilat and prednisolone. Examples of pharmacodynamic drug–disease interactions of concern to geriatricians include: anticholinergic drugs at doses tolerated by cognitively intact, non-Parkinsonian elders producing increased confusion and delirium in patients with dementia or Parkinson's disease; exacerbation of CHF by NSAID-induced water retention; increased claudication with beta blockers through unopposed $\alpha_1$-adrenergic vasoconstriction; worsening of stress urinary incontinence with diuretics or $\alpha_1$-antagonists such as terazosin or doxazosin; urinary retention in patients with benign prostatic hypertrophy treated with decongestants or anticholinergics; and worsening of constipation with calcium supplements, calcium channel blockers, anticholinergics, beta blockers or opioids.

*Drug–food interactions*  Most drug–food interactions affect drug or nutrient absorption. Food can reduce or increase drug absorption (Table 6). For some drugs food can reduce first-pass extraction or, by delaying gastric emptying, improve dissolution and absorption. When absorption is substantially affected by food, the drug should be consistently taken in either the fasted or the fed state, depending on the ability to tolerate taking the drug without food. Foods can also interact with drugs through other mechanisms, such as the induction or inhibition of certain cytochrome P450 isozymes (Table 1) or interference with the drug's mechanism of action, as with the reduction in warfarin anticoagulation when nutritional supplements containing vitamin K are taken.

Medications can also directly or indirectly impair nutritional status. Some drugs cause anorexia (for example digoxin, NSAIDs), dry mouth (for example anti-Parkinsonian drugs, beta blockers, tricyclic antidepressants, antihistamines), or altered taste perception (for example captopril, penicillamine), resulting in decreased oral intake. Proton-pump inhibitors and $H_2$ blockers may impair the absorption of protein-bound vitamin $B_{12}$. Phenytoin can increase the inactivation of vitamin D and cause folate deficiency, and furosemide can cause thiamine deficiency[45]. Poor dietry intake can enhance drug toxicity by providing inadequate levels of compounds needed for detoxification. For example, low glutathione levels result in increased susceptibility to acetaminophen toxicity at lower drug doses, and thiamine deficiency results in Wernicke–Korsakoff's psychosis when patients receive intravenous glucose.

*Multiple medications and drug–drug interactions*  Many drug–drug interactions involve induction or inhibition of cytochrome P450 isozymes (Table 2). Each inducing or inhibiting drug does not affect every isozyme; however, drugs are often metabolized by more than one isozyme. Induction can take days or weeks to reach maximum effect; inhibition occurs immediately. Smoking may cause less enzyme induction in elderly than in younger people; however, the induction of drug metabolism by phenytoin and inhibition by cimetidine is the same as in younger people. Pharmacokinetic drug–drug interactions can also interfere with drug absorption, protein binding, renal excretion or tubular secretion (Table 1).

Clinically significant protein binding interactions are less common than previously thought. They can occur only if a displacing drug (one that binds to the same site on the protein) reaches a high enough plasma concentration to compete for the majority of the binding sites. ADEs will then arise only if the drug being displaced has a narrow therapeutic index, such as warfarin. Initiation of therapy with a displacing drug such as salicylic acid or valproic acid results in a temporary increase in the concentration of warfarin. This will decrease as equilibrium is re-established, unless the added drug also affects warfarin metabolism, such as with sulfonamides or oral sulfonylurea hypoglycemics.

Other drug–drug interactions are pharmacodynamic in nature. Examples include the increased hypoglycemic effect that occurs when hypoglycemics taking sulfonylurea are given ACE inhibitors (probably due to an increased insulin effect), the decreased antihypertensive effect of many antihypertensives when NSAIDs are taken, and the increased risk of bleeding with NSAIDs and oral anticoagulants.

# References

1. Institute of Medicine. *To Err is Human: Building a Safer Health System*. Washington, DC: The National Academy of Medicine, 2000:26–48
2. Golden AG, Preston RA, Barnett SD, *et al*. Inappropriate medication prescribing in homebound older adults. *J Am Geriatr Soc* 1999;47:948–53
3. Leipzig RM. Pharmacology and appropriate prescribing. In Cobbs EL, Duthie EH, Murphy JB, eds. *Geriatrics Review Syllabus: A Core Curriculum in Geriatric Medicine*. Dubuque, IA: Kendall-Hunt Publishing, 1999:30–5
4. Darnell JC, Murray MD, Martz BL, Weinberger M. Medication use by ambulatory elderly: an in-home survey. *J Am Geriatr Soc* 1986;34:1–4
5. Ennis KJ, Reichard RA. Maximizing drug compliance in the elderly. Tips for staying on top

of your patients' medication use. *Postgrad Med* 1997;102:211–13, 218, 223–4

6. Salzman C. Medication compliance in the elderly. *J Clin Psychiatry* 1995;56:18–22; discussion 23

7. Hurwitz A, Brady DA, Schaal SE, *et al*. Gastric acidity in older adults. *J Am Med Assoc* 1997; 278:659–62

8. Campion EW, Avorn J, Reder VA, Olins NJ. Overmedication of the low-weight elderly. *Arch Intern Med* 1987;147:945–7

9. Katzung BG. Special aspects of geriatric pharmacology. In Katzung BG, ed. *Basic and Clinical Pharmacology*. New York: McGraw-Hill, 2001

10. Woodhouse K, Wynne HA. Age-related changes in hepatic function. Implications for drug therapy. *Drugs Aging* 1992;2:243–55

11. Lindeman RD, Tobin J, Shock NW. Longitudinal studies on the rate of decline in renal function with age. *J Am Geriatr Soc* 1985;33:278–85

12. Goldberg TH, Finkelstein MS. Difficulties in estimating glomerular filtration rate in the elderly. *Arch Intern Med* 1987;147:1430–3

13. Malmrose LC, Gray SL, Pieper CF, *et al*. Measured versus estimated creatinine clearance in a high-functioning elderly sample: MacArthur Foundation Study of Successful Aging. *J Am Geriatr Soc* 1993;41:715–21

14. Scott JC, Stanski DR. Decreased fentanyl and alfentanil dose requirements with age. A simultaneous pharmacokinetic and pharmacodynamic evaluation. *J Pharmacol Exp Ther* 1987; 240:159–66

15. Vestal RE, Wood AJ, Shand DG. Reduced beta-adrenoceptor sensitivity in the elderly. *Clin Pharmacol Ther* 1979;26:181–6

16. Reidenberg MM, Levy M, Warner H, *et al*. Relationship between diazepam dose, plasma level, age, and central nervous system depression. *Clin Pharmacol Ther* 1978;23:371–4

17. Shannon M. Predictors of major toxicity after theophylline overdose. *Ann Intern Med* 1993; 119:1161–7

18. Beers MH. Explicit criteria for determining potentially inappropriate medication use by the elderly. An update. *Arch Intern Med* 1997;157: 1531–6

19. Bikowski RM, Ripsin CM, Lorraine VL. Physician–patient congruence regarding medication regimens. *J Am Geriatr Soc* 2001;49: 1353–7

20. Fotherby MD. Withdrawal of antihypertensive therapy in the elderly. The issues. *Drugs Aging* 1995;6:436–44

21. Beard K. Adverse reactions as a cause of hospital admission in the aged. *Drugs Aging* 1992; 2:356–67

22. Morrow D, Leirer V, Altieri P, Tanke E. Elders' schema for taking medication: implications for instruction design. *J Gerontol* 1991;46:P378–85

23. Law R, Chalmers C. Medicines and elderly people: a general practice survey. *Br Med J* 1976;1:565–8

24. Gazmararian JA, Baker DW, Williams MV, *et al*. Health literacy among Medicare enrollees in a managed care organization. *J Am Med Assoc* 1999;281:545–51

25. Balkrishnan R. Predictors of medication adherence in the elderly. *Clin Ther* 1998;20:764–71

26. Fincke BG, Miller DR, Spiro A 3rd. The interaction of patient perception of overmedication with drug compliance and side effects. *J Gen Intern Med* 1998;13:182–5

27. Atkin PA, Finnegan TP, Ogle SJ, Shenfield GM. Functional ability of patients to manage medication packaging: a survey of geriatric inpatients. *Age Ageing* 1994;23:113–16

28. Col N, Fanale JE, Kronholm P. The role of medication noncompliance and adverse drug reactions in hospitalizations of the elderly. *Arch Intern Med* 1990;150:841–5

29. Cramer JA. Enhancing patient compliance in the elderly. Role of packaging aids and monitoring. *Drugs Aging* 1998;12:7–15

30. McLaughlin TJ, Gurwitz JH, Willison DJ, *et al*. Delayed thrombolytic treatment of older patients with acute myocardial infarction. *J Am Geriatr Soc* 1999;47:1222–8

31. Portenoy RK, Miransky J, Thaler HT, *et al*. Pain in ambulatory patients with lung or colon cancer. Prevalence, characteristics, and effect. *Cancer* 1992;70:1616–24

32. Morrison RS, Siu AL. A comparison of pain and its treatment in advanced dementia and cognitively intact patients with hip fracture. *J Pain Symptom Manage* 2000;19:240–8

33. McCormick D, Gurwitz JH, Goldberg RJ, Ansell J. Long-term anticoagulation therapy for atrial fibrillation in elderly patients: efficacy, risk, and current patterns of use. *J Thromb Thrombolysis* 1999;7:157–63

34. Gurwitz JH, Goldberg RJ, Chen Z, *et al*. Beta-blocker therapy in acute myocardial infarction: evidence for underutilization in the elderly. *Am J Med* 1992;93:605–10

35. McCormick D, Gurwitz JH, Lessard D, *et al*. Use of aspirin, beta-blockers, and lipid-lowering medications before recurrent acute myocardial infarction: missed opportunities for prevention? *Arch Intern Med* 1999;159: 561–7

36. Gurwitz JH, Avorn J. The ambiguous relation between aging and adverse drug reactions. *Ann Int Med* 1991;114:956–66

37. Weintraub M. Compliance in the elderly. *Clin Geriatr Med* 1990;6:445–52

38. Manasse HR Jr. Medication use in an imperfect world: drug misadventuring as an issue of

public policy, Part 1. *Am J Hosp Pharm* 1989; 46:929–44

39. Griffin JP, Weber JC. Voluntary systems of adverse reaction reporting – Part I. *Adverse Drug React Acute Poisoning Rev* 1985;4:213–30

40. Griffin JP, Weber JC. Voluntary systems of adverse reaction reporting – Part II. *Adverse Drug React Acute Poisoning Rev* 1986;5: 23–55

41. Cullen DJ, Bates DW, Small SD, *et al*. The incident reporting system does not detect adverse drug events: a problem for quality improvement. *Jt Comm J Qual Improv* 1995; 21:541–8

42. Phillips DP, Christenfeld N, Glynn LM. Increase in US medication-error deaths between 1983 and 1993. *Lancet* 1998;351:643–4

43. Burnum JF. Preventability of adverse drug reactions. *Ann Intern Med* 1976;85:80–1

44. Schneitman-McIntire O, Farnen TA, Gordon N, *et al*. Medication misadventures resulting in emergency department visits at an HMO medical center. *Am J Health Syst Pharm* 1996;53: 1416–22

45. Schumann K. Interactions between drugs and vitamins at advanced age. *Int J Vitam Nutr Res* 1999;69:173–8

46. Bertz RJ, Granneman GR. Use of *in vitro* and *in vivo* data to estimate the likelihood of metabolic pharmacokinetic interactions. *Clin Pharmacokinet* 1997;32:210–58

47. Aronoff GR, Berns JS, Brier ME, *et al*, eds. Drug prescribing in renal failure: dosing guidelines for adults. Fourth edn. Philadelphia: American College of Physicians, 1999

48. Leipzig RM. Avoiding adverse drug effects in elderly patients. *Cleve Clin J Med* 1998;65: 470–8

# 5

# Cognition in the geripause

*Karen L. Dahlman, Margaret C. Sewell and Richard C. Mohs*

## Introduction

Women outnumber men with every passing decade, and the risk of dementia dramatically increases with age. Therefore, it has become important for physicians in all specialties to understand the myriad emotional and physical factors that impact cognition in their female patients, so that they are better able to distinguish the benign from the pathological.

Cognitively, the period between the menopause and frank 'old age', for which the label 'geripause' is proposed, is regarded as a time during which most women continue to enjoy cognitive wellness even as they may experience some mild decline in certain cognitive functions, and worry more about the impact of 'senior moments' on their mental abilities. Geripausal women will often bring these worries to their doctors, who must be able to distinguish between the normal aging process and incipient dementia.

The first part of this chapter outlines what constitutes normal cognitive changes among women aged approximately 45–70, as well as physical, medical, and emotional factors that affect normal aging. The second part of the chapter reviews pathological cognitive changes. The final section discusses important assessment issues for the physician.

## Normal aging and cognition

The neuropsychology of the normal aging process is not fully understood. In addition to normal loss of hippocampal cells and expected brain atrophy, which begins around the age of 55, research suggests that cognitive slowing and changes in attentional ability account for some variance in memory function[1]. The age range 50–65 represents a time of fairly rapid cognitive alterations associated with normal aging[1].

Although many cognitive functions do decline as part of the normal aging process, the extent and pattern of loss varies greatly across individuals and across the specific cognitive domain being assessed. Generally speaking, well-rehearsed, over-learned activities are stable across the life span. For example, word-knowledge and reading ability do not diminish with aging. Other cognitive functions, including the speeded processing of novel information, complex problem solving, memory, mental flexibility and perceptual manipulation tasks are vulnerable to the aging process[2]. However, serious memory loss is not a normal consequence of aging and most older women continue to perform within normal limits on tests of cognitive function well into their eighties.

## Factors that affect normal aging

Substantial differences exist among individuals as they age. Cognitive functioning is modelled on a bell-shaped curve, with the vast majority of people falling in the normal range. Those individuals who are blessed with intelligence at the highest levels of the spectrum tend to decline relatively less with age as a group than those with a lower life-long baseline. The decline that is seen among those with lower life-long IQ is also more dramatic than that experienced by individuals in the higher ranges of intellectual functioning. Accordingly, functional impairment, the ability independently to perform both simple and complex activities of daily living at simple and more complex levels, will be experienced sooner and more acutely by those who start the aging process with fewer cognitive reserves[3].

Rowe and Kahn's reports[4,5] on successful aging suggest that three main components of the aging process must be met: low probability of disease and disease-related disability; high cognitive and physical functioning; and active engagement in life. Continuing engagement with life implies maintaining interpersonal relationships and productive activities. Research has shown that the social environment may be able to protect against cognitive declines in older individuals; specifically, individuals with greater emotional supports have better baseline performance on cognitive tests[6]. Associations between emotional vitality (defined as having a high sense of personal mastery, being happy, and having low depressive symptomatology and anxiety) have been documented across several different levels of physical disability[7,8], underlining the idea that emotional and social factors can mediate physical handicaps. One's life style, not just biological load (e.g. genetic factors), can affect healthy cognitive aging and longevity. Factors such as life-time occupation[9], socioeconomic status[1], education[10], physical activity[11], and leisure activity[12,13] may provide a cognitive 'reserve' that delays the onset of clinical manifestations of the disease. It is hypothesized that the mechanism may lie in preserving a set of skills that allow for better coping with the disabilities of an emerging dementia. Another theory is that leisure activities, learning and social interactions may produce structural and functional changes in the brain. For example, enhanced chronic neuronal activation associated with increased brain work, increased cerebral blood flow and increased glucose and oxygen metabolism may hinder the development of disease[13].

Emotional factors must be taken into account when interpreting cognitive changes in the geripausal woman. Depression, to take one example, is known to affect attention, concentration, memory, and motor speed and, unlike a primary memory disorder, is treatable. As depression remits, the cognitive symptoms of that disorder will gradually improve. If the cognitive complaints remain even after the depression has remitted, it is likely that a primary cognitive disorder is driving the clinical picture.

Research has demonstrated that estimates of life expectancy are more accurate when emotional and cognitive functioning are factored into the equation[14]. Depression is found in both men and women in later life, with little evidence for a 'female depression' syndrome. Increased prevalence of depression in females has been shown to be connected with greater exposure to risk factors such as being or becoming single, having lower educational levels, lower income, and one or more chronic physical illnesses or functional limitations[15]. Emotional vitality has been found to exist at all levels, even among the most disabled older community-dwelling women, and those women with adequate emotional supports are more likely to be emotionally vital than those women who lack social support[16]. Epidemiological research has shown that there is a peak in the onset of depressive illness during the perimenopausal years (ages 45–50)[17]. In patients with bipolar disorder, increased frequency of cycling may occur in the perimenopause[18] and, generally speaking, women with a history of affective disorders including a history of postpartum depression, premenstrual syndrome, or prior episodes of depression, are all at high risk for a depressive episode during the menopausal period[19–21].

Among the many factors that may affect cognitive function among older women, some are modifiable. One of these is bone mineral density (BMD), which is seen by some as a surrogate marker of cumulative estrogen exposure or endogenous estrogen. A large community-based study showed that women with osteoporosis have poorer cognitive function and increased risk for cognitive deterioration[22]. Because BMD is unlikely to affect cognition directly, perhaps the explanation is the inverse: poorer cognition could diminish physical activity, lead to weight loss and, in turn, affect BMD. However, this sample exclusively included participants who were ambulatory and community-dwelling. Therefore, it was suggested that low endogenous estrogen might underlie both relatively low BMD and poor cognitive functioning. As in many studies of the effects of hormone replacement therapy (HRT) on cognition, the data are difficult to interpret, because supplemental estrogen use is associated with women who are overall better educated, healthier and more compliant with medical advice than non-users[23–25].

Many studies have suggested that estrogen may be related to cognitive functioning in women, but the results of large-scale epidemiological investigations of postmenopausal women taking HRT have been inconsistent. Sherwin[26] has suggested that verbal memory might specifically be maintained with estrogen therapy after the menopause, and there is some evidence to support the idea that verbal functioning, if not verbal memory *per se*, is enhanced by HRT. For example, Grodstein and colleagues[27] found that verbal fluency, though not verbal memory, was significantly better among hormone users than non-users.

Some have observed that HRT might have a positive effect on cognitive function among those who are more disadvantaged; in a large urban, less well-educated, ethnically diverse sample of women, 'ever users' of estrogen performed better on cognitive measures than never users[28]. A study by Matthews and co-workers[29] has suggested that ever users of estrogen appear to be protected in some analyses from age-related declines in cognitive test scores, relative to never users, regardless of whether or not the women in these studies were taking estrogen at the time of the investigation. This suggests that those characteristics of women that led them to choose HRT in the first place may account for the pattern of results; specifically, the most potent protection for women against cognitive decline might be education.

Overall, however, few studies have provided clear evidence that cognition is globally enhanced among women who use hormones; in fact, many studies have suggested that HRT does not affect overall cognitive performance[11,30–32]. Many previous studies of estrogen and cognitive function have been relatively small, making conclusive identification of the effects of hormone therapy on intellectual functioning (in general or specifically with regard to duration of use and specific type of therapy used) very limited.

Other common medical conditions (for example, hypertension, diabetes, cerebrovascular disease) that may affect cognition in aging women are both numerous and well-known. For example, cardiovascular insufficiency in older individuals who have not suffered a major cardiac or vascular event such as stroke or heart attack has been shown significantly to impact performance on neuropsychological tests of executive functioning[33]. Nutritional requirements in aging women are different from those of younger women, which may result in deficiencies in cognitively critical substances such as vitamins $B_{12}$ and $B_6$ and folate[34]. Additionally, research has begun to document the beneficial effects of exercise, with a number of studies documenting a positive effect of fitness on cognitive speed and efficiency in those 55–70 years of age[35]. It has been suggested that the reason for this benefit is an increase in cerebral blood flow, which leads to better oxygenation of the brain. These factors must be taken into account when evaluating changes in the cognitive function of older women.

## Gender differences in the elderly

In a population-based study in the Netherlands, the oldest-old women were found to perform better than men on cognitive tests, in particular those measuring cognitive speed and memory[36]. Other research has shown that cognitive impairment without dementia has been found to occur with increased prevalence at higher rates in women[37].

A gender difference has been identified in the association between the APOE genotype and age-related cognitive decline, in that the APOE $\epsilon$4 allele is associated with normal age-related decline in cognitive functions in females between the ages of 70 and 80[38]. No such significant relationship between the APOE genotype and cognitive decline has been found in males.

Despite the popular myth that postmenopausal estrogen deficiency leads to decrements in memory performance in women, there has been little research to support this. A cross-sectional community-based study, for example, showed weak or absent gender differences in cognitive function declines with age, and failed to support the argument that estrogen deficiency is to blame for declines in cognitive functions in women[39].

## Pathological aging

### Mild cognitive impairment

Somewhere along the continuum from normal aging to dementia lies mild cognitive impairment (MCI), which is characterized by memory impairment beyond expectations for education and age, with other cognitive domains and overall functioning remaining intact. MCI represents a compelling area of research, because anywhere from 1 to 25% of patients with MCI may convert to Alzheimer's disease within 1 year compared with 1–2% among normal controls[40,41]. Neuropsychological testing is the only reliable way to distinguish MCI from normal aging or very mild Alzheimer's disease.

### Alzheimer's disease

It is estimated that 2.4 million Americans had a dementia diagnosis in 2000. An estimated 3.3 million in 2020 and 7.3 million in 2040 are expected[42]. In 1980, the prevalence of Alzheimer's disease in the USA was estimated to have been 11.3% of those 65 years of age and older. The public health impact of Alzheimer's disease will intensify as rapid growth of the oldest segment of the population continues.

Alzheimer's disease is an illness that causes progressive and irreversible cognitive impairment. It is characterized by an insidious and progressive decline in numerous areas of cognition that cause significant functional impairment. The cognitive functions that are usually affected in patients with Alzheimer's disease include memory (predominantly), orientation, language, problem-solving, visuospatial abilities, the ability to perform tasks (praxis), and social functioning. Changes in the brain tissue, including the formation of amyloid plaques and neurofibrillary tangles, and the eventual loss of brain cells, give rise to impairment of these mental functions. The illness is strongly associated with aging; it is rare before the age of 50 but increasingly prevalent above 65 years and may affect more than half the people who live into their nineties[43]. While the majority of cases of Alzheimer's disease are in older patients, approximately 5–10% of cases are in 'early onset', which occurs between the ages of 30 and 60.

The relationship between depression and Alzheimer's disease is complex, and the subject of much speculation and research. First-time major depressive episodes in the older patient may represent either a prodrome to Alzheimer's disease, a co-morbid condition with Alzheimer's disease, or a component of Alzheimer's disease itself[44]. Cognitive impairment associated with depression in older patients is sometimes referred to as 'pseudo-dementia' because the neuropsychological and behavioral profile (such as poor memory and attention, and the presence of apathy) closely mimics that found in primary memory disorders. However, the cognitive impairments associated with depression resolve as psychiatric symptoms remit (naturally or with therapeutic or psychopharmacological intervention). Dementia and depression may both be present in varying degrees. Careful questioning regarding the temporal order of depressive symptoms and memory loss can help tease this out. In other words, if depressive symptoms came first, it is more likely that the cognitive deficits that followed are related to depression than if memory loss is reported first and depressive symptoms afterwards.

Current diagnostic systems treat Alzheimer's disease in part as a diagnosis of exclusion;

however, recent evidence indicates that many patients 'excluded' by these criteria may have biological changes characteristic of Alzheimer's disease[45]. In many patients diagnosed with vascular dementia, autopsy revealed the presence of the plaques and tangles associated with Alzheimer's disease. Unless a dementia syndrome has a sudden onset following a discrete vascular event, co-morbid Alzheimer's disease should be considered and treated in addition to the management of vascular risk factors. This is supported by findings that a lower threshold of Alzheimer's pathology seems to exist to produce a clinical dementia syndrome, when cerebrovascular disease is also present[46].

## Assessment

While a definitive diagnosis of Alzheimer's disease is confirmed by examining brain tissue at autopsy, a clinical diagnosis by a physician may be made with a high degree of reliability[47]. In conjunction with a thorough history, physical examination, and mental status testing, other diagnostic procedures including laboratory tests, neuroimaging, and referral to a neuropsychologist, neurologist, or geriatric psychiatric specialist may help clarify the diagnosis. The most common diagnostic differentials are among normal aging, MCI, mild Alzheimer's disease, other dementias, or depression.

A thorough and sensitive interview with both the patient and, if possible, a family member, is invaluable when assessing the presence of cognitive impairment. Physicians and families alike tend to 'overdiagnose' normal aging. The geripausal woman is likely to complain of changes in memory or cognition and it is important to be able to distinguish between normal complaints in the 50–70-year-old woman from those symptoms that may be 'red flags' for the physician to initiate further evaluation. Common complaints in the geripausal woman, particularly if she is still in the workplace, include embarrassing but mild word-finding problems, misplacing objects and longer time needed to learn new information. Another common and realistic complaint of the geripausal woman is considerable difficulty, relative to her younger peers, with divided attention. The patient may say she used to be able to 'multi-task' and feel alarmed that she can now focus on only one task at a time. The physician needs to ask specific questions about memory loss, language changes, the handling of complex tasks, behavioral problems, and poor judgement. Since patients with very early dementia may be unaware of their symptoms or minimize their impact, an informant is helpful for a good history. Common 'red flags' are statements that the patient repeats questions, has difficulty balancing the checkbook or managing medications, buys repeat items at the store, becomes disoriented while driving, repeatedly forgets conversations, frequently uses the wrong word, or is difficult to understand. Often the geripausal woman is still working, and specific questions about occupational impairment must be addressed. Sensitive inquiry about other common causes of cognitive impairment are important; these include alcohol, drug, or medication abuse, and depression or anxiety symptoms.

The Mini-Mental State examination[48] is a widely used tool that provides a rapid screening of cognitive function, and should be part of any brief cognitive screen with patients. However, proposed cut-off scores for the 30-point instrument are not helpful, as the examination is sensitive to education level, English as a second language, sensory deficits, and tremor. For a gross detection of possible early dementia, difficulty with the three delayed recall items are the most sensitive marker. Despite its limitations, the Mini-Mental State examination is a valuable tool that provides an excellent marker for longitudinal comparison.

In addition to other diagnostic tools, neuropsychological testing is an effective and reliable way to aid in differential diagnosis between normal aging, MCI, early dementia and depression. A neuropsychological evaluation provides a valuable comparison base for future deterioration and medication monitoring, identifies the patient's strengths, and establishes the level of severity of the impairment.

## Conclusions

While the geripausal years represent a period of rapid cognitive changes, the vast majority of women remain cognitively intact well into old age. Physicians need to consider a multitude of factors, including nutrition, medical illness, exercise, lifestyle changes, psychological health, and family history in their holistic examination of the aging female patient. It is vital that a comprehensive assessment be performed so that early, significant clinical syndromes can be identified and potential interventions maximized. In addition to ongoing research efforts focused on the effects of hormone replacement treatments, large-scale initiatives are needed to examine the impact of oral contraceptives, socioeconomic variables and other modifiable factors in women's lives.

While the evidence for a beneficial effect of HRT on cognition remains inconclusive, it certainly causes no harm, in terms of either emotional or cognitive functions. There is no solid evidence for a 'female depression syndrome', nor is there empirical support for the idea of a universal menopausal detriment in cognitive ability.

# References

1. Lezak MD. *Neuropsychological Assessment*, 3rd edn. New York: Oxford University Press, 1995
2. Harvey PD, Dahlman KL. Neuropsychological evaluation of dementia. In Chalev A, ed. *Neuropsychological Assessment of Neuropsychiatric Disorders*. Washington, DC: American Psychiatric Press, 1999:329–72
3. Dahlman KL, Hoblyn J, Mohs RC. Cognitive changes in the menopause. In *The Menopause: Comprehensive Management*, 4th edn. 2000: 201–11
4. Rowe JW, Kahn RL. Usual and successful aging. *Science* 1987;237:143–8
5. Rowe JW, Kahn RL. Successful aging. *Gerontologist* 1997;37:433–40
6. Seeman TE, Lusignolo TM, Berkman, L. Social relationships, social support, and patterns of cognitive aging in healthy, high-functioning older adults: MacArthur studies of successful aging. *Health Psychol* 2001;20:243–55
7. Penninx BWJH, van Tilburg T, Deeg DJH, *et al*. Direct and buffer effects of social support and personal coping resources in individuals with arthritis. *Soc Sci Med* 1997;44: 393–402
8. Fitzpatrick F, Newman S, Archer R, Shipley, M. Social support, disability and depression: a longitudinal study of rheumatoid arthritis. *Soc Sci Med* 1991;33:605–11
9. Stern Y, Alexander GE, Prohovnik I, *et al*. Relationship between lifetime occupation and parietal flow: implications for a reserve against Alzheimer's disease pathology. *Neurology* 1995;45:55–60
10. Stern Y, Albert S, Tang M-X, Tsai W-Y. Rate of memory decline in AD is related to education and occupation: cognitive reserve? *Neurology* 1999;53:1942–2
11. Yaffe K, Barnes D, Nevitt M, *et al*. A prospective study of physical activity and cognitive decline in elderly women. *Arch Intern Med* 2001;161:1703–8
12. Everard KM, Lach HW, Fisher EB, Baum MC. Relationship of activity and social support to the functional health of older adults. *J Gerontol B Psychol Sci Soc Sci* 2000;55:S208–12
13. Scarmeas N, Levy G, Tang M-X, *et al*. Influence of leisure activity on the incidence of Alzheimer's disease. *Neurology* 2001;57: 2236–42
14. Gallo JJ, Schoen R, Jones R. Cognitive impairment and syndromal depression in estimates of active life expectancy: the 13-year follow-up of the Baltimore Epidemiologic Catchment Area sample. *Acta Psychiatr Scand* 2000; 101:265–73
15. Sonnenberg CM, Beekman ATF, Deeg DJH, van Tilburg W. Sex differences in late life depression. *Acta Psychiatr Scand* 2000;101: 286–92
16. Penninx BWJH, Gurualnik JM, Simonsick EM, *et al*. Emotional vitality among disabled older women: the women's health and aging study. *J Am Geriatr Soc* 1998;46:807–15
17. Weissman MW. Epidemiology of major depression in women. Presented at the *American Psychiatric Association Meeting*, New York, May 1996
18. Angst J. The course of affective disorders. II. Typology of bipolar manic-depressive illness. *Arch Psychiatr Nervankr* 1978;226: 65–72

19. Stewart DE, Boydell KM. Psychologic distress during menopause: associations across the reproductive life cycle. *Int Psychiatry Med* 1993;23:157–62

20. Avis NE, Brambilla D, McKinlay SM, Vass K. A longitudinal analysis of the association between menopause and depression. Results from the Massachusetts Women's Health Study. *Ann Epidemiol* 1994;4:214–20

21. Woods NF, Mitchell ES. Patterns of depressed mood in midlife women. Observations from the Seattle Midlife Women's Health Study. *Res Nurs Heath* 1996;19:111–23

22. Yaffe K, Browner W, Cauley J, *et al*. Association between bone mineral density and cognitive decline in older women. *J Am Geriatr Soc* 1999;47:1176–82

23. Egeland GM, Kuller LH, Matthews KA, *et al*. Premenopausal determinants of menopausal estrogen use. *Prev Med* 1991;20:343–9

24. Barrett-Connor E. Postmenopausal estrogen and prevention bias. *Ann Intern Med* 1991;115:455–6

25. Petitti DB. Coronary heart disease and estrogen replacement therapy. Can compliance bias explain the results of observational studies? *Ann Epidemiol* 1994;4:115–8

26. Sherwin BB. Cognitive assessment for postmenopausal women and general assessment of their mental health [Review]. *Psychopharmacol Bull* 1998;34:323–6

27. Grodstein F, Chen J, Pollen DA, *et al*. Postmenopausal hormone therapy and cognitive function in healthy older women. *J Am Geriatr Soc* 2000;48:746–52

28. Jacobs DM, Tang MX, Stern Y, *et al*. Cognitive function in nondemented older women who took estrogen after menopause. *Am Acad Neurol* 1998;50:368–73

29. Matthews K, Cauley J, Yaffe K, Zmuda JM. Estrogen replacement therapy and cognitive decline in older community women. *J Am Geriatr Soc* 1999;47:518–23

30. Hogervorst E, Boshuisen M, Riedel W, *et al*. The effect of hormone replacement therapy on cognitive function in elderly women. *Psychoneuroendocrinology* 1999;24:43–68

31. Henderson VW, Paganini-Hill A, Miller BL, *et al*. Estrogen for Alzheimer's disease in women. *Neurology* 2000;54:295–301

32. Fillenbaum GG, Hanlon JT, Landerman LR, Schmader KE. Impact of estrogen use on decline in cognitive function in a representative sample of older community-resident women. *Am J Epidemiol* 2001;153:137–44

33. Dywan J, Segalowitz SJ, Unsal A. Speed of information processing, health, and cognitive performance in older adults. *Dev Neuropsychol* 1992;8:473–90

34. Rosenberg IH, Miller JW. Nutritional factors in physical and cognitive functions of elderly people. *Am J Clin Nutr* 1992;55:1237–43

35. Dustman RE, Ruhling RO, Russell EM, *et al*. Aerobic exercise training and improved neuropsychological function of individuals. *Neurobiol aging* 1984;5:35–42

36. Van Exel E, Gussekloo J, deCraen AJM, *et al*. Cognitive function in the oldest old: women perform better than men. *J Neurol Neurosurg Psychiatry* 2001;71:29–32

37. Di Carlo A, Baldereschi M, Amaducci L, *et al*. Cognitive impairment without dementia in older people: prevalence, vascular risk factors, impact on disability. The Italian longitudinal study on aging. *J Am Geriatr Soc* 2000;48:774–82

38. Mortensen EL, Hogh P. A gender difference in the association between APOE genotype and age-related cognitive decline. *Neurology* 2001;57:89–95

39. Barrett-Connor E, Kritz-Silverstein D. Gender differences in cognitive function with age: The Rancho Bernardo Study. *J Am Geriatr Soc* 1999;47:159–64

40. Petersen RC, Smith GE, Waring SC, *et al*. Aging, memory, and mild cognitive impairment. *Int Psychogeriatr* 1997;9(Suppl 1):65–9

41. Petersen, RC, Smith GE, Waring SC, *et al*. Mild cognitive impairment: clinical characterization and outcome. *Arch Neurol* 1999;56:303–8

42. Evans DA, Estimated prevalence of Alzheimer's disease in the United States. *Milbank Q* 1990;68:267–89

43. Aisen P, Marin DB, Davis KL. *Alzheimer's Disease Questions and Answers*. Hampshire, UK: Merit Publishing International, 1997

44. Katz IR. Diagnosis and treatment of depression in patients with Alzheimer's disease and other dementias. *J Clin Psychiatry* 1998;59(Suppl 9): 38–44

45. Stewart R. Vascular dementia: a diagnosis running out of time. *Br J Psychiatry* 2002;180: 152–6

46. Snowdon DA, Dreiner LH, Mortimer JA, *et al*. Brain infarction and the clinical expression of Alzheimer's disease. *J Am Med Assoc* 1997; 277:813–17

47. Small GW, Rabins PV, Barry PP, *et al*. Diagnosis and treatment of Alzheimer's disease and related disorders. Consensus statement. *J Am Med Assoc* 1997;278:1363–71

48. Folstein MF, Folstein SE, McHugh PR. 'Minimental state': a practical method for grading the cognitive state of patients for the clinician. *J Psychiatr Res* 1975;12:189–98

# 6

# Sexuality in the geripause

*Bernard A. Eskin*

Sexuality after midlife has been described extensively in textbooks and both medical and health literature. Specific involvement of estrogen replacement therapy in the functional aspects has provided a strong impetus for research into the sexual effects in women throughout menopause and into the geripause. Particularly compelling is the suggestion from most literature that heterosexual intercourse continues and is hampered only by socio-economic factors, while cessation has been the mythical accepted expectation. The present mature woman is an educated, knowledgeable, active individual who desires to employ and achieve to maintain a significant quality of life.

## Demographics

We are assured that the counted population of the world is living longer. Currently, the average life expectancy is 78.9 and 72 years of age for women and men, respectively. By the year 2030, it is estimated that elderly people will make up approximately 17% of the total population of the USA[1]. The health-care profession must provide this growing population with a quality of life that would allow elderly people to enjoy living. Sexuality could play a role in the satisfaction evidently derived[2]. Hormonal transition in women involves a temporal decrease in the levels of both estrogens and androgens (most testosterone)[3,4]. The reduction of the latter is often associated with reduced sexual sensitivity, libido, and response[5,6].

Gradual changes in the genitourinary system associated with menopause include atrophic changes in the urethra, vulva, vagina, and neck of the bladder. Vaginal atrophy and diminished vaginal lubrication may interfere mechanically with sexual comfort and pleasure. In addition to these hormonal changes with aging, disease entities and associated medications may also negatively affect sexuality. Determining the impact of medications, both alone and in combination, on quality of life is essential to providing comprehensive care for elderly female patients.

In chronically ill patients, sexuality survives only as a memory but can become an ideal. Older women may fantasize a loving relationship and, as such, consider the alternatives to actual sex – hugging, body touch, kissing, as well as a sensual feeling of intimacy – as acceptable and desirable substitutes[7,8]. Recently, several behavior laboratories have begun subjective measurements and evaluations concerning these to determine whether they may serve as another mechanism for improving quality of life.

Perimenopausal active sexuality continues to be encouraged, when it can do no physical harm. However, there have been no attempts to follow a woman's sexual desires during the postmenopausal and geripausal phases. Our earlier preliminary studies showed a surprising decline in interest and desire for intimacy in those entering transition and premenopause[9]. Only recently has the older group been studied, and these results are enlightening[10].

## Homosexual activity

When defining sexuality in women, it is fundamentally important to define both heterosexual and homosexual activity. However, homosexual quality measurement has provided only limited information at this time, although an active program is in progress. Since actuarial histories for women indicate greater longevity than men, an increase in opportunities have been seen for gay female relationships to occur in older women. Minimal data have been published concerning the sexual outcomes of these encounters. Most of the data available in the elderly describe heterosexual responses.

## Heterosexual activity

Clinical sexuality is thought to decline acutely with advanced age. There has been much deliberation over the relative impact of menopause on sexual activity for women. Although those attending menopause and geripause clinics relate problems in sexual functioning, studies have shown that fewer than half of those complaining seek further treatment[11]. When treatment is obtained, the decrease in sexual response in considered often as an aberration of life stress, clinical depression, anxiety and psychological symptoms. Reductions in sexual function or physiology are never considered initially as the possible responsible factors.

Surprisingly, several studies have shown a lower sexual interest among peri- or premenopausal than menopausal women. Research among large general populations have not shown a clear association between menopause and steadily declining sexual function. An association between menopause status and active sex has been studied by interviewing general populations attracted commercially or singular patients with quality of life complaints through a medical program. Menopausal symptoms alone were not found to be causative for the dissatisfaction in most cases[12]. Most studies have suggested that menopausal conditions have an impact on some aspects of sexual functioning, such as physical changes that are prohibitive or uncomfortable during sexual intercourse[13]. Inconsistencies in results can be explained when a wide variation in interview techniques is used. Unfortunately, many variables exist that demean some of the results. Time frames used, women without partners and locale are often neglected in the analysis,

causing the study sample to be incomplete and the results faulty.

Outcomes for sexual function are measured by an extensive number of testing systems. These include, but are not limited to, satisfaction, sexuality, frequency of activity, form of activity (intercourse, masturbation, orgasm), sexual thoughts or fantasies, desire, and arousal[14]. Attitudes towards problems reaching orgasm, and difficulties, such as pain during intercourse, require more discreet questioning. Perhaps all of these are a characterization of libido, which has usually been defined to include sexual interest, arousal, desire, drive, motivation, and pleasure[15]. Fortunately, the sexual response cycle remains a most acceptable physiological measurement of the events and is the most universally understood[16,17]. Presentation of this acceptable basis for characterization of combined physical and mental activity has done much to provide diagnostic and treatment options.

Objectives to be addressed in this chapter are: the association between hormone-induced geripausal changes and sexual functioning; the physical and mental age-induced sexual restrictions; the contributions of health, psychosocial variables, sociodemographics, life style and partner limitations to various aspects of sexual functioning for women; and how the expectations are met in those actively sexual.

## Hormones in the geripause and sexuality

The impact of loss of reproduction on the sexuality and well-being of women, while frequently dismissed, remains indeterminate. Interestingly, the several worldwide cases where women over 55 years have acted as surrogates to carry their daughter's children have awakened many to the evidence of pseudo-reproductive responses to external hormonal stimulation. Ovulation had been noted earlier in women over 70 when bromergocryptine, a prolactin inhibitor, had been given[18]. This indicates that functional follicles may still exist in postmenopausal ovaries. Thus, sex hormone availability causes a theoretical resurgence of physical reproductive tissue activity. Whereas there is consensus that sexual interest and activity decline in women as they get older, consistent evidence is lacking that the menopause *per se*, or the hormonal changes associated with it, play a role in this decline. In comparison with age, menopause status makes only a small contribution. One study found menopausal status more important than age and two studies found menopausal status to be unrelated to sexuality[14,19,20].

The relation of hormonal changes associated with tissue changes in the menopause are of clinical importance in view of the widespread use of hormone replacement therapy. The overall impact of such exogenous hormones on women's sexuality and well-being is still unclear. Convincing individual evidence comes from placebo-controlled studies of women who have undergone surgical menopause (i.e. oophorectomy). In this group there is an acute fall in estrogens as compared to the gradual decline seen with natural menopause and with it an acute loss of desire. Most of the data show that, when immediate estrogen replacement is given, no loss of libido (desire) occurs, while therapy taken later may require longer 'down' time before improvement in libido responses occurs[21]. Post-surgery hospitalization often provides a means of determining the time for the return of desire.

Figure 2 in Chapter 3 shows the gradual decline seen in estrogen during the 'natural' menopause[22]. An apparent decrease below an individual threshold results in deficiency states such as amenorrhea, functional (or dysfunctional) uterine bleeding, and increasing endocervical and vaginal atrophy. Other evident changes described by our group and others show that elevated follicle stimulating hormone (FSH) and, later, luteinizing hormone (LH) will plateau and then begin (in early geripause) to decrease (Table 1). These changes in gonadotropin levels may cause the dramatic increases in atrophism seen in the reproductive system and other aging tissues[23–25]. The onset of geripausal symptoms begins when this reduction in FSH and LH occurs[23]. This is an important area for future clinical research.

**Table 1** Ratios of estrogen to gonadopropins in women during aging. Reproduced with permission from Eskin BA, Trivedi RA, Weidman C, Walter RE. Positive feedback disturbances and infertility in women over thirty. *Am J Gynecol Health* 1988; 11:110–17

| Age (years) | $E_2/LH$ Mean | SEM | $E_2/FSH$ Mean | SEM |
|---|---|---|---|---|
| 37–42 | 9.81 | 2 | 15.77 | 3.69 |
| 43–51 | 2.81 | 0.94 | 3.13 | 1.1 |
| 52–65 | 1.25 | 0.33 | 0.86 | 0.25 |
| > 65 | 0.44 | 0.09 | 0.25 | 0.05 |

$E_2$, estradiol; LH, luteinizing hormone; FSH, follicle stimulating hormone

Androgens have been described by many workers as maintaining sexual interest after surgical menopause[26,27]. It is believed that both testosterone and estradiol improve well-being and that the presence of estrogen may be required for androgenic action[28]. Unfortunately, the beneficial effects of testosterone, both on sexuality and on well-being, have shown the best results after the use of pharmacological levels[6]. This results in unacceptable (to most women) side-effects. These may consist of oily skin, acne, hirsutism and, in some severe cases, generalized virilization. The benefits of estradiol are seen at dose levels that are within or less than the physiological range. Unfortunately, recent long-term studies on the use of hormone replacement therapy have described serious complications (see chapter 10). Nevertheless, short-term use for sexual response may be a possibility, but will require further study.

There is general agreement that plasma estradiol levels fall substantially as a woman goes through the menopause, reflecting the decline in ovarian output of estradiol (Figure 2, Chapter 3). Thus, it becomes clear that several periods of hormonal change occur in women throughout menopause and geripause. It is apparent that there is a decreasing estrogen presence after menopause and, while the slope of descent (Figure 2, Chapter 3) is less than that seen in the premenopause, it is unrelenting. As already stated, at the time of the geripause, a particularly important event is the decrease in FSH after a variable plateau. LH begins its descent after FSH has fallen[23,24,27]. LH action on the adrenal steroid pathway is stimulatory, so that menopausal androgens have a stable relationship until the geripause. This absolute reduction in androgen may be the result of a decrease in LH with a simultaneous decrease in adrenal steroidogenesis. Estrogen in the form of estrone also decreases because of the limitations imposed by reduced aromatizing enzyme. Plasma binding-levels appear to be variable and hence it is difficult to presume any protein-binding activity changes[15].

As a result of these endocrine changes, the geripausal woman may require careful dose re-regulation for optimal results when hormonal replacement is indicated. In the geripause, the treatment to avoid severe atrophy of the vulva and vagina during sexual intercourse is most desirable. Our studies have shown that hormone replacement may be an effective method for both improving this physical problem and increasing sexual desire and arousal in the geripause[10].

If changes in sexuality are directly caused by the menopause, a direct association between hormone levels and sexual function would occur. However, most studies have not shown correlations between estradiol and sexual interest[14,15,19]. In one analysis, an association was noted between hormone levels (estradiol) and pain during or after intercourse, which were consistent with hormone levels[2,6]. Thus, hormone levels affect vaginal dryness and dyspareunia in many studies, with no direct relationship to sexual drive or interest[20,29]. Sexuality in the menopause appears to be a distillation of hormonal changes, the psychosocial impact of the loss of reproduction, condition of health, and the social changes that result from normal aging. Symptoms of perineal atrophy are listed in Table 2.

In summary, during the natural postmenopause/geripause, established evidence relating endogenous hormone levels to sexual behavior is both extremely limited and inconclusive. This is primarily the result of the restriction to univariate methods of analysis in most of the reports, and difficulty analyzing all the variables in the multivariate research.

**Table 2**  Symptoms of perineal atrophy

Itching in the vulvar area
Dyspareunia
Dryness in the vulva or vagina
Irritation in the vulva
Increased discharge
Pain with urination
Frequent urinary tract problems
Bleeding vaginally after intercourse
Fear of intercourse

Testosterone declines in early geripause compared with perimenopause without it being clear whether such decline is the result of aging, geripause, or both.

## The effects of aging

Evidence of an age-related decline in sexual interest and activity in women in the perimenopause and postmenopause has been suggested by several polls in the popular press. However, recent research suggests that a high proportion of postmenopausal women remain sexually active well into late life[30]. Age-related physiological changes do not render an active sexual relationship impossible or even necessarily difficult. In women, menopause terminates fertility and produces changes stemming from estrogen deficiency. The extent to which aging affects sexual function depends largely on psychological, pharmacological and illness-related factors. Also, importantly, age was related to only one outcome: difficulty in reaching orgasm. This may have been due in part to the narrow age range of the sample.

The sexual ages during the lifetime (Table 3) have been ably described and are particularly pertinent in women[31]. These stages have different biological, social, and psychological characteristics and potentials.

This life cycle fits well into the characteristic hormone patterns of estrogen. Middle age in women includes the menopausal transition through to postmenopause[31]. Notably, elderly women in the life cycle enter the early geripausal years with some remarkable sex hormone changes that influence the clinical findings that appear. The advanced elderly group contains

**Table 3** Lifetime sexual ages. Reproduced with permission from Levine SD. Woman's sexual capacities at midlife. In: Eskin BA, ed. *The Menopause: Comprehensive Management*, 4th edn. Carnforth, UK: Parthenon Publishing, 2000

*Childhood*: infancy to puberty
*Adolescence*: puberty to young adulthood
*Young adulthood*: approximate age 20 to mid-40s
*Middle age*: mid-40s to mid-60s
*Early elderly*: mid-60s to age 80
*Advanced elderly*: 80 and beyond

the late geripause, currently an extremely understudied group.

Using only subjective questionnaires, menopausal women reported significantly lowered sexual desire and the belief that interest in sexual activity declines with age[33]. Several reports from these women stated that they recognized a sudden decrease in sexual arousal compared with an earlier decade in the premenopause. These specific associations were markedly variable, depending on whether the data were unadjusted (direct data only) or multivariate (using all social and medical variants) in analyses. In the unadjusted analyses, postmenopausal women reported a significant decrease in sexual desire, while adjusted data showed some postmenopausal enhancement.

When multiple regression analyses were compared in several studies on premenopausal, perimenopausal and postmenopausal women, those in the perimenopause had the least desire. Finding an association between interest in sexual activity and the hormonal changes in the menopause and geripause is confounding because of the multivariates involved. When a careful study in Sweden of 567 women aged 38, 46, 50, and 54 was performed, a progressive decline in sexual interest occurred across all menopausal stages. Compared with pre- and perimenopausal women, postmenopausal women reported lower sexual interest during the previous 5 years of the perimenopause[34].

Several cross-sectional studies on aging were carried out to determine whether the woman's age *per se*, was responsible for the loss of sexual desire and/or arousal. Patients from several clinics were surveyed[14]. These researchers found that, while perimenopausal women indicated that their sexual interest was lower than in the premenopause, postmenopausal women had completely mixed opinions. Again, in these studies the selection of patients was by age, utilizing a median of 51 years as menopausal[14,15,19]. Interestingly, women in the postmenopause, the years following one menopausal year, indicated a greater and increasing interest in sexuality compared with the perimenopausal groups. It would appear that age is not in itself a cause of lack of interest, and that the multivariate factor of an approaching menopause (perimenopause) is influential. In the postmenopause and geripause, when conditions may be stabilized, sexuality seems to return or at least plateau.

On the other hand, a direct association between menopausal status and sexual dysfunction was reported in the age group of 35–59 years, described in two general practices in England[35]. Unfortunately, sexual interest was considered as part of the sexual dysfunction complex, which consisted of impaired interest in sexual activity, frequency of orgasm, dyspareunia and vaginal dryness.

In all of the surveys of geripausal women the pattern that sex was not desired or was unacceptable was challenged. Most referred to health as the factor most seriously affecting the loss of this activity. The age-old considerations of religious beliefs and family pressures seemed less important. Opportunity continued to be a problem to many. Medically, most early geripausal women stated that they were able to continue physically with sexual intercourse. Local therapy was indicated in a minor number of individuals. In most cases these women are under gynecological care and, if no abnormalities are detected, sexual activity is permissible. No medical evidence seems to contraindicate their participation because of age.

## Multivariate contributions

The variables associated with menopausal health and activity are obviously critical to the results obtained. In several studies, postmenopausal status did not seem to be related to the following factors: frequency of sexual intercourse; satisfaction with one's sexual relationship;

difficulty reaching orgasm; and pain during or after intercourse[14]. Most important for therapy, estrogen was effective in reducing dyspareunia in multivariate analysis[10].

Psychosocial factors seem to hold more importance than ovarian function or secretion in determining the sexual function of older women. These have included the availability of a partner, previous sexual behavior and enjoyment, marital relationships, mental health, general physical health, stress, expectations, and male partner problems[3,14]. During the postmenopause and most of the geripause there is a further decrease in ovarian hormone production and vaginal tissue turgor, both of which increase the incidence of dyspareunia and difficulty with insertion. It is less clear how menopausal estrogen affects sexual loss of interest or libido. As previously stated, few multivariable studies have been performed to include the considerable range of psychological, social, and health conditions this represents. Significant predictors of low sexual desire were low frequency of sexual intercourse, being single, poor physical fitness, lower social status, and anticipation of decreased sexuality[18]. Additionally, we know little about the singular contributions of these factors on sexual functioning; most of the information is anecdotal.

Separating arousal and desire in postmenopausal and geripausal women has recently been attempted. Sexual *arousal* was studied[10,15], but a relation between these states and sexual arousal showed inconsistent results. Additionally no association between menopause status and frequency of sexual intercourse, satisfaction, difficulty reaching orgasm, and pain during or after intercourse has been described[15]. No association was seen between menopause status and sexual *desire* in multivariate regressions in women at menopause[18]. By not using marital status as a single factor in the study, obvious differences occurred.

Sexual satisfaction did not differ by menopausal status, and no correlation between menopausal status and orgasm was seen in well-controlled studies[15]. Compared with pre- and perimenopausal women, postmenopausal women reported lower frequency of intercourse, but improved capacity for orgasm[3]. Studies of women in geripausal ages were not found in the older literature and appear only recently[10]. On the other hand, feelings for partner, sexual responsivity, frequency of sexual intercourse, and libido seemed to persist where there was a stable relationship[36]. However, some studies have shown that stimulation increases with short-term or new partners. Higher sexual function was recorded among widowed or separated/divorced women in a sample of postmenopausal women who had partners[30]. The quality of the marital relationships were quite strongly related to frequency of sexual intercourse and quality of sexual activity[35].

When dealing with psychological symptomatology the presence of dysfunctional sexual problems became evident, particularly in the menopause. These conditions led to lower satisfaction, frequency, and desire[17]. Diminished sexual function is a well-known symptom of depression, and recent work has accredited the use of antidepressants as an important mechanism for improving desire and arousal. Psychiatric status and marital adjustment were two variables having direct effects on sexual functioning[36].

At 65, the age of onset of geripause, a remarkable change in health status begins, although sexuality may remain active. Levels of physical health are extremely variable according to location, financial status and activity level. Lack of proper health conditions reduces the number of women who can be physically sexual, but those women who participate and/or enjoy closeness do not show the social inhibitions that were seen in previous generations. The few studies in the literature of women in the geripause indicate that they are sexually active and interested[10].

## Outcomes and expectations

In dealing with the measures of quality of life, many useful activities can be described and are presented in other chapters. Improved sexuality affects both psychological and medical quality. However, few studies have been performed concerning the physical results and satisfaction of women who do have sexual activity. There are several self-reporting gauges of female sexual function that seem effective only for large-scale clinical trials[36,39]. These research techniques are difficult to individualize with patients. Sexual activity decreases quantitatively with age and, as indicated, possibly as a result of estrogen deficiency[40,41]. While the loss of some sexual responses are the result of aging, desire and arousal may be restored by hormones[35,42]. Gynecological evidence that dyspareunia is often the result of a severely atrophied introitus has become a reasonable cause for discontinuation of intercourse[6,43] with few dissenters[13]. In a large sample, it was seen that postmenopausal/geripausal women were more likely to report unusual pain on intercourse[44].

In our studies of menopausal and geripausal women, we reversed the usual design. Only those women who were in stable relationships and had sexual intercourse at least three times a month were successively evaluated in medical practice. Multivariate analyses would be required statistically mostly for those women who were not in a stable sexual relationship who were not included. Desire has already reached at least a threshold level when there is intercourse.

Sexual and gynecological modalities were compared during menopause and geripause for those women who chose to take hormone replacement and those who did not. The use of hormone replacement plausibly maintained adequate turgor of the perineum and vagina, reducing dyspareunia[20,29]. Lubrication in the form of gels, creams and ointments continues to be an important ancillary therapeutic for sexually active women. These were not required as frequently in both menopause and early geripause when hormone replacement therapy was taken. Finally, through direct questioning, the patients stated that both desire and arousal were improved[10]. Thus, if medically feasible, giving replacement of reproductive hormones (estrogen and progesterone or estrogen alone) seems to provide a means of maintaining desire and arousal.

In light of the need for estrogen, still to be determined is whether there are specific doses of hormone replacement that result in the best perineal–vulvovaginal turgidity and other tissue needs for the individual. Women taking hormone therapy required less lubrication and at a later date. When hormone therapy is contraindicated for medical and/or psychological reasons, suitable substitutes may be considered. These alternatives are described in Chapter 10. Similarly, recent alternative medications have often been shown to be effective under certain circumstances. It is evident that individual problems in achieving a satisfying sexual response need to be met. When sildenafil citrate is used successfully for the male, on intercourse, traumatic tissue changes may result in a woman who has an atrophic perineum[45]. The use of hormone replacement may prevent this serious problem and lubrication would provide easier entry. Advice, derived from her sexual response history and pelvic examination, can provide improvement in the quality of a postmenopausal/geripausal woman's sex life and comfort. Thus, personalized therapy should be provided for the patient.

It appears that women who are using hormones are more likely to be sexually active and have better general and sexual health. The hormone treatment is effective in reducing vulvovaginal atrophy and ensuing sexual discomfort. In several subjective evaluations, women on hormone replacement showed greater sexual desire, arousal and satisfaction. These women require less lubrication and the need for lubrication occurred later. Neither hyterectomy nor mild-to-moderate vaginal discharge appeared to modify any of these findings[10].

Psychologically, women who were sexually active appeared to have reduced depression and anxiety. Similarly, therapeutic use of antidepressants was effective in improving sexual desire, showing evidence of satisfaction. The use of both anticonvulsive and antipsychotic therapies, however, were not statistically effective.

## Conclusions

Sexuality in the postmenopause and geripause has been investigated utilizing several subjective techniques. These women appear to have an increase in sexual *desire* over those in the perimenopause. *Arousal*, while somewhat less than in the premenopause, continues to remain at a functional level. However, many variables may override these conclusions. Evidently, the major problems are general health, psychological well-being, availability of a partner, and the circumstances of life style (e.g. housing, freedom, privacy). Age is not an evident factor in either desire or arousal. Endocrinologically, the reduction of sex hormones (estrogen, progesterone and testosterone) does not appear to cause the discontinuation of sexual activity, once initiated, or decrease satisfaction. Hormone replacement, psychosocial therapy, and ancillary medication by the health professional can improve the sexuality and sexual function of the active mature woman.

# References

1. Gelfand MM. Sexuality among older women. *J Women's Health Gender-Based Med* 2000; 19:515–20
2. Michael RT, Gagnon JH, Lawmann EO, *et al. Sex in America*. Boston, MA: Little Brown, 1994
3. Longcope C. Hormone dynamics at the menopause. *Ann NY Acad Sci* 1990;592:21–30
4. Zumoff B, Strain G, Miller L, Rosner W. Twenty-four-hour mean plasma testosterone concentration declines with age in normal premenopausal women. *J Clin Endocrinol Metab* 1995;80:1429–30
5. Sherwin BB, Gelfand MM. The role of androgen in the maintenance of sexual functioning in oophorectomized women. *Psychosom Med* 1987;49:397–409
6. Bancroft J, Cawood EH. Androgens and the menopause. *Clin Endocrinal* 1996;45:577–87
7. Masters WH, Johnson VE, Kolodny RC. *On Sex and Human Loving*. New York: Little, Brown, 1982
8. Meston CM. Aging and sexuality. *West J Med* 1977;167:285–90
9. Eskin BA. Sex and the gynecologic patient. In Oaks WW, Melchiode GA, Ficher IV, eds. *Sex and the Life Cycle*. New York: Grune and Stratton, 1976:199–212
10. Eskin BA. Hormone replacement on sexuality in the postmenopause and geripause. *Obstet Gynecol* 2001;97:525–6
11. Berkman LF. The role of social relations in health promotion. *Psychosom Med* 1995;57:245–54
12. Garamszegi C, Dinnerstein L, Dudley E, *et al.* Menopausal status: subjectively and objectively defined. *J Psychosom Obstet Gynecol* 1998;19:165–73
13. Laan E,van Lunsen RH. Hormones and sexuality in postmenopausal women: a psychophysiological study. *J Psychosom Obstet Gynecol* 1997;18:126–33
14. Avis NE, Stellato MA, Crawford S, *et al.* Is there an association between menopausal status and sexual functioning? *Menopause* 2000;7: 297–309
15. Cawood EHH, Bancroft J. Steroid hormones, the menopause, sexuality, and well-being of women. *Psychol Med* 1996;26:925–36
16. Masters WH, Johnson VE. *Human Sexuality Response*. Boston, MA: Little Brown, 1996
17. Basson R, Berman J, Burnett A, *et al.* Report of the international consensus development conference on female sexual of dysfunction: definitions and classifications. *J Urol* 2000;163: 888–96
18. Shifren JL, Schiff I. The aging ovary., *J Women's Health Gender-Based Med* 2000;9:53–7
19. Dennerstein L, Dudley E, Berger H. Are changes in sexual functioning during midlife due to aging or menopause? *Fertil Steril* 2001;76:456–60
20. Sarrel PM. Sexuality and menopause. *Obstet Gynecol* 1990;75:526–31
21. Guzick DS, Hoeger K. Sex, hormones and hysterectomies. *N Engl J Med* 2000;343: 730–11
22. Eskin BA. Epilogue. In Eskin BA, ed. *The Menopause: Comprehensive Management*, 4th edn. Carnforth, UK: Parthenon Publishing, 2000:299–302
23. Eskin BA, Trivedi RA, Weideman C, Walker RE. Positive feedback disturbances and infertility in women over thirty. *Am J Gynecol Health* 1988;11:110–17
24. Sherman BM, West JH, Korenman SG. The menopausal transition: analysis of LH, FSH, estradiol, and progesterone concentrations during menstrual cycles of older women. *J Clin Endocrinol Metab* 1976;42:629–36
25. Korenman SG. Menopausal endocrinology and management. *Arch Intern Med* 1982;142: 1131–6
26. Shifren JL, Braunstein GD, Simon JA, *et al.* Transdermal testosterone treatment of women with impaired sexual function after oophorectomy. *N Engl J Med* 2000;343:682–8

27. Burger HG, Dudley EC, Cui J, et al. A prospective longitudinal study of serum testosterone, dehydroepiandrosterone sulfate, and sex hormone-binding globulin levels through the menopause transition. *J Clin Endocrinol Metab* 2000;25:2832–8

28. Sherwin BB, Gelfand MM. Sex steroids and affect in the surgical menopause: a double-blind cross-over study. *Psychoneuroendocrinology* 1995;10:325–35

29. Burger HG. The endocrinology of the menopause. *Maturitas* 1992;23:129–36

30. Greendale GH, Hogan P, Shumaker S. Sexual functioning in postmenopausal women; the PEPI trial. *J Women's Health* 1996;5:445–58

31. Levine SD. Woman's sexual capacities at midlife. In: Eskin BA, ed. *The Menopause: Comprehensive Management*, 4th edn. Carnforth, UK: Parthenon Publishing, 2000

32. Eskin BA. Sexual aging. In Ficher M, Fishkin RE, Jacobs JA. *Sexual Arousal*. Springfield: Charles C. Thomas, 1983

33. Levine SD. *Sexuality in Midlife*. New York: Plenum, 1998

34. Hallstrom T. Sexuality in the climacteric. *Clin Obstet Gynecol* 1977;4:227–39

35. Osborn M, Hawton K, Garth D. Sexual dysfunction among middle-aged women in the community. *Br Med J* 1988;296:959–62

36. Dennerstein L, Dudley EC, Hopper JL, Burger H. Sexuality, hormones and the menopause transition. *Maturitas* 1997;26:83–93

37. Leiblum S, Bachmann G, Kemman E, et al. Vaginal atrophy in the postmenopausal woman: the importance of sexual activity and hormones. *J Am Med Assoc* 1983;249:2195–8

38. Hawton K, Gath D, Day A. Sexual function in a community. *Arch Sex Behav* 1994;23: 375–95

39. Taylor JF, Rosen RV, Lieblum SR. Self-report assessment in female sexual function: psychometric evaluation of the brief index of sexual functioning for women. *Arch Sex Behav* 1994;23:627–43

40. Pfeiffer E, Davis GC. Determination of sexual behavior in middle and old age. *J Am Geriatric Soc* 1997;20:151–8

41. Hallstrom OT. *Mental Disorders and Sexuality in the Climacteric*. Gothenburg: Scandinavian University Books, 1973

42. Koster A, Grade K. Sexual desire and menopause development: a prospective study. *Maturitas* 1993;16:49–60

43. Sarrel PM. Effects of hormone replacement therapy on sexual psychophysiology and behavior in the postmenopause. *J Women's Health Gender-Based Med* 2000;9:525–32

44. Dennerstein L, Dudley E, Burger H. Well-being and the menopausal transition. *J Psychosom Obstet Gynecol* 1997;18:95–101

45. Goldstein I, Rosen R, Padma-Nathan H, et al. Sildenafil in the treatment of erectile dysfunction. *N Engl J Med* 1992;338:1397–404

# 7

# Gynecological changes of the geripause

*Brian M. Berger*

## Introduction

Long postmenopausal life-spans distinguish humans from all other primates[1]. The continuing growth of female life expectancy has resulted in a marked increase of women in years beyond the menopause. Women can nowadays expect to live one-third of their lives in a potential hormonal deficiency state. Women over 50 comprise 17% of the total population of any country in the modern Western world[2]. This pattern may have evolved with mother–child food sharing, a practice that allowed aging females to enhance their daughters' fertility, thereby increasing selection against senescence. Other apes live no longer than 50 years. That is, they become frail with age so that all physiological systems fail in tandem. This threshold defines maximum life span, a parameter that can be used to estimate other life history averages. In humans, maximum life span is nearly 100 years, but fertility and other systems in women universally end in approximately half that time, well in advance of other aspects of physiological frailty. Still unknown is how natural selection came to favor this distinctly human 'postreproductive' component of life history with long postmenopausal life spans[3].

## Pituitary and ovarian changes with reproductive aging

Reproductive aging in women is closely tied to the loss of ovarian follicles through atresia. The sentinel endocrinological finding is the monotropic rise of follicle stimulating hormone (FSH), associated with a decline in ovarian inhibin B secretion. Fertility becomes significantly compromised long before overt clinical signs occur, such as cycle irregularity. Compromised fertility is primarily related to oocyte dysfunction. The relationships, if any, between the monotropic FSH rise, accelerated follicular atresia, shortened follicular phase, and oocyte quality remain to be determined. The next phase of reproductive aging is the perimenopause. Lack of predictability is the rule with regard to the nature and duration of the perimenopause. Long cycles are interspersed with short ones, and intermittent ovulatory cycles are intermingled with periods that are hormonally indistinct from the postmenopausal state. Even after the last menstrual period, evidence of intermittent ovarian estradiol production may still be detected. Although fertility is severely compromised during the perimenopause, ovulation may occur without warning and contraception must be practiced if pregnancy is not desired.

## Gynecological symptoms of the menopause

Hot flushes are the most common symptom of the climacteric. The symptoms are characteristic of a heat-dissipation response and consist of sweating on the face, neck and chest, as well as peripheral vasodilatation. Although hot flushes clearly accompany the estrogen withdrawal at menopause, estrogen alone is not responsible, since levels do not differ between symptomatic and asymptomatic women. Vasomotor symptoms affect more than half of the female population around the menopause, with a mean duration of 2–3 years[4]. While not as common as the vasomotor symptoms, urogenital atrophy is experienced by 15% of premenopausal women, 10–40% of postmenopausal women and 10–25% of women receiving systemic hormone therapy. The most common symptoms are dryness, burning, pruritus, irritation and dyspareunia. Estrogen loss is the largest single cause, but drugs and chemical sensitivities are also responsible.

## Hormone replacement therapy for gynecological changes

One of the most complex and difficult healthcare decisions that women face is whether to use postmenopausal hormone replacement therapy (HRT)[5]. The belief that HRT has an overall beneficial effect on cardiovascular disease comes from the results of prospective cohort studies. Recently, results from two long-term prospective trials have cast doubt on the previously supposed benefits of HRT on coronary heart disease (CHD). The Women's Health Initiative[6] was discontinued after only 5.2 years (the study had been planned for 8.5 years) after it showed that absolute excess risks per 10 000 person-years attributable to estrogen plus progestin were seven more CHD events, eight more strokes, eight more PEs, and eight more invasive breast cancers. Absolute risk reductions per 10 000 person-years were six fewer colorectal cancers and five fewer hip fractures. The absolute excess risk of events included in the global index was 19 per 10 000 person-years. The investigators concluded that the risk–benefit profile found in this trial is not consistent with the requirements for a viable intervention for primary prevention of chronic diseases, and that this regimen should not be initiated or continued for primary prevention of CHD. The Heart and Estrogen/progestin Replacement Study follow-up (HERS II) showed that treatment for 6.8 years with estrogen plus progestin in older women with coronary disease increased the rates of venous thromboembolism and biliary tract surgery[7]. In addition, after 6.8 years, hormone therapy

did not reduce risk of cardiovascular events in women with CHD[8]. In summary, these trials suggest that the benefits of HRT include prevention of osteoporotic fractures and colorectal cancer, while prevention of dementia is uncertain. Harms include CHD, stroke, thromboembolic events, breast cancer with 5 or more years of use, and cholecystitis.

Estrogen replacement therapy (ERT) or HRT is the treatment of choice for symptomatic relief in postmenopausal women. Guidelines and analyses of the benefits and risks of HRT, the details of which are beyond the scope of this chapter, are available for clinicians who counsel women about the use of postmenopausal hormones[9]. Some of these were developed before the results of large-scale, randomized trials became available. However, even those published since the HERS data became available do not offer consistent and explicit guidance. All guidelines recommend that the risk–benefit assessment should be individualized, but only some still emphasize the importance of coronary heart disease in the equation.

Dosages prescribed for menopausal symptoms or to prevent osteoporosis (and, potentially, other conditions) can restore the vagina to premenopausal physiology and relieve symptoms. There is strong evidence, including data from randomized clinical trials, that estrogen therapy is a highly effective approach to controlling vasomotor and genitourinary symptoms. The decision to initiate ERT/HRT must be individualized according to each woman's needs[9]. Other approaches – such as the use of clonidine, selective serotonin-reuptake inhibitors, or vitamin E or the consumption of soy-based products or other phytoestrogens – may also offer relief from vasomotor symptoms, although they appear to be less effective than HRT.

## Hormone replacement therapy for urogenital symptoms

A meta-analysis of estrogen therapy in the management of urogenital atrophy in postmenopausal women evaluated the efficacy of estrogen therapy in the treatment of post-menopausal women with symptoms and signs associated with urogenital atrophy. Of the 77 relevant articles reviewed, nine contained ten randomized controlled trials. Meta-analysis of these using the Stouffer method revealed a statistically significant benefit of estrogen therapy for all outcomes studied. In 54 uncontrolled case series, the patients' symptoms were treated by 24 different treatment modalities. All routes of administration appeared to be effective and maximum benefit was obtained between 1 and 3 months after the start of treatment. As expected, the least systemic absorption of estrogen was seen with estriol (administered orally or vaginally), then vaginal estradiol as measured by pretherapy and post-therapy serum estradiol and estrone. They concluded that estrogen is efficacious in the treatment of urogenital atrophy, and low-dose vaginal estradiol preparations are as effective as systemic estrogen therapy in the treatment of urogenital atrophy in postmenopausal women[10].

## Local versus systemic treatment options

When used to treat vasomotor symptoms, HRT has been shown to be cost effective[11]. However, this cost-effectiveness was reduced if the number of office procedures and visits to the clinic were increased owing to systemic side-effects. Although systemic HRT is frequently used for the treatment of urogenital atrophy, recent attention has also focused on local delivery of estrogen to the affected urogenital tissue[12]. Locally applied HRT is a method by which systemic side-effects can be reduced or eliminated and cost effectiveness increased. In addition, concomitant progestins, which are necessary for women with an intact uterus to minimize or eliminate estrogen-induced endometrial cancer[13] may not be necessary with vaginal rings and vaginal tablets. If ERT is given only to treat urogenital atrophy, estrogen creams one or two times per week may prevent recurrence after symptoms are resolved. Progestins may also not be required for occasional estrogen cream use.

Rioux and colleagues examined the efficacy and safety of 25 µg 17β-estradiol vaginal tablets (Vagifem®) compared with 1.25 mg conjugated equine estrogen vaginal cream (Premarin Vaginal Cream®) for the relief of menopause-derived atrophic vaginitis resulting from estrogen deficiency[14]. In a multicenter, open-label, randomized, parallel-group study, 159 menopausal women were treated for 24 weeks with either vaginal tablets or vaginal cream. Composite scores of vaginal symptoms (dryness, soreness, and irritation) demonstrated that both treatments provided equivalent relief of the symptoms of atrophic vaginitis. Fewer patients who were using the vaginal tablets experienced endometrial proliferation or hyperplasia than patients who were using the vaginal cream. Significantly more patients who were using the vaginal tablets rated their medication favorably than did patients who were using the vaginal cream ($p \leq 0.001$). Patients who were receiving the vaginal tablets also had a lower incidence of patient withdrawal (10 vs. 32%). Treatment regimens with 25 µg 17β-estradiol vaginal tablets and with 1.25 mg conjugated equine estrogen vaginal cream were equivalent in relieving symptoms of atrophic vaginitis. The vaginal tablets demonstrated a localized effect without appreciable systemic estradiol increases or estrogenic side-effects.

A study examining the efficacy and acceptability of a continuous low-dose estradiol-releasing vaginal ring with conjugated equine estrogen vaginal cream in the treatment of postmenopausal urogenital atrophy examined 194 postmenopausal women with symptoms and signs of urogenital atrophy. They were randomized on a 2 : 1 basis to 12 weeks of treatment with an estrogen vaginal ring or an estrogen cream. Equivalence (95% CI) was demonstrated between the two treatments for relief of vaginal dryness and dyspareunia, resolution of atrophic signs, improvement in vaginal mucosal maturation indices and reduction in vaginal pH. No significant difference was demonstrated in the endometrial response to a progestin challenge test, and equivalence was demonstrated in the incidence of intercurrent bleeding episodes. The vaginal ring was significantly more acceptable than the cream ($p < 0.0001$), and was preferred to the cream ($p < 0.001$)[15].

## Sexual function and the menopause

Urogenital symptoms associated with estrogen loss can occur episodically throughout a woman's life (e.g. during lactation, during treatment with gonadotropin releasing hormone (GnRH) agonists, etc.) but they are most common and chronic in duration in postmenopausal women. These urogenital complaints can be associated with a diminished frequency of all forms of sexual behavior[16]. Complaints associated with urogenital aging include vaginal dryness, irritation, and pressure, vaginal discharge and infection, vulvovaginal pruritis, dyspareunia, post-coital bleeding, urinary frequency, urgency and incontinence, and recurrent urinary tract infections. Although these symptoms have affected women for centuries, they are now becoming more widely recognized by health professionals and society in general because of the increased life expectancy, the acceptance of open discussion of this topic, and the advent of effective therapy. Urogenital aging is a public health issue because of its high prevalence and because early detection and pharmacological intervention may prevent the development of serious conditions such as uterine prolapse and urinary incontinence. The risk of uterovaginal prolapse also increases with the number of vaginal births and is higher in overweight women[17].

Few studies have examined the long-term effects of hormone deficiency on sexual response. Eskin studied 30 women treated with estrogen alone or combined estrogen and progestin, and 30 parallel controls, aged 53–80 years, over 3 months. Geripause transition was observed after age 64.4 years. Women treated with HRT were compared with controls: discomfort was less ($p < 0.01$); less lubricant was necessary ($p < 0.001$); fewer women discontinued vaginal intercourse (16%); and desire and arousal continued to be present ($p < 0.02$). Orgasmic responses through intercourse or masturbation were diverse (not significant). This preliminary study indicated a positive effect of HRT on maintaining desire and arousal during geripause: prolongation of tissue protection was evident[18].

The ovaries provide approximately half the circulating testosterone in premenopausal women. Testosterone production continues into the postmenopausal years and presumably contributes to the normal sexual function in the postmenopause. After bilateral oophorectomy, many women report impaired sexual functioning despite estrogen replacement. In women who have undergone oophorectomy and hysterectomy, transdermal testosterone improves sexual function and psychological well-being. Shifren and colleagues evaluated the effects of transdermal testosterone in women who had impaired sexual function after surgically induced menopause[19]. The mean ($\pm$ SD) serum free testosterone concentration increased from $1.2 \pm 0.8$ pg/ml ($4.2 \pm 2.8$ pmol/l) during placebo treatment to $3.9 \pm 2.4$ pg/ml ($13.5 \pm 8.3$ pmol/l) and $5.9 \pm 4.8$ pg/ml ($20.5 \pm 16.6$ pmol/l) during treatment with 150 and 300 µg of testosterone per day, respectively (normal range, 1.3–6.8 pg/ml (4.5–23.6 pmol/l)). Despite an appreciable placebo response, the higher testosterone dose resulted in further increases in scores for frequency of sexual activity and pleasure–orgasm in the Brief Index of Sexual Functioning for Women ($p = 0.03$ for both comparisons with placebo).

Vaginal anatomy does not appear to be related to sexual function in women. Weber and co-workers[20] looked at 104 women presenting for gynecologic care (mean age 55.8 years) and performed measurements of vaginal caliber and length, and grading of vulvovaginal atrophy. Current sexual activity was not associated with differences in vaginal length or introital caliber. Among 73 sexually active women, 30 had one or both symptoms of dyspareunia and vaginal dryness, and 43 had neither symptom. Menopausal status, current use of estrogen, introital caliber and vaginal length were not different in women with dyspareunia, vaginal dryness, or both compared with women having neither symptom. Premenopausal women with dyspareunia, vaginal dryness, or both had significantly higher global sexual function scores, reflecting worse sexual function, compared with premenopausal women without these symptoms ($0.61 \pm 0.16$ vs. $0.46 \pm 0.15$, respectively; $p = 0.02$); however, there was no significant difference in postmenopausal women ($0.6 \pm 0.12$ vs. $0.61 \pm 0.12$)[20].

## Non-pharmacological treatment of urogenital symptoms

Menopause does not always need to be treated pharmacologically. Life style changes, such as quitting smoking, increasing physical activity, and maintaining a healthy diet, may be useful in controlling symptoms and preventing chronic disease. Vaginal moisturizers provide longer relief by changing the fluid content of the endothelium and lowering the vaginal pH. Vaginal lubricants provide short-term relief. Women with contraindications to ERT/HRT could use lubricants for intercourse-related dryness or moisturizers for more continuous relief.

Non-hormonal methods may also be effective at treating the vaginal symptoms of estrogen deficiency. A study was performed comparing dienoestrol (Cilag), an estrogenic vaginal cream versus Replens®, a moisturizing vaginal gel. Replens was given three times a week during the 12 weeks of the study, while dienoestrol was administered daily during the first 2 weeks and thereafter three times a week. Vaginal dryness index, itching, irritation, dyspareunia, pH, and safety were evaluated every week during the first month and every month thereafter. Both treatments had a significant increase on the vaginal dryness index as early as the first week of treatment, and the hormonal compound was significantly better than the non-hormonal compound. All symptoms such as itching, irritation and dyspareunia significantly decreased or disappeared without any difference between the two treatments[21].

The lay press promotes agrimony, black cohosh, chaste tree, dong quai, witch hazel, and phytoestrogens for vaginal dryness and dyspareunia; however, no evidence exists to support these specific claims. Pharmacists should be actively involved in identifying, preventing, and treating urogenital atrophy[22].

## Diagnosing clinically significant hormone deficiency

Notelovitz[23] has reported a simple diagnostic test and the effect of the route of hormone administration. A preliminary double-blinded study in 67 symptomatic postmenopausal women confirmed: that atrophic vaginitis was associated with an increase in the lateral wall vaginal pH; that this was paralleled by similar changes in pH in the urethra; and that locally applied vaginal conjugated estrogen cream normalized the pH in the vagina and urethra. Thus, the testing of the vaginal pH serves both as a surrogate for evaluating urethral pH and as a monitor of compliance with treatment[23].

In another study, by Davila and associates[24], 69 women presenting for routine out-patient gynecological care were asked to complete a five-item questionnaire regarding the presence and severity (0–3) of vaginal atrophy symptoms. They underwent a pelvic examination recording vaginal mucosal changes and severity (0–3), including pH. Symptom scores were poorly correlated with age (0.35) and physical findings (0.35) but not with vaginal sidewall cytological maturation index (–0.04). The authors concluded that, although urogenital atrophy occurs universally after menopause, most elderly women are minimally symptomatic. Symptoms alone should not guide initiation of therapy[24].

## Fertility in the menopause

A dramatic increase in the numbers of US women with impaired fecundity has occurred over the past decade. This is largely due to the 'baby-boom' cohort of women, many of whom delayed childbearing, reaching their later and less fecund reproductive years. A recent study projected that the number of women experiencing infertility will range from 5.4 to 7.7 million in 2025, with the most likely number being just under 6.5 million. This is a substantial revision (upward) in the number of infertile women, largely a result of the increase in the observed percentage of infertile women in 1995. This increase in both rates and numbers has made advanced age the leading cause of infertility in the USA.

Female life expectancy is higher at birth and at age 65 than the corresponding male life expectancies in the USA – and in most developed countries. Current estimates project that women will live an average of 90 years by the year 2020. However, while women are living longer than ever before, the age of menopause has not changed, occurring at approximately 51 years in the USA. Ages of menopause and of the preceding reproductive events such as the beginning of subfertility and infertility are likely to be dictated by the process of follicle depletion leading to loss of oocyte quantity and quality. To some extent this process is influenced by life-style factors such as smoking, and possibly also by the use of oral contraceptives.

Aging in women, and in particular, the effect of decreased ovarian reserve and possibly uterine senescence, cause a decreased natural fecundity rate, and adversely affect the success rates of fertility therapy in women over the age of 35. Studies of women in oocyte-donation programs have established reduced oocyte competence as the major cause of declining fertility with age, although inadequate endometrial function can also be a contributing factor. Most research has emphasized the importance of chromosomal abnormalities because of the well-established increase in aneuploidy with increasing maternal age, but little is known about the underlying cellular and molecular mechanisms. The unusual case of successful pregnancy achieved by oocyte donation in a woman > 60 years of age demonstrates that the uterus is capable of supporting nidation and subsequent gestation for many years beyond natural menopause[25]. It also shows that other aspects of human physiology are capable of adapting to the stresses and changes of pregnancy sufficiently well to achieve a normal birth at the age of 63 years[26].

## Conclusion

HRT has been proposed for the prevention and treatment of many chronic conditions, ranging from osteoporosis, heart disease, urinary incontinence and Alzheimer's disease. With the exception of osteoporosis, however, many of the suggested benefits remain controversial. Part of the controversy stems from the relative absence of randomized controlled trials, particularly those enrolling sufficient numbers of elderly women. In addition, highly variable levels of estrogens are present in nearly all postmenopausal women, even at advanced ages. Similar to other endocrine systems, estrogen deficiency and the need for its replacement are, therefore, likely to be relative rather than absolute[27,28]. Because many markers of estrogen deficiency exhibit overlap between risk groups, their clinical usefulness as predictors of frailty, disability, and response to HRT has been limited. Future studies will need to focus not only on the use of highly variable circulating serum estrogen levels but also on markers of overall estrogenic effects at the level of individual target tissues.

# References

1. Hawkes K, O'Connell JF, Jones NG, *et al.* Grandmothering, menopause, and the evolution of human life histories. *Proc Natl Acad Sci USA* 1998;95:1336–9
2. Thomas F, Renaud F, Benefice E, *et al.* International variability of ages at menarche and menopause: patterns and main determinants. *Hum Biol* 2001;73:271–90
3. Hill K, Boesch C, Goodall J, *et al.* Mortality rates among wild chimpanzees. *J Hum Evol* 2001;40:437–50
4. Freedman RR. Physiology of hot flashes. *Am J Hum Biol* 2001;13:453–64
5. Nawaz H, Katz DL. American College of Preventive Medicine Practice Policy Statement: perimeno-pausal and postmenopausal hormone replacement therapy. *Am J Prev Med* 1999;17:250–4
6. Writing Group for the women's Health Initiative Investigators. Risks and benefits of estrogen plus progestin in healthy postmenopausal women: principal results from the Women's Health

Initiative randomized controlled trial. *J Am Med Assoc* 2002;288:321–33

7. Hulley S, Furberg C, Barrett-Connor E, *et al.* HERS Research Group. Noncardiovascular disease outcomes during 6.8 years of hormone therapy: Heart and Estrogen/progestin Replacement Study follow-up (HERS II). *J Am Med Assoc* 2002;288:58–66

8. Grady D, Herrington D, Bittner WV, *et al.* HERS Research Group. Cardiovascular disease outcomes during 6.8 years of hormone therapy: Heart and Estrogen/progestin Replacement Study follow-up (HERS II). *J Am Med Assoc* 2002;288:49–57

9. The North American Menopause Society. A decision tree for the use of estrogen replacement therapy or hormone replacement therapy in postmenopausal women: consensus opinion. *Menopause* 2000;7:76–86

10. Cardozo L, Bachmann G, McClish D, *et al.* Meta-analysis of estrogen therapy in the management of urogenital atrophy in postmenopausal women: second report of the Hormones and Urogenital Therapy Committee. *Obstet Gynecol* 1998;92:722–7

11. Townsend J, Buxton M. Cost effectiveness scenario analysis for a proposed trial of hormone replacement therapy. *Health Policy* 1997;39: 181–94

12. Bachmann G. Urogenital ageing: an old problem newly recognized. *Maturitas* 1995; 22(Suppl):S1–5

13. Grady D, Gebretsadik T, Kerlikowske K, *et al.* Hormone replacement therapy and endometrial cancer risk: a meta-analysis. *Obstet Gynecol* 1995;85:304–13

14. Rioux JE, Devlin C, Gelfand MM, *et al.* 17beta-estradiol vaginal tablet versus conjugated equine estrogen vaginal cream to relieve menopausal atrophic vaginitis. *Menopause* 2000;7:156–61

15. Ayton RA, Darling GM, Murkies AL, *et al.* A comparative study of safety and efficacy of continuous low dose oestradiol released from a vaginal ring compared with conjugated equine oestrogen vaginal cream in the treatment of postmenopausal urogenital atrophy. *Br J Obstet Gynaecol* 1996;103:351–8

16. Sarrel PM. Effects of hormone replacement therapy on sexual psychophysiology and behavior in postmenopause. *J Womens Health Gender-Based Med* 2000;9(Suppl 1):S25–32

17. Risk factors for genital prolapse in non-hysterectomized women around menopause. Results from a large cross-sectional study in menopausal clinics in Italy. Progetto Menopausa Italia Study Group. *Eur J Obstet Gynecol Reprod Biol* 2000;93:135–40

18. Eskin BA. Hormone replacement therapy and sexual response in postmenopause and geripause. *Obstet Gynecol* 2001;97(4 Suppl 1):S25

19. Shifren JL, Braunstein GD, Simon JA, *et al.* Transdermal testosterone treatment in women with impaired sexual function after oophorectomy. *N Engl J Med* 2000;343:682–8

20. Weber AM, Walters MD, Schover LR, Mitchinson A. Vaginal anatomy and sexual function. *Obstet Gynecol* 1995;86:946–9

21. Bygdeman M, Swahn ML. Replens versus dienoestrol cream in the symptomatic treatment of vaginal atrophy in postmenopausal women. *Maturitas* 1996;23:259–63

22. Willhite LA, O'Connell MB. Urogenital atrophy: prevention and treatment. *Pharmacotherapy* 2001;21:464–80

23. Notelovitz M. Estrogen therapy in the management of problems associated with urogenital ageing: a simple diagnostic test and the effect of the route of hormone administration. *Maturitas* 1995;22(Suppl):S31–3

24. Davila GW, Karapanagiotou I, Woodhouse S, *et al.* Are women with urogenital atrophy symptomatic? *Obstet Gynecol* 2001;97(4 Suppl 1): S48

25. Paulson RJ, Thornton MH, Francis MM, Salvador HS. Successful pregnancy in a 63-year-old woman. *Fertil Steril* 1997;67:949–51

26. Sauer MV, Paulson RJ, Lobo RA. Oocyte donation to women of advanced reproductive age: pregnancy results and obstetrical outcomes in patients 45 years and older. *Hum Reprod* 1996;11:2540–3

27. Suzuki N, Yano T, Nakazawa N, *et al.* A possible role of estrone produced in adipose tissues in modulating postmenopausal bone density. *Maturitas* 1995;22:9–12

28. Tchernof A, Poehlman ET, Despres JP. Body fat distribution, the menopause transition, and hormone replacement therapy. *Diabetes Metab* 2000;26:12–20

# Part II
# Care of the Older Patient

# 8

# Approach to the elderly patient

*Bruce R. Troen*

There is a tremendous amount of variation in the manner in which individuals age and respond to illness. Consequently, knowledge of a patient's baseline function and health is critical for accurate diagnosis and therapy. Problems that merit special attention in the elderly are listed in Table 1. There is often altered presentation of disease in the elderly; severe or life-threatening illnesses may be manifest by vague, non-specific, or even trivial symptoms. Such symptoms may represent an abrupt change in the patient's health. For example, the patient could cease to go shopping, refuse to arise from bed, or fall more often than usual. Non-specific symptoms that may represent specific illnesses include confusion, self-neglect, falling, incontinence, apathy, anorexia, dyspnea, and fatigue. Furthermore, symptoms that appear to represent illness within one organ system can actually indicate change in another. Delirium in the elderly infrequently results from acute central nervous system pathology. It is most commonly a sign of systemic illness that is secondarily affecting the brain. Delirium is also a much more common harbinger of physical illness in older people than are fever, pain, or tachycardia. Many presentations of pathology represent change in the older patient's homeostatic reserve and could also reflect changes in sensitivity to pain and other stimuli (for example, in a patient with acute and/or chronic cognitive impairment). Examples of altered presentations of specific illnesses in the elderly include: depression without sadness; infectious disease without leukocytosis, fever, or tachycardia; silent surgical abdomen; silent malignancy ('mass without symptoms'); myocardial infarction without

**Table 1** Common issues in the elderly

Function
Polypharmacy
Ambulation
Cognition
Depression
Urinary incontinence
Constipation
Alcohol
Elder mistreatment

chest pain; non-dyspneic pulmonary edema; and apathetic thyrotoxicosis. Often the elderly will not volunteer information about symptoms, owing to misconceptions about normal age-related changes versus disease-related phenomena. These 'hidden illnesses' in the elderly include sexual dysfunction, depression, incontinence, musculoskeletal stiffness, hearing loss, and dementia. To ferret out these problems, and also alcoholism in the elderly, requires proactive questioning by physicians and other health-care workers. Because a specific disease approach may not allow for accurate diagnoses in the elderly, it is often more useful to consider the presenting problem, such as those grouped under the 'I's of Geriatrics' (Table 2). Of particular note is iatrogenesis, because of the advantages and disadvantages that must be weighed in proceeding with diagnosis and treatment, particularly in frail older individuals.

## History

Obtaining a history from an older patient may take more time and require eliciting information from family members and friends. Nevertheless,

**Table 2** The I's of Geriatrics. Aadapted with permission from Kane RL, Ouslander JG, Abrass IB. *Clinical Implications of the Aging Process. Essentials of Clinical Geriatrics.* New York: McGraw-Hill Health Professions Division, 1999: 3–18

Iatrogenesis
Immobility
Immune deficiency
Impairment of vision/hearing
Impotence
Impoverishment
Inanition (malnutrition)
Incoherence
Incontinence
Infection
Insomnia
Instability
Institutionalization
Intellectual impairment
Irritable colon
Isolation (depression)

**Table 3** Activities of daily living (basic self-care) and instrumental activities of daily living (community interactions)

*Activities of daily living*
(mnemonic – 'DEATH')
Dressing
Eating
Ambulating
Toileting
Hygiene

*Instrumental activities of daily living*
(mnemonic – 'SHAFT')
Shopping
Housework
Accounting
Food preparation
Transportation

the patient should remain the primary source, barring advanced cognitive impairment. If a patient's responses are inappropriate and/or inconsistent, then evaluation of cognitive status should be undertaken (see below). The initial interview should be conducted with the patient dressed, seated and facing you at eye level. Given changes in vision, hearing and speech discrimination, it is important to talk directly without jargon to the patient and ensure that the patient understands. This includes allowing enough time for the older patient to respond. It is critical to obtain a thorough medication history, including over-the-counter medications and home remedies. Adverse drug reactions and interactions are particularly common among the elderly and are directly proportional to the number of medications being taken, because of the high incidence of disease. Age alone is not an independent predictor of adverse drug reactions[1]. It is helpful to have the patient bring all of his or her medicine to the physician's office ('brown bag' technique). It is essential to determine the patient's compliance and perceived effects of the medications. Special emphasis also needs to be placed on social history,

health-care maintenance, functional capabilities, nutritional history, alcohol consumption, and the review of systems. Explicit inquiries about urinary signs and symptoms (especially incontinence for women and hesitancy for men) should be included in the review of systems. Functional assessment includes determination of activities of daily living (ADL) and instrumental activities of daily living (IADL) (Table 3)[2,3]. For those patients who depend upon a caregiver, screening for elder mistreatment should be considered[4]. Elder abuse includes physical neglect, psychological abuse and/or neglect, financial or material abuse/neglect, or violation of personal rights.

## Physical examination

For very frail patients, multiple sessions for a complete physical examination may be required. If back pain, deformity, or significant arthritis exist, time in the supine position may need to be limited. This is particularly pertinent for osteoporotic and/or arthritic patients undergoing pelvic examination. During general observation of the patient and assessment of vital signs, special attention should be given to the presence of ADL deficits, poor hygiene, disheveled appearance, systolic hypertension, orthostatic hypotension, and the patient's

**Table 4** Geriatric principles. Reproduced with permission from Rosenblatt D. *Geriatric Gems.* Ann Arbour, USA: University of Michigan Geriatrics Center, 1995

---

Assess each patient individually
Assess cognitive and functional status
Disease often presents atypically
Disease often presents as a change in functional
  status
Rule out organic causes of behavioral changes first
Pathogenesis of symptoms is often multifactorial
An ounce of prevention is worth a pound of cure
Beware of iatrogenesis
Take a holistic approach
Be the patient's advocate
Do not be ageist

---

weight. The timed 'Get Up & Go' test helps to determine functional mobility[5]. The patient is asked to rise from a seating position, walk 3 m, turn around, and return to sit in the chair. A time of less than 20 s suggests good mobility, whereas times over 30 s suggest potential problems. During this test, the patient's gait should be assessed. Lower extremity function in the elderly (balance, gait, strength, and endurance) can predict short-term mortality and nursing home admission[6]. Visual and aural acuity should be assessed. Decreased hearing can occur as a result of wax accumulation in the ear. The skin should be assessed for ulcers and neoplasms in sun-exposed areas. Cardio-vascular palpation is less reliable when kypho-scoliosis exists. Systolic murmurs associated with benign aortic sclerosis are common. However, diastolic murmurs and the presence of an $S_3$ gallop are always important and merit further consideration and work-up. Arterial insufficiency results in hair loss, bruits and decreased pulses, whereas venous disease more commonly leads to stasis, skin changes and edema. A baseline pulmonary examination is particularly important, since rales may not indicate infectious disease or congestive heart failure. Breast masses may be easier to palpate, owing to lack of estrogenic stimulation. If the patient is unable to lie flat, the abdomen may appear falsely distended. There can be a palpable liver edge without hepatomegaly, and peritoneal signs

may be blunt or even absent in the frail elderly. Often one can palpate a distended bladder, aortic aneurysm, and even a sigmoid colon fecal impaction. A rectal examination can assess fecal impaction and sacral reflexes, and can obtain stool for hemoccult testing. A speculum examination of the vagina may be painful and difficult, owing to the absence of estrogen. Extremities should be examined for arthritis and deformities. It is also important to assess toes and toenails. A 'Mini-Mental Status' examination should be performed in all older patients to establish a baseline. A documented mental status will help to determine the acuity of any change and, therefore, the necessary work-up. The Folstein Mini-Mental Status' Examination[7] remains the bulwark in screening for dementia and delirium, although other tools such as the clock drawing and time and change tests have shown promise in recent studies[8,9]. Behavioral changes and/or sadness should prompt screening for depression, using the Geriatric Depression Scale[10] or explicitly asking the patient about sadness/depression[11].

Health care providers face the challenge of incorporating a geriatric database into their care of the elderly and not falling prey to the myth of hopelessness in treating older patients. Indeed, there is likely to be greater success for some preventive strategies, owing to increased risks of disease faced by the elderly. Furthermore, since the elderly can manifest dramatic symptoms and signs in response to relatively minor perturbations in their physiology, targeted therapies that produce small 'objective' improvements in an organ system can lead to dramatic benefits for the patient. A proactive approach that incorporates the 'Geriatric Principles' in Table 4 will begin to lay the foundation for enhanced care of patients in the geripause. The following chapters will provide some approaches to a selection of geriatric diseases and syndromes. While the approach is not all-encompassing, the goal is to provide paradigms to evaluate and manage some of the most pressing and widespread problems experienced by elderly patients and thereby enhance their quality of life.

# References

1. Denham MJ. Adverse drug reactions. *Br Med Bull* 1990;46:53–62
2. Katz S, Downs TD, Cash HR, Grotz RC. Progress in development of the index of ADL. *Gerontologist* 1970;10:20–30
3. Lawton MP, Brody EM. Assessment of older people: self-maintaining and instrumental activities of daily living. *Gerontologist* 1969;9:179–86
4. Swagerty DL Jr, Takahashi PY, Evans JM. Elder mistreatment. *Am Farm Physician* 1999;59:2804–8
5. Podsiadlo D, Richardson S. The timed 'Up & Go': a test of basic functional mobility for frail elderly persons. *J Am Geriatr Soc* 1991;39:142–8
6. Guralnik JM, Simonstick EM, Ferrucci L, *et al.* A short physical performance battery assessing lower extremity function: association with self-reported disability and prediction of mortality and nursing home admission. *J Gerontol* 1994;49:M85–94
7. Folstein MF, Folstein SE, McHugh PR. 'Mini-mental state'. A practical method for grading the cognitive state of patients for the clinician. *J Psychiatr Res* 1975;12:189–98
8. Esteban-Santillan C, Praditsuwan R, Ueda H, Geldmacher DS. Clock drawing test in very mild Alzheimer's disease. *J Am Geriatr Soc* 1998;46:1266–9
9. Froehilich TE, Robinson JT, Inouye SK. Screening for dementia in the outpatient setting: the time and change test. *J Am Geriatr Soc* 1998;46:1506–11
10. Yesavage JA, Brink TL, Rose TL, *et al.* Development and validation of a geriatric depression screening scale: a preliminary report. *J Psychiatr Res* 1982;17:37–49
11. Mahoney J, Drinka TJ, Abler R, *et al.* Screening for depression: single question versus GDS [see comments]. *J Am Geriatr Soc* 1994;42:1006–8
12. Kane RL, Ouslander JG, Abrass IB. *Clinical Implications of the Aging Process. Essentials of Clinical Geriatrics.* New York: McGraw-Hill Health Professions Division, 1999:3–18
13. Rosenblatt D. *Geriatric Gems.* Ann Arbor, MI: University of Michigan Geriatrics Center, 1995

# 9

# Functional assessment in the geripause

*Frederick T. Sherman*

An older woman's functional status is the most important consideration in the initial geriatric assessment. Functional status is primarily determined by physical and/or cognitive impairments. Medical illness, affective disorders, lack of social supports, and economic and environmental factors cause further deterioration, worsening overall function. Declining functional status is often a marker for undetected underlying conditions. Performing an assessment that reveals these problems is challenging, because certain syndromes and conditions manifest differently in the geriatric patient than in the middle-aged or younger adult. This effort, however, can be streamlined by using brief, easily remembered screening tools that are tailor-made for the primary care setting. Systematic screening for common geriatric conditions, generally indicated for women over 70 years of age, can help reduce the chance that a problem will go untreated and worsen with time[1,2]. These geriatric conditions go beyond the standard history and physical examination and include screens for delirium, dementia, depression, polypharmacy and adverse drug reactions, vision and hearing impairments, decline in general physical performance, psychosocial needs, urinary incontinence, and malnutrition.

While the brief screens discussed in this chapter are designed to be utilized by the individual clinician in an office setting, they are seldom diagnostic. Rather, a positive screen should lead the clinician to further evaluation, definitive diagnosis, and treatment. Brief, office-based geriatric screens often lead to medical, psychiatric, or rehabilitation interventions that result in maintenance or improvement of functional status. Small, incremental gains can produce

**Table 1** The DEEP-IN mnemonic for geriatric functional assessment. Reproduced with permission from Sherman FT. Functional assessment: easy-to-use screening tools speed initial office work-up. *Geriatrics* 2001;56:36–40

| | |
|---|---|
| D | Delirium, dementia, depression, drugs |
| E | Eyes (vision impairment) |
| E | Ears (hearing impairment) |
| P | Physical performance, 'phalls' (falls), psychosocial |
| I | Incontinence (urinary) |
| N | Nutrition |

significant positive effects for older adults and their families, allowing both to function at their highest levels in the living settings they prefer.

This chapter describes how to use a series of office-based screening tests, using the easily remembered mnemonic 'DEEP-IN', designed to streamline initial assessment of the older woman. The mnemonic DEEP-IN (Table 1) can help physicians quickly identify older adults who are frail or at high risk for frailty[1]. These screens will lead to the diagnosis and treatment of conditions that undermine physical and cognitive status, independence, and quality of life.

## DEEP-IN

The screens suggested by the mnemonic are not diagnostic, but their results can indicate which patients may benefit from further testing or intervention. The 'D' in the mnemonic represents delirium, dementia, depression, and drugs. The subsequent categories are 'EE' for eyes and ears, 'P' for physical performance, 'phalls' (falls), and psychosocial issues, 'I' for incontinence (urinary), and 'N' for nutrition.

## Delirium

For cases of suspected delirium in an older adult, a good rule of thumb is to consider any change in mental status to be delirium until proved otherwise. This is particularly true if the episode occurs when a patient is in the emergency department, the hospital, a nursing home, or an assisted living setting. The Confusion Assessment Method[4] can be used to identify the presence of delirium in a patient who meets the first two criteria below, and either of the other two (3 or 4):

(1) *Acute onset and fluctuating course.* Is there evidence of an acute change in mental status, and does the behavior come and go?

(2) *Inattention.* Does the patient have difficulty focusing attention? Is the patient easily distracted or having difficulty following what is being said?

(3) *Disorganized thinking.* Is the patient's speech rambling or irrelevant, or switching from one subject to the next?

(4) *An altered level of consciousness.* A normal patient should be alert; any other assessment of the patient's level of consciousness – for example, lethargic, stupor, or hyperalert – is abnormal.

Middle-aged adults experiencing a delirium, such as from alcohol withdrawal, typically exhibit a hyperkinetic, hyperalert delirium. In older persons, however, a delirium tends to be 'quiet'. Marked by lethargy and difficulty responding to stimuli, the delirium is hypokinetic and hypoalert. Causes include: drugs; electrolyte imbalance; organ-specific illnesses such as lung, liver, cardiac, and renal disease; common infections such as pneumonia, gallbladder sepsis, and urinary tract infections; and pain.

### Lingering delirium

Most clinicians presume that an episode of delirium is totally reversible, based on their observations of younger adults. The recovery from a delirium in older adults, however, may be prolonged and never fully resolve. One important study looked at the outcomes of 325 hospitalized older patients with delirium who were admitted from either the community or a long-term care facility[5]. Delirium symptoms completely resolved in only 4% of patients at hospital discharge, in 20% after 3 months and in an additional 17% after 6 months. The average length of hospitalization was 19 days for patients with delirium, compared with 7 days for those without. Finally, older patients with delirium had a seven-fold increased risk for nursing home placement. Thus, when counseling the family of a patient with delirium, it is important for physicians to discuss potential outcomes frankly and realistically. Complete resolution of delirium is often a slow process; in some cases, it can take months or years.

## Dementia

Although the Folstein Mini-Mental State Examination (MMSE), a 30-item interviewer-administered assessment, is widely used to screen older adults for dementia, it takes, on average, 9 minutes to perform and the result may be difficult to interpret, particularly in patients with little education or impaired vision. Briefer screens for cognitive impairment will allow the clinician to determine whether the MMSE or further testing needs to be performed. Although many brief tools are available, the five discussed below evaluate recent memory, verbal fluency, and constructional abilities. Each takes less than 1 minute to administer and the busy clinician can choose to use one as his standard screen or alternate among the screening tools (Table 2). While not diagnostic of dementia, positive results on any of these screens should lead to the administration of the MMSE.

### Three-item recall

To conduct this test, tell the patient that you are going to name three objects (e.g. ball, flag,

**Table 2** Five screening tests for dementia

Three-item recall
Animal naming test
Clock completion test
Four IADL score
7-minute battery

and tree) and that you want her to remember them so that she can recite them 1 minute later. Recall of all three items suggests a low probability of dementia, whereas recall of only one or two is associated with a moderate increase in the odds of dementia[6].

## Animal-naming test

This screen is used to gauge impairment in verbal fluency and semantic memory which are often impaired in early dementia, particularly Alzheimer's disease. To perform the test, simply ask the patient to name as many animals as she can in 1 minute. The typical response of a patient with Alzheimer's disease would be: 'dog, cat, cow, [long pause] dog...' Then the patient's attention will drift off, and she will lose focus and not name any more animals. Normal older adults with a high school education can usually name 18 different animals within 1 min. Anything less than 12 is abnormal and correlates well with an MMSE score of less than 23. Animal-naming test scores can vary depending on the patient's age and level of education, but 18 and 12 are generally good cut-off points for normal and abnormal results, respectively[7].

## Clock completion test

The clock completion test (CCT) evaluates non-dominant parietal lobe function, which is often diminished in early-stage Alzheimer's disease, about the same time as the recent memory and language impairments occur. To perform this test, give the patient a blank sheet of paper with a 3-inch diameter circle copied on it. Ask her to put the numbers 1–12 in the circle just as they would appear on a standard clock face. Patients with dementia tend to

bunch the numbers together, usually placing most of them on the right half of the circle. The most accurate way to score this test is to section the clock face into quadrants after the patient has completed the task (Figure 1).

The patient's entries in the first three quadrants are scored as either 0 (normal) or 1 (abnormal). The fourth quadrant (9–11), which is the most sensitive indicator of dementia, is scored as either 0 (normal) or 4 (abnormal). On a properly performed examination, the fourth quadrant will have three numbers in it, usually 9–11[8]. If the fourth quadrant is abnormal, i.e. having less than or more than three numbers, there is a high chance of dementia and further definitive testing is indicated. Add up the scores of the four quadrants (maximum, 7). Any score of 4 or more is a good indication of the presence of dementia. Because of the high number of points assigned to it, results from the fourth quadrant alone are often diagnostic.

The CCT was validated in a study that compared its results with those using a standard mental status test[8]. The investigators retrospectively reviewed the results of clock-drawing tests taken from 76 consecutive outpatients, aged 55–92 (mean, 76), of whom 40 had dementia. The researchers found the CCT to be a reliable method of identifying dementia, with sensitivity of 87% and specificity of 82%. The CCT, however, was not found to be an accurate indicator of the severity of dementia[8]. Therefore, a patient who scores 6 is not necessarily more cognitively impaired than a patient who scores 4.

## Four instrumental activities of daily living score

Although there are seven recognized instrumental activities of daily living (IADL), the Four IADL Score[9] assesses the following four activities that are associated with independent living:

(1) Money management;

(2) Medication management;

(3) Telephone use; and

(4) Traveling.

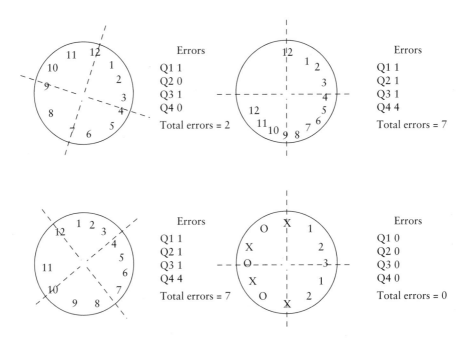

**Figure 1** The clock completion test begins by asking the patient to write the numbers 1–12 in a 3-inch circle so that the result represents a standard clock face. The dotted lines illustrate the sectioning of the clock face into four equal quadrants (Q1, Q2 Q3, and Q4) based on the digit that best represents the 12 of a correctly completed clock. The quadrant error scores flank each of the clocks. As the clock in the bottom right hand corner shows, positioning of the digits, rather than listing the correct clock face numbers, is the focus of the test. Reproduced with permission from Watson YI, Arfken CA, Birge SJ. Clock completion: an objective screening test for dementia. *J Am Geriatr Soc* 1993;41:1235–40

If your patient is physically able to perform these IADL but needs assistance because of cognitive impairment, suspect a developing dementia. It is important to ask the primary caregiver, because patients with mild cognitive impairment often do not realize the extent of their disability and deny any functional impairment. Simply asking a family member or friend whether the patient needs assistance is all that is required to administer the test. The more IADL that are impaired in a community-residing older person, the greater the probability that dementia will develop within 1 year.

### Seven-minute battery

The 7-minute neurocognitive battery (also the 7-minute screen) consists of four sets of questions that focus on orientation to time and date, memory, visuospatial skills, and verbal fluency. Three of its four tests are versions of the three-item recall, animal-naming test, and CCT mentioned above. The 7-minute screen is clinically appealing because it: can be administered and scored in approximately 7 minutes and 40 seconds (hence the screen name); can be administered in the out-patient setting by a trained assistant; has a sensitivity of 92% and specificity of 96% for detecting Alzheimer's disease[10].

For more information on the 7-minute screen, visit http://www.7minutescreen.com.

### Depression

Depression is no more common in older adults than in middle-aged or younger populations, but it can be more devastating. Suicidal acts are the most extreme consequence of depression in older persons. An older Caucasion man who verbalizes suicidal intent is at highest risk for carrying out a self-destructive act. Older male patients who do commit suicide tend to use violent, aggressive measures. Therefore, statements

**Table 3** Five-item version of the Geriatric Depression Scale. Reproduced with permission from Hoyl MT, Alessi CA, Harker JO, *et al.* Development and testing of a five-item version of the Geriatric Depression Scale. *J Am Geriatr Soc* 1999;47:873–8

1. Are you basically satisfied with your life?
2. Do you often get bored?
3. Do you often feel helpless?
4. Do you prefer to stay home rather than going out and doing new things?
5. Do you feel pretty worthless the way you are now?

Positive answers for depression screening are 'yes' to questions 2–5 and 'no' to question 1. A score of 0–1 positive answers suggests that the patient is not depressed; scores of 2 or higher indicate possible depression.

Sensitivity, 97%; specificity, 85%; positive predictive value, 85%; negative predictive value, 97%

of intent should be taken seriously. The depression screen should begin with a single question: 'Do you often feel sad or depressed?' The sensitivity and specificity of this single question are 85 and 65%, respectively, in predicting depression. If the patient answers affirmatively, further screening can be performed using the five-item Geriatric Depression Scale (Table 3)[11].

If results of either or both tests are positive, the primary care physician should perform a thorough interview that evaluates neurovegetative signs including insomnia, appetite disturbances, weight loss, and anhedonia. Antidepressant therapy and referral for psychotherapy should be initiated. Failure of antidepressants or the expressions of suicidal thoughts warrant referral to a psychiatrist.

## Drugs

Any older patient who is taking more than four prescribed drugs has an increased risk for falls. Long-acting benzodiazepines have also been associated with cognitive impairment and falls in older adults. One way of remembering drugs that are particularly prone to cause adverse drug reactions and poor functional outcomes

in the elderly, such as falls, delirium, and/or incontinence, is to be wary of any drug class that starts with 'anti'. Antipsychotics, antidepressants, antihypertensives, anti-inflammatories, antianxiety and anti-insomnia medications, while commonly used in the elderly, should be reviewed at each visit by the clinician. When using medications in the elderly, 'start low', increase slowly, watching for side-effects, but 'be prepared to go to full therapeutic dose' so as not to undertreat the older adult for fear of adverse side-effects. Over-the-counter agents and alternative or complementary supplements can also pose risks for adverse reactions and drug–drug interactions when used with prescription agents. Most importantly, always ask the older adult to bring in all their prescribed and non-prescribed medications at each visit for a medication review.

## Ears (hearing impairment)

Hearing impairment affects about one-third of adults over the age of 65 years and can lead to social isolation, accidents, depression, and the appearance of cognitive impairment. The older adult who asks you to repeat yourself during the history taking, stares intensely at your face while you are interviewing them so as to 'face read', or fails to follow your directions during the physical examination, should be considered to have a hearing deficit. Before performing any brief hearing test, check the patient's ear canals for cerumen and remove it with a curette or aural syringe. Rarely, cerumen removal alone will totally resolve hearing impairment. While two simple screens are available to detect hearing impairment, the simple whisper test requires no equipment, takes less than a minute to perform, and has a high sensitivity and specificity.

## Whisper test

To perform this screen, sit or stand directly in front of and about 18 inches (45 cm) across from the patient. Explain that you are going to whisper some numbers, then ask the patient to close her eyes. After exhaling to standardize the loudness of your voice, whisper four random

**Table 4**  Physical performance tests

Single chair-rise
Three chair-rises in rapid succession (timed)
Timed rapid gait
Timed 'up & go'
Three static stances
Functional reach

numbers from 1–9 at 1-second intervals. Ask the patient to repeat all the numbers you whispered. A patient who does not hear at least two of the numbers fails the test, which has a sensitivity of 80–100% and specificity of 80–90%.

### Audioscope

A more costly, yet slightly more accurate, alternative screen to the simple whisper test, is the audioscope test. The audioscope delivers four high-frequency (500, 1000, 2000, and 4000 Hz) tones at approximately 40 dB. A patient unable to discern the 1000- or 2000-Hz tone in either or both ears is considered to have a hearing impairment. Sensitivity and specificity of audioscope testing are 94 and 72%, respectively (roughly comparable with the whisper test).

### Eyes (vision impairment)

Because cataracts, glaucoma, age-related macular degeneration, and diabetic retinopathy occur most commonly in the elderly, it is imperative to administer a simple screen for visual impairment. The screen consists of two parts: a simple question, which, if positive, leads to testing each eye with a Snellen eye chart. The question is: 'Because of your eyesight, do you have any difficulty driving, watching television, reading, or performing any other daily activity?' If the patient answers 'Yes', then test each eye while wearing corrective lenses with the Snellen eye chart 20 feet (6 m) from the patient. A smaller hand-held version can be placed 14 inches (35 cm) from the patient. Patients fail this visual screen if they are unable to read all the letters on the 20/40 line. Referral to an optician, optometrist, or ophthalmologist is indicated if the patient answers 'Yes' to the question and fails the vision screen.

### Physical performance

Poor physical performance and cognitive dysfunction are intimately linked, both contributing, in an additive fashion, to impaired performance of basic activities of daily living (ADL). Quick, easily administered, office-based physical performance testing can identify patients at risk for losing any ADL and living alone. The tests (summarized in Table 4) will also confirm or refute the patient's and caregiver's assessments of physical performance, and help identify patients at high risk for loss of independent function. Specific screens include: a single chair rise and timed chair rises; rapid gait; timed 'up and go' (TUG); and functional reach.

### Chair rise(s)

The first step in this screen is making sure the patient can safely rise from and sit down in a chair without using their arms. The single chair-rise test begins with the patient seated with hands folded on their lap. They are then asked to stand up and sit down. A patient passes the test by rising and sitting without using their arms for assistance. A patient who cannot rise and sit without using their hands has about a 40% chance of developing an ADL impairment within 1 year if no intervention is initiated[12].

For patients who are able to do a single chair rise, the second step is the quantitative or timed three-chair-rise test. Simply ask the patient to stand up and sit down three times (without using her arms) while you time the activity. Taking longer than 10 seconds significantly increases the risk of ADL impairment over the next 12 months. Typically, bathing and dressing are the first ADL to be lost. You can perform the timed rapid gait test too, which also predicts ADL impairment in the next year.

### Timed rapid gait test

This timed test requires an unobstructed 10-foot (3-m) path in the office, examination

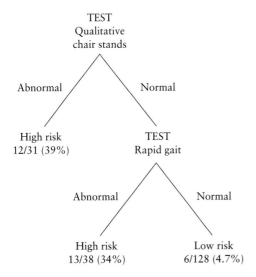

TEST
Qualitative
chair stands

Abnormal / \ Normal

High risk
12/31 (39%)

TEST
Rapid gait

Abnormal / \ Normal

High risk
13/38 (34%)

Low risk
6/128 (4.7%)

**Figure 2** Assessment strategy to determine risk of activities of daily living dependence among older adults with mild-to-moderate cognitive impairment. Adapted with permission from Gill TM, Richardson ED, Tinetti ME. Evaluating the risk of dependence in activities of daily living among community-living older adults with mild to moderate cognitive impairment. *J Gerontol A Biol Sci Med Sci* 1995;50:M235–41

room, or hallway and a watch with a second hand. Ask the standing patient to walk 10 feet, turn, and walk back as quickly as possible. Patients who routinely use canes or other assistive devices should also use them during testing. Those who complete the test within 10 seconds are likely to remain stable in ADL status for at least 1 year. Patients who complete both the timed rapid gait test and the three chair-rises in less than 10 seconds have a 95% chance of maintaining ADL stability over the next year (Figure 2)[13].

## Falls ('phalls')

Since approximately one-third of older community-residing women will fall in any given year, it is important to perform a brief falls risk assessment[13]. The first phase of a falls risk assessment consists of asking the patient about any history of falls. Adults reporting a fall within the past year are at increased risk

for recurrent falls and should undergo a brief balance and gait assessment. If the patient has no history of falls, one of the three following performance tests can be administered. If results of any are positive, the patient is at increased risk of falling and should be referred to a falls prevention program.

(1) *Timed 'up and go' test.* A patient rises from a chair, walks 10 feet, turns around, walks back to the chair, and sits down again. If completion of the task takes longer than 15 seconds, the patient is at increased risk for falls[14,15]. The clinician should walk with the patient, watching her, particularly when turning, to make sure she does not become unsteady.

(2) *Static balance.* Testing for static (standing) balance can also predict fall risk. The patient is asked to assume three consecutive standing stances, keeping eyes open and hands at their sides: side-by-side stance (feet parallel and touching); semi-tandem stance (feet parallel with the heal of one foot next to the first metatarsal–phalangeal joint of the other); and tandem stance (one foot directly in front of the other). Patients unable to hold a side-by-side stance for 10 seconds are at high risk of falling. Those who cannot hold a semi-tandem stance for 10 seconds are at moderate risk of falling and those who can hold a tandem stance for 10 seconds are at low risk of falling.

(3) *Functional reach.* This screen requires a wooden yardstick (ruler) and some Velcro to adhere the yardstick to the wall at the patient's shoulder height. Functional reach is the amount of distance, in inches, that the patient's arm can move along the yardstick while bending forward at the waist with their feet kept stationary[16]. The patient's risk of falling within the next 6 months is significantly higher if s/he cannot reach 10 inches (25 cm). A functional reach of 6–10 inches doubles the risk of recurrent falling in 6 months, while a functional reach of less than 6 inches (15 cm) quadruples the risk.

## Psychosocial

Screening for psychosocial issues including the need for family (e.g. working daughters or sons) or paid caregivers (e.g. home health aides or the visiting nurse) that allow the older adult to remain at home is important. It is important to determine the degree of caregiver stress or 'burnout' by asking the caregiver whether s/he is stressed, anxious, depressed, or sleep deprived, and whether s/he is attending to his/her own medical and psychological needs. The clinician should look for depression and/or anxiety in the caregiver, since these are signs of caregiver burnout. The discussion and completion of advance directives are critical to the long-term functioning of older women as well as assuring them that their plans for future medical care will be carried out, if they should lose capacity to make informed decisions.

## Urinary incontinence

Urinary incontinence is a common, under-reported condition in the elderly woman. Embarrassment over discussing urinary incontinence with a male physician as well as the misbelief that urinary incontinence is a normal part of female aging often leads to the usage of pads to deal with urinary incontinence. Proactive screening for urinary incontinence involves asking two simple questions: 'In the past year, have you ever lost your urine and gotten wet? If yes, then, 'Have you lost urine on at least six separate days?' A 'yes' answer to both of these questions indicates that the patient has a high probability (79% for women and 76% for men) of having urinary incontinence when a urological evaluation is performed. The evaluation should look for acute, potentially reversible causes of urinary incontinence including stool impaction, drug side-effects, urinary tract infection, or delirium, and chronic, treatable causes including stress, urge, or mixed causes[17].

## Nutrition

Clinical malnutrition in the elderly includes both obesity, common among community-residing elderly, and protein energy under-nutrition, more common among hospitalized and institutionalized older adults. Simple screens for both types of nutritional disorders include: a question about weight loss; and measurements of weight and height and calculation of the body mass index. The screening question is: 'Have you lost 10 pounds over the past 6 months without trying to do so?' Any patient who answers 'yes' is at an increased risk of mortality over the next 4 years. If the older patient weighs less than 100 lb (45 kg), mortality, driven by underlying medical or psychiatric problems, rises significantly. Answering 'yes' to the single question or a weight less than 100 lb requires further investigation. Other possible indicators of malnutrition are a body mass index $< 22 \text{ kg/m}^2$ or $> 30 \text{ kg/m}^2$.

Approximately 75% of all cases of dangerous weight loss are linked to disease, whereas the remainder are associated with difficulties in obtaining food, chewing or swallowing problems, and poor oral hygiene.

## Conclusion

Delirium, dementia, depression, polypharmacy, hearing and vision deterioration, physical performance, urinary incontinence, and malnutrition are key considerations in the initial assessment of the older patient. Functional assessment need not be time-consuming. How well an older person can perform ADL can be gauged quickly and effectively using screening tools that can be administered in the office setting. The mnemonic DEEP-IN is easy to remember, and the screens it represents are easy to administer. Integrating DEEP-IN into the initial and periodic patient assessment can help identify problems that would be missed during a routine evaluation.

# References

1. Moore AA, Siu AL. Screening for common problems in ambulatory elderly: clinical confirmation of a screening instrument. *Am J Med* 1996;100:438–43

2. Ruben D. Principles of geriatric assessment. In Hazzard WR, *et al.* eds. *Principles of Geriatric Medicine and Gerontology*, 4th edn. New York: McGraw-Hill, 1999:467–81

3. Sherman FT. Functional assessment: easy-to-use screening tools speed initial office work-up. *Geriatrics* 2001;56:36–40

4. Inouye SK, van Dyck CH, Alessi CA, *et al.* Clarifying confusion: the confusion assessment method. A new method for detection of delirium. *Ann Intern Med* 1990;113:941–8

5. Levkoff SE, Evans DA, Liptzin B, *et al.* Delirium: the occurrence and persistence of symptoms among elderly hospitalized patients. *Arch Intern Med* 1992;152:334–40

6. Siu AL. Screening for dementia and investigating its causes. *Ann Intern Med* 1991;115:122–32

7. Morris JC, Heyman A, Mohs RC, *et al.* The Consortium to Establish a Registry for Alzheimer's Disease (CERAD). Part I. Clinical and neuropsychological assessment of Alzheimer's disease. *Neurology* 1989;39:1159–65

8. Watson YI, Arfken CL, Birge SJ. Clock completion: an objective screening test for dementia. *J Am Geriatr Soc* 1993;41:1235–40

9. Barberger-Gateau P, Dartigues JF, Letenneur L. Four Instrumental Activities of Daily Living Score as a predictor of one-year incident dementia. *Age Ageing* 1993;22:457–63

10. Solomon PR, Hirschoff A, Kelly B, *et al.* A 7-minute neurocognitive screening battery highly sensitive to Alzheimer's disease. *Arch Neurol* 1998;55:349–55

11. Hoyl MT, Alessi CA, Harker JO, *et al.* Development and testing of a five-item version of the Geriatric Depression Scale. *J Am Geriatr Soc* 1999;47:873–8

12. Gill TM, Richardson ED, Tinetti ME. Evaluating the risk of dependence in activities of daily living among community-living older adults with mild to moderate cognitive impairment. *J Gerontol A Biol Sci Med Sci* 1995;50:M235–41

13. Perell KL, Nelson A, Goldman RL, *et al.* Fall risk assessment measures: an analytic review. *J Gerontol Med Sci* 2001;56A:M761–6

14. Podsadlo D, Richardson S. The timed 'UP and Go': a test of basic functional mobility for frail elderly person. *J Am Geriatr Soc* 1991;39:142

15. Shumway-Cook A, Brauer S, Woollacott MH. Predicting the probability for falls in community-dwelling older adults using the timed up and go test. *Phys Ther* 2000;80:896–903

16. Duncan PW, Wiener DK, Chandler J, Studentski S. Functional reach: a new clinical measure of balance. *J Gerontol Med Sci* 1990;45A:M192–7

17. Ouslander J. Urinary incontinence. In Osterweil D, Brummel-Smith K, Beck JC, eds. *Comprehensive Geriatric Assessment*. New York: McGraw-Hill, 2000:555–72

# 10

# Therapies of the geripause: hormone replacement and modifications

*Bernard A. Eskin*

## Objectives

The objectives of this chapter are to present specific knowledge of how treatment for geripausal women may differ from that given to younger patients. The basic concepts of the pharmacology of gerontology are knowledgeably presented in Chapter 4. While aging is not gender-driven, this chapter pertains to what therapeutic challenges are specific for women who are postmenopausal and entering the geripausal period of life. In males, there is no evident reproductive change in the early fifties age group. However, in women cessation of reproduction and loss of an effective steroid (estrogen), has major general and specific effects on growth, development, metabolism, and quality of health. By the geripause, a woman has been without estrogen for at least a decade and gender differences may not be as contrasting.

This chapter concerns the more specific therapies for the woman in postmenopause/geripause that relate to her age. These medications, and the replacement hormones that are appropriate and useful, are discussed.

## General therapeutics

General medical therapies for the geripausal woman have not been remarkably modified from those given to younger patients. The therapeutic requirements for the increasing cardiac, pulmonary, gastrointestinal, and neurological diseases that occur are being carefully re-assessed by many gerontologists, who have preferred until recently to undertreat those over 65 years of age[1,2]. There was the belief that older patients required a lower dose than younger patients for many conditions. This concept, which has been acceptable for a majority of therapies, is certainly not universal. Undertreatment, which has been casually used, has resulted in serious chronicity and complications[3]. Outdated life charts have been employed which have resulted in improper expectations for the patient and, often, might have caused the physician to use low and inadequate dose levels[4].

Evaluating specific changes in therapy in general medicine for the present gerontological patient is beyond the scope of this textbook. However, several of the contributors describe treatments to which they adhere and special methods used in the elderly for various complaints.

## Inappropriate medical use

There has been growing evidence that some medications are not effective for the geripausal patient and actually may be a health hazard[5]. Inappropriate medication use is a major patient safety concern, especially in the elderly population[6-9]. Many researchers have documented widespread unacceptable medication use by elderly persons in hospitals[10], nursing homes[11-13], board and care facilities[14], physician office practices[15,16], hospital out-patient departments[17], and homebound elderly[18], with the estimated prevalence of potentially

**Table 1** Estimates by an expert panel of potentially inappropriate medication use in the United States by generic name. Reproduced from US Food and Drug Administration. *Guidelines for the Study of Drugs Likely to be Used in the Elderly*. Rockville, USA: Food and Drug Administration Center for Drug Evaluation and Research, 1999[4]

| *Always avoid* | *Rarely appropriate* | *Some indications* |
|---|---|---|
| Barbiturates* | Chlordiazepoxide | Amitriptyline |
| Flurazepam | Diazepam | Doxepin |
| Meprobamate | Propoxyphene | Indomethacin |
| Chlorpropamide | Carisoprodol | Dipyridamole |
| Meperidine | Chlorzoxazone | Ticlopidine |
| Pentazocine | Cyclobenzaprine | Methyldopa |
| Trimethobenzamide | Metaxalone | Reserpine |
| Belladonna alkaloids | Methocarbamol | Disopyramide |
| Dicyclomine | | Oxybutynin |
| Hyoscyamine | | Chlorpheniramine |
| Propantheline | | Cyproheptadine |
| | | Diphenhydramine |
| | | Hydroxyzine |
| | | Promethazine |

*Includes butabarbital, secobarbital, and pentobarbital

improper use ranging from 12 to 40%. Two studies have examined inappropriate medication use in the community-dwelling elderly using population-based nationally representative surveys. Using the National Medical Expenditure Survey (NMES), Willcox and co-workers[19] estimated that 23.5% of the community-dwelling elderly in the USA (6.64 million people) used at least one of 20 inappropriate medications in 1987. Using the Medicare Current Beneficiary Survey (MCBS), the General Accounting Office[20] estimated that 17.5% (5.2 million) of the community-dwelling elderly used at least one of the same 20 inappropriate medications in 1992. At this time, many unacceptable treatments for the elderly exist[5].

Most studies of inappropriate medication use on elderly patients, including the two nationally representative studies, use explicit criteria developed in 1991 by Beers and colleagues[21] for nursing home patients. Although generally accepted by the medical community[7] and expert opinion, the Beers criteria continue to be questioned. The explicit criteria expressed cannot completely capture all factors that define appropriate prescription decision making[22]. Some drugs on the Beers criteria

may be justified in the given circumstance because the benefits outweigh the risk for a specific patient. Beers[23] agreed that there are limitations to both the sensitivity and specificity of the criteria presented; however, these criteria may be considered a screening test for assessing inappropriate use.

The available national estimates from the most recent Medical Expenditure Panel Survey-1996 (MEPS) of potentially inappropriate medication use among the community-dwelling elderly populations have been reported[5]. These estimates use updated criteria specifically designed to be applied to community-dwelling individuals[18]. Because of ongoing controversy surrounding the Beers criteria[17], a panel was convened with expertise in geriatrics, pharmacoepidemiology, and pharmacy to identify a subset of these drugs that should be avoided. The panel was instructed to identify any clinical indications for use of the listed drugs as of 1996. In comparing previously published findings with their own data, they examined trends over a 10-year period. Only those factors that could be associated with inappropriate medication use among elderly patients were considered. Most of the products that were selected by these expert panels are relevant of general gerontological and medical practices, as noted in Table 1[5]. Although some hormonal therapies are included in this report[24], details of hormone replacement therapies more appropriate for postmenopausal and geripausal women will be presented in this chapter.

## Replacement therapies

Replacement therapies are given as substitutes for biological or hormonal secretions that are reduced or lost during the aging process. A deficiency or inadequacy may result from the loss and eventually cause an abnormality or disease process.

Many replacement therapies are available for the elderly. The most evident are those needed for hormone deficiencies (e.g. insulin, thyroid, etc.). These occur through either aging or reduction of secretion from the atrophy of the endocrine glands. If tissue and cellular growth continue, there is often a reduction in the effectiveness of many secretions shown by decreased metabolic function. This is often caused by decreased receptor availability or response at the target organs. Additionally, some endocrine gland stimulators develop a reduced rate of effectiveness because of receptor loss at the endocrine cells. This requires enhancement by exogenous replacement.

Supplements, such as vitamins, elements and macronutrients have been used to replace or maintain tissue with recommended dietary allowances established by medical and governmental agencies. Specific US recommendations made for vitamin and mineral replacement are presented in Table 2. A popular source of desired food intake is described in the 'food pyramid' (Figure 1), showing the daily dietary requirements suggested by the United States government (USDA).

## General hormone replacement treatment

The most effective replacement therapies (see Chapter 3) have been those related to hormone loss from the thyroid, adrenal, pancreas (insulin), and pituitary. These have been briefly discussed. Correlating the endocrine diagnoses and dose–response results becomes particularly important in the aging patient since the highest proportion of hormonal deficiency diseases occur in senior patients. Basically these conditions are easier to treat in the older individual; however, there is an increase in other medical problems in the elderly that require attention to be certain that they are not complicated by the replacement treatment.

Since this textbook is particularly directed to women in the postmenopause and geripause, the present use of sex hormone replacement therapies and the large, sometimes ambiguous, literature that has accumulated will be emphasized. Geripausal women are being studied primarily for continuation of therapy. A realignment of dose responses specifically for this age group is actively in progress.

## Sex hormone replacement therapy

By the time a women enters the geripause she has been well initiated into the many problems that a decreasing estrogen level can cause. In the premenopause (see Figure 2, Chapter 3) these problems have included dysfunctional uterine bleeding with cyclic uterine cramps and depression. Hot flushes or vascular instability, generally considered a hypothalamic effect, may begin in the thirties, but may be reduced or completely gone by 65. Osteoporosis or osteopenia is usually monitored by dual-energy X-ray absorptiometry (DEXA)[26,27] and/or other examinations during the postmenopause. Atrophic vulvovaginitis and severe dryness of the perineum may become uncomfortable with itching and burning or sexual pain (dyspareunia) when the woman reaches late postmenopause[28,29]. Reduced cognition is the first sign of neurological change and becomes evident during early premenopause. However, later in the perimenopause the loss becomes consistent and relentless through postmenopause and geripause[30,31].

In most cases, general menopausal symptoms due to reduced estrogen are inseparable from those seen in aging. Many women have discussed initial interest and decisions concerning

**Table 2** Dietary reference intakes for older adults (compiled by the National Policy and Resource Center on Nutrition and Aging, Florida International University; revised 18 December 2001. Values excerpted with permission from Institute of Medicine. *Dietary Reference Intakes: Applications in Dietary Assessment*, 2000[25])

*Vitamins and elements*

| | Vitamin A (μg)[b,c] | Vitamin C (mg) | Vitamin D (μg)[d,e] | Vitamin E (mg)[f,g,h] | Vitamin K (μg) | Thiamin (mg) | Riboflavin (mg) | Niacin (mg)[h,i] | Vitamin B₆ (mg) | Folate (μg)[h,i] |
|---|---|---|---|---|---|---|---|---|---|---|
| **RDA or AI\*** | | | | | | | | | | |
| *Age 51–70* | | | | | | | | | | |
| Male | 900 | 90 | 10* | 15 | 120* | 1.2 | 1.3 | 16 | 1.7 | 400 |
| Female | 700 | 75 | 10* | 15 | 90* | 1.1 | 1.1 | 14 | 1.5 | 400 |
| *Age 70+* | | | | | | | | | | |
| Male | 900 | 90 | 15* | 15 | 120* | 1.2 | 1.3 | 16 | 1.7 | 400 |
| Female | 700 | 75 | 15* | 15 | 90* | 1.1 | 1.1 | 14 | 1.5 | 400 |
| *Tolerable upper intake levels (UL)[a]* | | | | | | | | | | |
| *Age 51–70* | | | | | | | | | | |
| Male | 3000 | 2000 | 50 | 1000 | ND | ND | ND | 35 | 100 | 1000 |
| Female | 3000 | 2000 | 50 | 1000 | ND | ND | ND | 35 | 100 | 1000 |
| *Age 70+* | | | | | | | | | | |
| Male | 3000 | 2000 | 50 | 1000 | ND | ND | ND | 35 | 100 | 1000 |
| Female | 3000 | 2000 | 50 | 1000 | ND | ND | ND | 35 | 100 | 1000 |

| | Vitamin B₁₂ (μg)[k] | Pantothenic acid (mg) | Biotin (μg) | Choline (mg)[l] | Boron (mg) | Calcium (mg) | Chromium (μg) | Copper (μg) | Fluoride (mg) | Lodine (μg) |
|---|---|---|---|---|---|---|---|---|---|---|
| **RDA or AI\*** | | | | | | | | | | |
| *Age 51–70* | | | | | | | | | | |
| Male | 2.4 | 5* | 30* | 550* | ND | 1200* | 30* | 900 | 4* | 150 |
| Female | 2.4 | 5* | 30* | 425* | ND | 1200* | 30* | 900 | 3* | 150 |
| *Age 70+* | | | | | | | | | | |
| Male | 2.4 | 5* | 30* | 550* | ND | 1200* | 30* | 900 | 4* | 150 |
| Female | 2.4 | 5* | 30* | 425* | ND | 1200* | 30* | 900 | 3* | 150 |

*(Continued)*

**Table 2** Continued

| | Vitamin B$_{12}$ (µg)[k] | Pantothenic acid (mg) | Biotin (µg) | Choline (mg)[l] | Calcium (mg) | Boron (mg) | Chromium (µg) | Copper (µg) | Fluoride (mg) | Iodine (µg) |
|---|---|---|---|---|---|---|---|---|---|---|
| *Tolerable upper intake levels** | | | | | | | | | | |
| Age 51–70 | | | | | | | | | | |
| Male | ND | ND | ND | 3500 | 2500 | 20 | ND | 10000 | 10 | 1100 |
| Female | ND | ND | ND | 3500 | 2500 | 20 | ND | 10000 | 10 | 1100 |
| Age 70+ | | | | | | | | | | |
| Male | ND | ND | ND | 3500 | 2500 | 20 | ND | 10000 | 10 | 1100 |
| Female | ND | ND | ND | 3500 | 2500 | 20 | ND | 10000 | 10 | 1100 |

*Elements and macronutrients*

| | Iron (mg) | Magnesium (mg)[m] | Manganese (mg) | Molybdenum (mg) | Nickel (mg) | Phosphorus (mg) | Selenium (µg) | Vanadium (mg)[n] | Zinc (mg)[n] |
|---|---|---|---|---|---|---|---|---|---|
| *RDA or AI** | | | | | | | | | |
| Age 51–70 | | | | | | | | | |
| Male | 8 | 420 | 2.3* | 45 | ND | 700 | 55 | ND | 11 |
| Female | 8 | 320 | 1.8* | 45 | ND | 700 | 55 | ND | 8 |
| Age 70+ | | | | | | | | | |
| Male | 8 | 420 | 2.3* | 45 | ND | 700 | 55 | ND | 11 |
| Female | 8 | 320 | 1.8* | 45 | ND | 700 | 55 | ND | 8 |
| *Tolerable upper intake levels (UL)* | | | | | | | | | |
| Age 51–70 | | | | | | | | | |
| Male | 45 | 350 | 11 | 2000 | 1 | 4000 | 400 | 1.8 | 40 |
| Female | 45 | 350 | 11 | 2000 | 1 | 4000 | 400 | 1.8 | 40 |
| Age 70+ | | | | | | | | | |
| Male | 45 | 350 | 11 | 2000 | 1 | 3000 | 400 | 1.8 | 40 |
| Female | 45 | 350 | 11 | 2000 | 1 | 3000 | 400 | 1.8 | 40 |

(Continued)

**Table 2** Continued

| | Energy (Kcal) | Protein (g) | Carbohy-drates² | Total fat² | Saturated fat² | Cholesterol (mg) | Sodium (mg) | Fiber (g)³ |
|---|---|---|---|---|---|---|---|---|
| *1989 RDAs for age 51+* | | | | | | | | |
| Male | 2300 | 63 | >55% | <30% | <10% | <300 | <2400 | 20–35 |
| Female | 1900 | 50 | >55% | <30% | <10% | <300 | <2400 | 20–35 |
| | | | | | | per day | per day | per day |

[1]The 1989 RDAs are used as no new Dietary Reference Intakes have been established for energy and protein, and other macronutrients

[2]The Food and Nutrition Board's Committee on Diet and Health recommendations base intake on the per cent of total calories in the diet (NCR, 1989)

[3]The National Cancer Institute and American Dietetic Association recommend 20–35 g dietary fiber daily (ADA, 1997)

ND, values not determined. This table (taken from the DRI reports, see www.nap.edu) presents the recommended dietary allowances (RDAs) in bold type and adequate intakes (AIs) in ordinary type followd by an asterisk (*). RDAs and AIs may both be used as goals for individual intake. RDAs are set to meet the needs of almost all (97–98%) individuals in a group. The AI for life stage and gender groups (other than healthy, breast-fed infants) is believed to cover needs of all individuals in the group, but lack of data or uncertainty in the data prevent being able to specify with confidence the percentage of individuals covered by this intake

[a]UL = The maximum level of daily nutrient intake that is likely to pose no risk of adverse effects. Unless otherwise especified, the UL represents total intake from food, water, and supplements. Owing to lack of suitable data, ULs could not be established for vitamin K, thiamin, riboflavin, vitamin B₁₂, pantothenic acid, biotin, or carotenoids. In the absence of ULs, extra caution may be warranted in consuming levels above recommended intakes

[b]As retinal activity equivalents (RAEs). 1 RAE =1 µg retinal, 12 µg β-carotene, or 24 µg β-cryptoxanthin. To calculate RAEs from the REs of provitamin A carotenoids in foods, divide the REs by 2. For performed vitamin A in foods or supplements and for provitamin A carotenoids in supplements, 1 RE = 1 RAE

[c]ULs – As preformed vitamin A only

[d]cholecalciferol. 1 µg cholecalciferol = 40 IU vitamin D

[e]In the absence of adequate exposure to sunlight

[f]as alpha-tocopherol. Alpha-tocopherol includes RRR-alpha-tocopherol, the only form of alpha-tocopherol that occurs naturally in foods, and the 2R-steroisomeric forms of alpha-tocopherol (RRR-, RSR-, RRS-, and RSS-alpha-tocopherol) that occur in fortified foods and supplements. It does not include the 2S-stereoisomeric forms of alpha-tocopherol (SRR-, SSR-, SRS-, SSS-alpha-tocopherol), also found in fortified foods and supplements

[g]ULs – as alpha-tocopherol; applies to any form of supplemental alpha-tocopherol

[h]The ULs for vitamin E, niacin, and folate apply to synthetic forms obtained from supplements, fortified foods, or a combination of the two

[i]As niacin equivalents (NE). 1 mg of niacin = 60 mg of tryptophan: 0–6 months = performed niacin (not NE)

[j]As dietary folate equivalents (DFE). 1 DFE = 1 µg food folate = 0.6 µg of folic acid from fortified food ar as a supplement consumed with food = 0.5 µg of a supplement taken on an empty stomach

[k]Because 10–30% of older people may malabsorb food-bound B₁₂, it is advisable for those older than 50 years to meet their RDA mainly by consuming foods fortified with B₁₂ or a supplemrnt containing B₁₂

[l]Although Als have been set for choline, there are few data to assess whether a dietary supply of choline is needed at all stages of the life cycle, and it may be that the choline requirment can be met by endogenous synthesis at some of these stages

[m]The ULs for magnesium represent intake from a pharmacological agent only and do not include intake from food and water

[n]Although vanadium in food has not been shown to cause adverse effects in humans, there is no justification for adding vanadium to food and vanadium supplements should be used with caution. The UL is based on adverse effects in laboratory animals and these data could be used to set a UL for adults but not children or adolescents

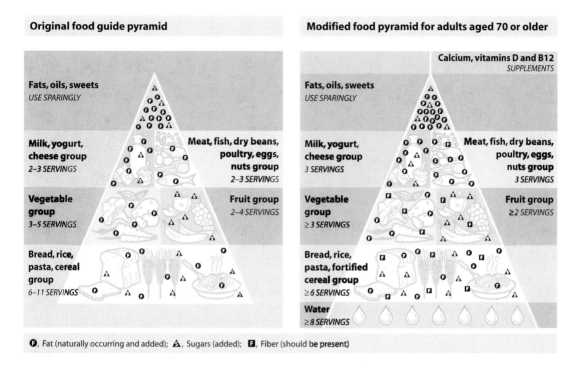

**Figure 1**  The pyramid scheme for geripausal women

the use of estrogen replacement therapy (ERT) while undergoing these transitions. Initially, treatment with estrogen (ERT) or combined sex hormones (hormone replacement therapy; HRT) in a given population may be as high as 40%; however, those continuing estrogen replacement may be reduced to less than 15% by the onset of geripause[32]. Either complications or side-effects reduce the numbers; while other patients are satisfied with other treatments or deny the importance of the symptoms that they are having. Therefore, each woman singularly tries to maintain her own level of expectation.

As previously described throughout this textbook, the medical need for any therapy during geripause differs with the intensity of the symptoms. Most relevant are those concerning the skin, breast and perineal atrophy, bone loss leading to frailty, neurological

deficits, and cognitive failures. Decisions concerning treatment must be made on the basis of effectiveness as opposed to undesirable complications. Recent modifications have been made concerning the dosage and delivery of the hormones used[33]. More specific tissue responses have been noted with certain combinations and pharmaceuticals. Alternative medications have becomes available and may be suitable for some.

## Estrogen physiology

Estradiol ($E_2$), estrone ($E_1$) and estriol ($E_3$) are the only three natural estrogens present in significant quantities in the human female. The action of estrogens is measured by the level of receptor responses on the $\alpha$ estrogen receptor. Estradiol is the most potent, naturally occurring ovarian and placental estrogen in humans; estrone is an oxidation product of estradiol; and estriol (much weaker) is produced by hydroxylation of estrogen and primarily identified with pregnancy. Comparing these basic steroids: estradiol is three to four times more chemically active than estrone and estriol. The biological estrogenic potency of estradiol is about 12 times that of estrone and 80 times that of estriol.

In the postmenopause, estrogen continues to be produced in peripheral tissue by chemical transformation of androgens, while meager progesterone release occurs. As presented in Table 3, estrogen decreases gradually during the perimenopause, but then rapidly decreases in the postmenopause. Significant changes in the gonadotropins are evident, with follicle stimulating hormone (FSH) persistently high throughout the early postmenopause and decreasing with the onset of geripause. Luteinizing hormone (LH) remains moderately elevated after FSH has risen, but never reaches the elevations seen during the ovulatory surge in reproductive women. LH also decreases after geripause. This drop in both gonadotropins symbolizes and defines the changes of phase. The full endocrine significance of these reductions remains unknown. They may represent a failing or aging hypophyseal–pituitary axis, as described in basic neuroendocrine research[34].

Therefore, the use of estrogen replacement during postmenopause/geripause requires further analysis. A need for use of estrogen for reproduction after 50 years of age seems redundant since these inactive ovaries would not produce the required functional ova. However, the presence of active estrogen receptors in many target organs throughout the body appears to make the total loss of estrogen seem premature[35]. Whether this loss of estrogen is protective or prematurely destructive in women remains a point for conjecture.

The loss of menses is considered by many as a measure of aging in women. Menopause is considered as the termination of reproduction and not related to the general aging process. Geriatric aging is similar in men and women with no advantage evident to men. Since estrogen is the prime sex steroid that is deficient, the

**Table 3** Average estrogen levels from transition (data approximate; averaged from multiple laboratory sources)

| Life stage (years) | Average estrogen levels (pg/ml) |
| --- | --- |
| 36–42 | 30–600 pg/ml* |
| 42–52 | 0–200 pg/ml |
| 52–65 | < 20 pg/ml |
| > 65 | < 10 pg/ml |

*Dependent on ovulatory activity

questions remain: 'What effect does this loss have on women postmenopausally and into the geripause?' and 'What evidence is there that replacement of the estrogen delays the aging process?'

## Estrogen replacement therapy or hormone replacement therapy?

In the late 1960s, replacement treatment with the available oral estrogen compounds alone was considered a boon to the menopausal woman. These consisted of conjugated estrogens (equine or synthetic) and estradiol (ethinyl, esterified, estropipate, or valerate). While investigations of long-term use were not available, the products were placed on the market and extremely successful. Within ten years, it was evident that the morbidity for endometrial pathology – both hyperplasia and carcinoma – rose significantly in women taking the estrogen replacement. Even at restricted and lowered doses, the endometrial abnormalities persisted. The major benefits noted while taking estrogen were reductions in hot flushes and increased turgidity of the vulva and vaginal tissues. Other health advantages were suggested from short-term trials and recorded patient trends. However, the evidence from endometrial abnormalities was compelling and popularity of this estrogen alone treatment in women with uteri was severely diminished. Eventually this therapy was generally discontinued after 1976.

Shortly thereafter, a series of clinical trials began that utilized 'cyclic' therapy and consisted of estrogen on a monthly basis with oral progestins added during the second half of a projected 28-day 'cycle'[24]. Progestins are steroids derived synthetically from androgens that have biological effects similar to progesterone; oral progesterone was not available. Initially this was suggested to all menopausal patients, presumably to reduce breast abnormalities. Surprisingly, breast disease was not a significant factor when estrogen was given alone. For that reason, this combination of estrogen and progestin (HRT) was given only to those women who had uteri as a protection against endometrial hyperplasia or carcinoma; and estrogen alone (ERT) was recommended for women who had undergone hysterectomies.

During the early 1990s, estrogen and progesterone were available together continuously as well as cyclically. Throughout these years since the re-establishment of HRT, either cyclically or continuously, there have been re-evaluations of these dosing factors. No conclusive differences in clinical results were recognized comparing these methods of treatment. Nevertheless, several product studies showed that HRT seemed to result in a higher breast cancer risk than ERT alone. The recent studies using continuous HRT compared with ERT clearly indicate this fact and have resulted in the discontinuation of one arm of a long-term study, the Women's Health Initiative (WHI), but only for the continuous HRT. The study with women on ERT, who are without uteri, continues.

It appears from clinical trials and several basic research studies that ERT is capable of improving certain cardiac conditions and profiles. This was initially considered to be due to improved cholesterol status, but appears to be due mainly to other mechanisms related to cardiovascular function (Chapter 12). Additionally, bone demineralization has been carefully evaluated and the positive effect of estrogen in preventing osteopenia and osteoporosis has been validated (Chapter 13). However, beyond these results, consideration of menopausal–geripausal women on estrogen replacement becomes seriously complex and time-related.

## Key benefits of hormone replacement therapy: known and conditional

Numerous commercially available estrogen replacement agents have achieved United States regulatory approval, based on scientific evidence (Table 4), and are indicated for alleviation of vasomotor dysfunctions (hot flushes)[28], improvement of genital atrophy[24], and prevention of bone demineralization[27,36,37]. However these statistical findings were obtained in short-term clinical trials, where hormone replacement was given to patients to prevent or treat those symptoms. There are side-effects, contraindications and complications for these drug therapies. There may be additional potential risks associated with estrogen replacement, including thrombolism[38–40], endometrial cancer[41], breast cancer[42–44], and ovarian cancer[45].

Particularly difficult to assess is the effect of HRT/ERT on breast cancer. Since the incidence of breast cancer increases with age in all women, evaluation of the effects with hormone therapies require careful statistical review[46]. Recent studies have shown dose–response evidence that lower doses reduced breast disease. Additionally, the use of estrogen–progestin combinations appears to increase the risk beyond that seen with estrogen alone[47].

A series of new long-term trials have begun and are continuing which are aimed to provide definitive characterization of the desirable action and the level of complications for HRT and ERT. These trials are HERS (Heart and Estrogen Replacement Study)[48], ERA (Estrogen Replacement and Arteriosclerosis)[49], and the WHI[50]. Those results that have been either presented or published to date have produced findings concerning long-term cardioprotective effects with replacement therapy. Both ERA and HERS deal with the response to already existing heart disease and provide some consistent evidence of a prophylactic effect for coronary heart disease if the patient has been on an acceptable dosage of HRT for more than 2, but no longer than 5, years.

Unproven general benefits of hormone replacement (Table 4) derived from trials

**Table 4** Key benefits of hormone replacement therapy: known and conditional

*Known*
1. Improves osteopenia/osteoporosis
2. Improves central nervous system function
3. Reduces genitourinary atrophy
4. Decreases hot flushes

*Unknown*
1. Reduces cardiovascular disease risk
2. Reduces colon cancer risk
3. Controls psychiatric illnesses
4. Improves lipoprotein profile
5. Improves sleep disturbances
6. Reduces tooth loss
7. Reduces age-related macular degeneration
8. Lessens Alzheimer's disease
9. Reduces cataracts

Order given of importance to geripausal women

include improved cognitive function[51–54], protection against colorectal cancer[55] and cardiovascular diseases[56], lessening of psychiatric illnesses (including Alzheimer's disease)[57], improvement of lipoprotein profile, and protection against cataracts[58]. These findings show that the relative risk for the diseases stated is reduced in the various clinical trials that were used. They have not yet been considered to be clinically proven and remain only tentative.

## Pharmacologic replacement options

There is no single, ideal, standard therapeutic regimen for hormone replacement throughout the menopausal transition. In addition, there are a variety of estrogen or estrogen and progestin compounds available that may be used as a single agent or in combination, at various dose levels, and administered by various routes (oral, transdermal, and vaginal). Commonly used and commercially available estrogen agents are listed in Table 5, which is a sampling of the many pharmaceutical products available on the market. Table 6 provides a number of the alternative medications and suggested therapies that can be purchased by the patient. There has been some difficulty in terminology for describing 'natural' estrogen from plant or animal sources. Most pharmacologists consider 'natural' estrogens as those that are produced endogenously. The final usefulness of an estrogen preparation is generally considered to be based on its biological effectiveness.

In singling out the postmenopausal/geripausal woman, a serious matter is the dose of the hormone that is given[14]. Several reviews present the problems involved as the woman ages. Particularly appealing is the reduction in incidence of thromboses, breast tenderness and dysfunctional uterine bleeding that it allows with minimal therapy[14,33,59,60]. As a woman goes through the postmenopause and geripause, the incidence of chronic diseases such as diabetes, cardiovascular disease, and neurological problems, increases. Therefore, the patient can be given the lowest dose that specifically improves her menopausal problem. The use of low replacement-hormones would diminish any undesirable effect. This availability of useful dose levels is an asset.

A considerable amount of time and effort has been spent studying single product evidence for many of the symptoms. Generally most of the medications used have relatively similar effects, although they may vary according to dosage and delivery system. Clinicians choose doses that accommodate the needs of the individual postmenopausal or geripausal woman according to the standards such as height and weight (body mass index, BMI) or dose–response expectations. It is most gratifying that many varied doses of the medications are now available for the prescribing physician. Treatment should be limited to the needs of the patient and, since there are many dosage variations, therapy can be further adjusted for the patient according to the endpoint desired.

The use of combination estrogen and progestogen therapies is generally required for those women who still have a uterus (with or without adnexae), since abnormal endometrial responses may occur, even after several years of atrophy. Hyperplasia or adenosis of the endometrial cells is often seen with irregular bleeding or shedding. This was particularly evident when unopposed estrogen was given. Cyclic or combination medications prevent

**Table 5** Hormone replacement/osteoporosis therapies

| Brand | Compound | Dose |
|---|---|---|
| *Hormone replacement – transdermal system* | | |
| Alora | estradiol | 0.05 mg/24 hours twice a week |
| Esclim | | |
| Estraderm | | |
| Vivelle | | |
| Vivelle-DOT | | 0.0375 mg/24 hours twice a week |
| | | 0.05 mg/24 hours twice a week |
| | | 0.075 mg/24 hours twice a week |
| | | 0.1 mg/24 hours twice a week |
| Climara | | 0.025 mg/24 hours once a week |
| | | 0.05 mg/24 hours once a week |
| | | 0.075 mg/24 hours once a week |
| | | 0.1 mg/24 hours once a week |
| Combipatch | estradiol | 0.05 mg 0.14 mg/24 hours twice a week |
| | norethindrone | 0.05 mg 0.25 mg /24 hours twice a week |
| | | |
| *Oral therapy/estrogen – cyclic* | | |
| Cenestin | synthetic conjugated estrogens A | 0.625 mg daily |
| | | 1.25 mg daily |
| Estinyl | ethinyl estradiol | 0.02 mg daily |
| | | 0.05 mg daily |
| Estrace | estradiol | 1 mg daily |
| | | 2 mg daily |
| Estratab | esterified estrogens | 0.625 mg daily |
| Ogen | estropipate | 0.625 mg daily |
| Ortho-Est | | 1.25 mg daily |
| Premarin | conjugated estrogens | 0.625 mg daily |
| | | 1.25 mg daily |
| | | |
| *Progestins – cyclic* | | |
| Prometrium | progesterone | 200 mg at bedtime, 12-day for cycle |
| Provera | medroxyprogesterone | 2.5 mg daily |
| | | 5 mg daily |
| | | 10 mg daily |
| *Oral combination products* | | |
| Activella | estradiol | 1 mg/0.5 mg daily |
| | norethindrone | |
| Estratest | esterified estrogens | 1.25 mg/2.5 mg daily |
| Estratest H.S. | methyltestosterone | 0.625 mg/1.25 mg daily |
| FemHRT 1/5 | norethindrone | 1 mg/5 µg daily |
| | ethinyl estradiol | |
| Ortho-Prefest | estradiol | 1 mg/0 mg daily for 3 days, alternating |
| | norgestimate | 1 mg/0.09 mg daily for 3 days |
| Premphase (Cyclic) | conjugated estrogens | 0.625 mg/0 mg daily for 14 days |
| | medroxyprogesterone | 0.625 mg/5 mg daily for 14 days |
| Prempro (Continuous) | conjugated estrogens | 0.625 mg/2.5 mg daily |
| | medroxyprogesterone | 0.625 mg/5 mg daily |
| | | |
| *Vaginal estrogens* | | |
| Estrace | estradiol 0.1 mg/g | 1 g 1–3 times a week |
| Ogen | estropipate 1.5 mg/g | 1 g 1–3 times a week |
| Premarin (vaginal) | conjugated estrogens 0.625 mg/g | 1 g 1–3 times a week |

*(Continued)*

**Table 5** Continued

| Brand | Compound | Dose |
|---|---|---|
| Estring | estradiol 0.0075 mg/24 hours | 1 ring every 3 months |
| Vagifem | estradiol | 0.025 mg/tablet, 1 tablet vaginally twice a week |
| *Osteoporosis therapy/prevention* | | |
| Actonel | risedronate | 5 mg daily |
| Evista | raloxifene | 60 mg daily |
| Fosamax | alendronate | 5 mg daily |
| | | 10 mg daily |
| | | 35 mg once a week |
| | | 70 mg once a week |
| Miacalcin | calcitonin – salmon | 100 IU subcutaneously or intramuscularly daily |
| | | 200 IU nasally daily |
| Citracal + D | calcium citrate vitamin D | 5 tablets daily |
| Oscal 500 + D | calcium carbonate vitamin D | 3 tablets daily |

**Table 6** Alternative menopausal medications

*Creams, gels*
Pro-Gest® (progesterone cream)
Phytoestrogen cream (isoflavones in gel base)

*Oral medications*
Phytoestrogens (generic)
  isoflavones
    genistein
    biochanin
    daidzein
    formononetin
Promensil

*Botanicals*
  St John's wort
  black cohosh
  *Ginkgo biloba*
  ginseng
  chasteberry (monk's pepper)
  evening primorse
  dong quai
  valerian root

these changes and the endometrial carcinoma rate in women on HRT is below that in untreated controls[16].

The use of testosterone 'replacement' still remains difficult to accept. Recent journal articles on sexuality have indicated increased desire and satisfaction[52]. However, side-effects for androgens remain the same: i.e. masculinizng changes in skin, hair, and occasionally the vulvar area. Androgens as metabolic steroids may increase musculoskeletal hyperactivity and tone, a factor not fully understood in aging and under investigation for the elderly woman. Sexuality and the use of replacement hormones is discussed in Chapter 6.

## Delivery systems

The delivery systems used are of prime importance. Often, delivery techniques have been varied to provide an improvement in personal convenience. Oral medications can be given singly or in a combination daily regimen with elimination of monthly bleeding. New patches have an extended effective life of 1–2 weeks and some contain both estrogen and progesterone simultaneously, thus eliminating cyclic therapy. Vaginal rings and body creams/gels/oils containing adequate therapeutic levels have become available. Long-acting rings are placed in the vagina and provide timed sex steroid replacement therapy. Each of these methods may permit a desirable effect with therapeutic efficiency.

There has been evidence that women taking oral HRT/ERT may experience a greater risk of gallbladder disease than seen with patches. This statistical reduction seen with patches is probably due to the reduction in concentration of estrogen degradation by the liver and gallbladder during initial venous bypass after absorption.

## Alternative medications in the menopause

Many alternative medications have been suggested medically and by health advocates for postmenopausal and geripausal women, particularly for those with specific symptoms that may be related to sex hormone loss. A short list of the natural therapies that are taken appears in Table 6. Often patients who may not be candidates for HRT or selective estrogen receptor modulators (SERM) therapy will seek relief using alternative medications, which may be herbal or plant-derived. These forms may also carry contraindications or side-effects, which need to be explained to the woman.

The isoflavones as well as certain phyto-estrogens have been utilized with some success[55]. The botanicals (herbs) may show severe side-effects and need careful patient directions and dosage adjustment. In most cases, the purity of the product must be carefully investigated as well.

While not considered an alternative type of medication, several drugs are appropriately recommended for use with certain menopausal symptoms. These include effective medications for osteoporosis treatment and prevention, also listed in Table 5. Some have shown successful responses when used as indicated and even when administered in intervals for up to a year[60]. Osteoporosis and bone problems are discussed in Chapter 13.

Therapies for vascular instability (hot flushes) include some of those listed in Table 6 as well as several psychopharmaceutical products. Most women in the late menopause and geripause do not suffer hot flushes. When the symptom recurs, a medical evaluation by a neurologist is often useful. Some of the SERM medications listed have recently been shown to have a positive effect on flushes.

**Table 7** Contraindications to hormone replacement therapy

Progestogens/estrogens should not be used in individuals with any of the following conditions or circumstances:

(1) Known or suspected pregnancy, including use for missed abortion or diagnostic test for pregnancy. Progestin or estrogen may cause fetal harm when administered to a pregnant woman

(2) Known or suspected cancer of the breast

(3) Known or suspected estrogen-dependent neoplasia

(4) Undiagnosed abnormal genital bleeding

(5) Active or history of thrombophlebitis or thromboembolic disorders

(6) Known sensitivity to estrogen- and/or progestin-containing products

## The down side of replacement

Like most therapies, there are specific contraindications, side-effects, and complications when any sex hormones are administered. Table 7 and 8 list and briefly describe contraindications and complications that may be encountered. These facts must be clearly explained to the patient before treatment. Careful screening is recommended with physician office visits at least twice a year in most circumstances. When deciding upon the best care, the likelihood of complications occurring in the patient, from her history, must be weighed against the value of the treatment.

There has been described the possibility of reducing doses of both ERT and HRT while maintaining effective replacement for certain of the accepted and non-labelled uses. Most prominent is the potential of lower incidences of side-effects, mainly bleeding and breast discomfort. The benefits of these lower doses in retaining bone mineral density, favoring lipid–cholesterol metabolism, preventing dysfunctional uterine bleeding and breast pain, controlling vasomotor symptoms, and reducing vulvovaginal atrophy, are being evaluated in clinical trials.

**Table 8** Complications with hormone replacement therapy

*Induction of malignant neoplasms*
*Endometrial cancer*
The reported endometrial cancer risk among users of unopposed estrogen in about 2- to 14-fold greater than in non-users, and appears to be dependent on duration of treatment and on estrogen dose. Most studies show no significant increased risk associated with the use of estrogens for less than 1 year. The greatest risk appears to be associated with prolonged use, with increased risks of 15- to 24-fold for use of 5–10 years or more, and this risk has been shown to presist for at least 15 years after cessation of estrogen treatment.
*Breast cancer*
While the majority of studies have not shown an increased risk of breast cancer in women who have ever used estrogen replacement therapy, some have reported a moderately increased risk (relative risks of 1.3–2) in those taking higher doses or those taking lower doses for a prolonged period of time, especially in excess of 10 years. The effect of added progestins on the risk of breast cancer is unknown.

*Gallbladder disease*
A 2- to 4-fold increase in the risk of gallbladder disease requiring surgery in women receiving postmenopausal estrogen has been reported.

*Hypercalcemia*
Administration of estrogens may lead to severe hypercalcemia in patients with breast cancer and bone metastases.

*Pregnancy*
Use in pregnancy is not recommended.

*Venous thromboembolism*
Five epidemiological studies have found an increased risk of venous thromboembolism (VTE) in users of estrogen replacement therapy (ERT) who did not have predisposing conditions for VTE, such as a history of cardiovascular disease or a recent history of pregnancy, surgery, trauma, or serious illness. The increased risk was found only in current ERT users; it did not persist in former users. The risk appeared to be higher in the first year of use and decreased thereafter. The findings were similar for ERT alone or with added progestin and pertain to commonly used oral and transdermal doses, with a possible dose-dependent effect on risk. The studies found the VTE risk to be about 1 case per 10 000 women per year among women not using ERT and without predisposing conditions. The risk in current ERT users was increased to 2–3 cases per 10 000 women per year.

*Visual disturbances*
Medication should be discontinued pending examination if there is a sudden partial or complete loss of vision, or if there is a sudden onset of proptosis, diplopia or migraine. If examination reveals papilledema or retinal vascular lessions, medication should be withdrawn.

This provides an important area for specificity of symptoms. Since the menopausal problems are not universal in women, both dosage and product employed may be tailored to the need. Certainly both side-effects and complications would be reduced.

## Outcomes from the HERS II and WHI studies

As noted previously in this chapter, a series of long-term studies were started between 1993 and 1998[50,61–63]. These were large-scale placebo-controlled studies primarily concerned with the effectiveness of HRT at reducing risk of and prevention of chronic diseases in women. Primary emphasis was on cardiovascular disease, but other age-related problems such as osteoporosis, colorectal cancer, ovarian cancer, breast cancer, and hip fractures were tabulated. This trial used the most popular HRT, which consists of conjugated equine estrogens (Premarin®) and medroxyprogesterone acetate (Provera®) together in a continuous single tablet form (Prempro®) daily (see Table 5). This investigation dealt with the

**Table 9** Relative and absolute risk or benefit seen in the estrogen-plus-progestin arm of the Women's Health Initiative study ($n = 16\ 608$, placebo and study drug). Adapted with permission from Writing Group for the Women's Health Initiative Investigators. Risks and benefits of estrogen plus progestin in healthy post-menopausal women: principal results from the Women's Health Initiative randomised controlled trial. J Am Med Assoc 2002;288:321–33[62]

| Health Event | Relative risk vs. placebo group at 5.2 years | Increased absolute risk per 10 000 women/year | Increased absolute benefit per 10 000 women/year | Total number of cases |
|---|---|---|---|---|
| Heart attacks (CHD) | 1.29 | 7 | | 286 |
| Strokes | 1.41 | 8 | | 212 |
| Breast cancer | 1.26 | 8 | | 290 |
| Pulmonary embolism | 2.13 | 8 | | 101 |
| Colorectal cancer | 0.63 | | 6 | 112 |
| Hip fractures | 0.66 | | 5 | 106 |
| Endometrial cancer | 0.83 | | * | 47 |
| Death due to other causes | 0.92 | | * | 331 |

*Increased absolute benefit per 10 000 women/year – not recorded; CHD, coronary heart disease

prevention of coronary heart disease (CHD) in menopausal/geripausal women (average age 71 years) who had previously had CHD. The HERS writing group concluded that 'HRT should not be used to reduce the risk of CHD events in women with CHD'. The specificity of the experimental medications used was not included in this statement, which obviously is a major factor[61].

The WHI, a joint trial with National Institutes of Health (NIH) assistance, was initiated with the purpose to show whether this same HRT had a preventive effect in CHD on a *healthy*, somewhat younger group of menopausal/geripausal women, ranging in age from 50 to 79[62]. The WHI placebo-controlled trial in centers throughout the United States utilized both ERT (estrogen alone) and HRT for comparison, and thus permitted a determination of the effectiveness of estrogen alone on the tissues studied. After 5.2 years (mean) of treatment, the HRT series was discontinued because the overall health risks that were encountered exceeded the benefits obtained. A markedly increased invasive breast cancer rate in menopausal/geripausal women was the most salient problem. Conclusions from this research stated that HRT regimens 'should not be initiated or continued for providing prevention of CHD'. The ERT trial continues and will complete the full-term study in 2005, since no significant adverse effects were seen which would warrant termination[62].

Relative and absolute risk or benefit of the continuous combined (HRT) arm of the WHI study is presented in Table 9. These are the general results obtained after 5.2 years of the study. The data shows that the endometrial cancer risk is reduced and is actually favorable. The improvement in colorectal cancer risk over placebos is beneficial. Both of these positive factors may be useful in treatment decisions where genetic or historic vulnerability might exist. The clinical effect on bone is shown by a reduction in hip fracture risk[63].

However, these results are damaging for the use of HRT when CHD is involved. The unexpected rise in strokes and pulmonary emboli, while previously identified in the complications, may be higher in the WHI group. Whether other progestins or biological progesterone may be safer when substituted remains to be proven. Adequate trials, focused on this problem, are necessary.

## The use of estrogen in postmenopausal/geripausal women

Throughout this textbook, references have been made to the increased longevity for women found in all developed countries in the 21st century. Projections for 2010 show that a life expectancy of 81 years for women and 74 years for men is likely. However, quality of life (QoL) reports have shown that women have twice the medical abnormalities of men prior to their deaths. This accounts for major health-care utilization in older women. Post-menopausal women will reach 1.2 billion worldwide by 2030 with 47 million new menopausal women each year[50]. Thus, the geripause population grows by leaps and bounds as the years go on.

Prescription plan data reveal that 35% of women aged 40–60 are most likely to use HRT. This level declines (15%) in those older than 65 (the geripause) and falls further (7%) in women older than 80. Improving the hormone dosage given by reducing the medication to the minimum needed by the individual is a reasonable advancement. The reasons for the change in interest is fear of other potential medical problems with aging, which may further complicate the woman's life. Therefore, the weight of evidence on benefits versus difficulties in this aging population must be accounted for.

Since the HERS and WHI (HRT arm) studies have been released, the cardiovascular and breast cancer risks with HRT become significant factors for many women who have endometrium. The time elements implied in these studies indicate that both conditions increase after 5 years. Genetic and legacy history would specifically provide a negative condition for some women. While the absolute risks do not appear large, they are significant and a decision to use hormone therapy would require careful review of alternative treatments.

The acute use for hot flushes and other usually fleeting symptoms of estrogen deprivation require only short-term therapy. However, major problems for geripausal/postmenopausal women are long term. These include osteopenia, osteoporosis, and fracture, as well as cardiovascular events. HRT has not been seen to improve CHD.

Perineal turgor, which effects vulvar, urethral, and vaginal normalcy is improved with estrogen treatment. The result is comfort, urinary competency, and effective sexuality. Utilization to prevent Alzheimer's disease and cognitive loss has been demonstrated, but not proven. Thus, these requirements will rely on the personal needs of the perimenopausal/geripausal woman.

ERT remains potentially effective without significant difficulty; however, we await further data from the WHI program. A recent study derived from the 1979–98 cohort study of former participants in the Breast Cancer Detection Demonstration Project, a breast screening program, concluded that ERT, but not HRT, users – particularly for 10 or more years – were at significantly increased risk for ovarian cancer[64]. Additionally, there has been some consideration concerning the use of other progestogen products, rather than medroxy-progesterone acetate used in the WHI trials in HRT. This may provide another means of continuing the use of estrogen with reduced risk. Obviously, these products would require substantial clinical trials for further proof.

Thus, with her physician, the postmenopausal/geripausal patient desiring long-term HRT must decide whether HRT is a tolerable mode of treatment. What alternatives can be used? Alternative medications are described; but the effectiveness of these therapies is often questionable.

## Quality of life

Recent studies on QoL have been mostly connected with the HERS project. This study group used a 'QoL questionnaire' that uniquely assessed functional capacity, emotional health, vitality, and depression. Hormone therapy seemed to have mixed results in these women (aged 50–80). The effects on improving their QoL depended on the presence of existing menopausal symptoms[57]. Unfortunately, the HERS population was an unhealthy population, since they had survived a cardiovascular incident. Editorials have indicated that no final decisions can be made at this time, since few studies include the QoL and emotional status of women on estrogen therapy.

## Conclusions

Physicians and medical institutions have provided care that has successfully resulted in longevity with improved physical health. Enriched quality of life continues to be an elusive but desirable goal. Replacement therapies remain potential mechanisms for promoting and maintaining good health in the aging individual, and need to continue to be tenaciously investigated.

# References

1. Rochon PA, Gurwitz JH. Prescribing for seniors, neither too much or too little. *J Am Med Assoc* 1999;252:113–15
2. Rochon PA, Anderson GM, Tu JM, *et al.* Age and gender-related use of the low dose drug therapy: the need to manufacture 'seniors' doses. *J Am Geriatr Soc* 1999;47:954–9
3. Barron HV, Viskin S, Lundstrom RJ, *et al.* Beta-blocker dasage and mortality after myocardial infarction. *Arch Intern Med* 1998;158:449–53
4. US Food and Drug Administration. *Guidelines for the Study of Drugs Likely to be Used in the Elderly.* Rockville, MD: Food and Drug Administration Center for Drug Evaluation and Research, 1999
5. Zhan C, Sangl J, Bierman AS, *et al.* Potentially inappropriate medication use in the community-dwelling elderly. *J Am Med Assoc* 2001;286:2823–9
6. Lindley C, Tuly M, Parmasothy V, Tallis R. Inappropriate medication is a major cause of adverse drug reactions in elderly patients. *Age Aging* 1992;21:294–300
7. Gurwitz J. Suboptimal medication use in the elderly, the tip of the iceberg. *J Am Med Assoc* 1994;272:316–17
8. Nash D, Keoning J, Chatterton M. *Why the Elderly Need Individual and Pharmaceutical Care.* Philadelphia, PA: Office of Health Policy and Clinical Outcomes, Thomas Jefferson University, 2000
9. Institute of Medicine. *To Err is Human: Building a Safer Health System.* Washington, DC: National Academy Press, 1999
10. Gosney W, Tallis R. Prescription of contraindicated and interacting drugs in elderly patients admitted to the hospital. *Lancet* 1984;2:564–7
11. Ray W, Federspie C, Schaffner W. A study of antipsychotic drug use in nursing homes: epidemiologic evidence suggesting misuse. *Am J Public Health* 1980;70:485–91
12. Beers MH, Ouslander JH, Fingold SF, *et al.* Inappropriate medication prescribing in skilled nursing facilities. *Ann Intern Med* 1992;117:684–9
13. Williams B, Betley C. Inappropriate use of nonpsychotrophic medications in nursing homes. *J Am Geriatr Soc* 1995;43:513–19
14. Spore D, Mor V, Larrat P, *et al.* Inappropriate drug prescriptions for elderly residents of board and care facilities. *Am J Public Health* 1997;87:404–9
15. Aparasu R, Fliginger S. Inappropriate medication prescribing for the elderly by office-based physicians. *Ann Pharmacother* 1997;31:823–9
16. Mort JR, Aparasu RR. Prescribing potentially inappropriate psychotropic medications to the ambulatory elderly. *Arch Intern Med* 2000;160:2825–31
17. Aparasu R, Sitzman S. Inappropriate prescribing for elderly outpatients. *Am J Health syst Pharm* 1999;56:433–9
18. Golden A, Preston R, Barnet S, *et al.* Inappropriate medication prescribing in homebound older adults. *J Am Geriatr Soc* 1999;47:948–53
19. Wilcox SW, Himmelstein D, Woolhandler S. Inappropriate drug prescribing for the community-dwelling elderly. *J Am Med Assoc* 1994;272:292–6
20. *Prescription Drugs and the Elderly. Many Still Receive Potentially Harmful Drugs Despite Recent Improvement.* Washington, DC: US General Accounting Office, 1995
21. Beers MH, Ouslander JC, Rolingher I, *et al.* Explicit criteria for determining inappropriate medication use in nursing homes. *Arch Intern Med* 1991;151:1825–32
22. Anderson G. Beers M, Kerluk K. Auditing prescription practice using exploit criteria and computerized drug benefit claims data. *J Eval Clin Pract* 1997:3:283–94
23. Beers MH. Exploit criteria for determining potentially inappropriate medication use by the elderly: an update. *Arch Intern Med* 1997;157;1531–6
24. Gambrell RD, Natrajan RK. Hormone replacement therapy. In Eskin BA, ed. *The Menopause: Comprehensive Management*, 4th edn. Carnforth, UK: Parthenon Publishing, 2000:257–73

25. Institute of Medicine. *Dietary Reference Intakes: Applications in Dietary Assessment*, 2000
26. Siris ES, Miller PD, Barrett-Conner E, *et al.* Identification and fracture outcomes of undiagnosed low BMD in postmenopausal women. National Osteoporosis Risk Assessment. *J Am Med Assoc* 2001;286:2815–22
27. Cauley JA, Seeley DJ, Ensrud K, *et al.* Estrogen replacement therapy and fractures in older women. *Ann Intern Med* 1995;122:9–16
28. American College of Obstetricians and Gynecologists. ACOG Educational Bulletin No. 247. ACOG, 1998
29. Campbell S, Whitehead M. Oestrogen therapy and the menstrual syndrome. *Clin Obstet Gynaecol* 1997;4:31–47
30. Honjo H, Tanaka K, Kashiwagi T. Senile dementia – Alzheimer's type and estrogen. *Horm Metab Res* 1995;27:204–7
31. Henderson VW, Paganimi-Hill A, Emanuel CK, *et al.* Estrogen replacement therapy in older women. *Arch Neurol* 1994;51:896–900
32. Carr BR. HRT management: the American experience. *Eur J Obstet Gynecol Reprod Biol* 1996;64(Suppl):S17–20
33. Andrews WC. Trend to lower doses of ERT/HRT for the management of menopause. *ACOG Clin Rev* 2001;6:1–16
34. Eskin BA, Trivedi RA, Weideman CA, Walker RF. Positive feedback disturbances and infertility in women over thirty. *Am J Gynecol Health* 1988;2:110
35. Roth GS. Hormone receptor changes during adulthood and senescence: significance for aging research. *Fed Proc* 1979;38:910
36. Campbell S. Whitehead M. Oestrogen therapy and the menstrual syndrome. *Clin Obstet Gynaecol* 1977;4:31–47
37. Vellareal DT. Osteopenic effects of HRT in physically frail, elderly women. *J Am Med Assoc* 2001;286:815–20
38. Daly E, Vessey MP, Hawkins MM, *et al.* Risk of venous thromboembolism in users of hormone replacement therapy. *Lancet* 1996;348:977–80
39. Grodstein F, Stampfer MJ, Goldhaber SZ, *et al.* Prospective study of exogenous hormones and risk of pulmonary embolism in women. *Lancet* 1996;348:983–7
40. Jack H, Derby LE, Myers MW, *et al.* Risk of hospital admission for idiopathic venous thromboembolism among users of postmenopausal oestrogens. *Lancet* 1996;348:981–3
41. The Writing Group for the PEPI trial. Effects of hormone replacement therapy on endometrial histology in postmenopausal women. *J Am Med Assoc* 1996;275:370–5
42. Colditz GA, Hankinson SE, Hunter DJ, *et al.* The use of estrogens and progestins and the risk of breast cancer in prostmenopausal women. *N Engl J Med* 1995;332:1589–93
43. Cauley JA, Seeley DJ, Ensrud K, *et al.* Estrogen replacement therapy and fractures in older women. *Ann Intern Med* 1995;122:9–16
44. Roth GS. Hormone receptor changes during adulthood and senescence: significance for aging research. *Fed Proc* 1979;38:910
45. Altkorn D, Vokes T. Treatment of postmenopausal osteoporosis. *J Am Med Assoc* 2001;285:1415–17
46. Eskin BA. Endocrinology of the breast. In Eskin BA, Asbell SO, Jardines L, eds. *Breast Disease for the Primary Care Physician*. Carnforth, UK: Parthenon Publishing, 1999
47. Scharirer C, Lubin J, Troisi R, *et al.* Menopausal estrogen and estrogen–progestin replacement therapy and breast cancer risk. *J Am Med Assoc* 2000;283:485–91
48. Hulley S, Grady D, Bush T, *et al.* Randomized trial of estrogen plus progestin for secondary prevention of coronary heart disease in postmenopausal women. *J Am Med Assoc* 1985;280:608–13
49. Herrington DM, Reboussin DM, Brosnilian KB, *et al.* Effects of estrogen replacement on the progression of coronary artery atherosclerosis. *N Engl J of Med* 2000;343:522–9
50. The Women's Health Initiative Study Group. Design of the Women's Health Initiative Clinical Trial and Observational Study. *Control Clin Trials* 1998;19:61–109
51. Kampen DL, Sherwin BB. Estrogen use and verbal memory in healthy postmenopausal women. *Obstet Gynecol* 1994;83:979–83
52. Sherwin BB. Estrogen and/or androgen replacement therapy and cognitive functioning in surgically menopausal women. *Psychoneuroendocrinology* 1988;13:345–57
53. Fillit H, Weinred H, Cholst I, *et al.* Observations in a preliminary open trial of estradiol therapy for senile dementia – Alzheimer's type. *Psychoneuroendocrinology* 1986;11:337–45
54. Funk JL, Morter KF, Meyer JS. Effects of estrogen replacement therapy on cerebral perfusion and cognition among postmenopausal women. *Dementia* 1991;1:268–72
55. Henderson VW, Paganini-Hill A, Emanuel CK, *et al.* Estrogen replacement therapy in older women. *Arch Neurol* 1994;51:896–900
56. Grodstein F, *et al.* A prospective observational study of postmenopausal hormone therapy and primary prevention of cardiovascular disease. *Ann Intern Med* 2000;133:933–41

57. Honjo H, Tanaka K, Kashiwagi T, *et al*. Senile dementia – Alzheimer's type and estrogen. *Horm Metab Res* 1955;27:204–7

58. Freeman EE, *et al*. Hormone replacement may protect against cataracts. *Arch Ophthalmol* 2001;199:1687–92

59. Speroff L, Whitcomb RW, Kempfers NJ, *et al*. Efficacy and local tolerance of a low-dose 7-day matrix estradiol transdermal system in the treatment of menopausal vasomotor symptoms. *Obstet Gynecol* 1996;88:587–92

60. Reid IR, Brown JP, Burkhardt P, *et al*. Intravenous zoledronic acid in postmenopausal women with low bone minteral density. *N Engl J Med* 2002;346:653–61

61. Grady D, Herrington D, Bittner V, *et al*. for the HERS Research Group. Heart and estrogen/progestin replacement study follow-up (HERS II): Part 1. Cardiovascular outcomes during 6.8 years of hormone therapy. *J Am Med Assoc* 2002;288:49–57

62. Writing Group for the Women's Health Initiative Investigators. Risks and benefits of estrogen plus progestin in healthy post-menopausal women: principal results from the Women's Health Initiative randomized controlled trial. *J Am Med Assoc* 2002;288:321–33

63. Hulley S, Furberg C, Barrett-Connor E, *et al*. for the HERS Research Group. Heart and estrogen/progestin replacement study follow-up (HERS II): Part 2. Non-cardiovascular outcomes during 6.8 years of hormone therapy. *J Am Med Assoc* 2002;288:58–66

64. Lacey JV, Mink PJ, Lubin JH, *et al*. Menopausal hormone replacement therapy and risk of ovarian cancer. *J Am Med Assoc* 2002;288:334–41

# 11

# Neuromuscular conditions: definition and epidemiology of falls and gait disorders

*Neil Alexander*

## Falls

A fall is a sudden, unintentional change in position causing an individual to land at a lower level on an object, or the ground. Since the majority of falls are not associated with syncope, most investigators exclude falls associated with loss of consciousness (such as from a seizure) although loss of consciousness may occur following the fall. Other overwhelming events, such as sustaining a violent blow or sudden onset of paralysis, are also not as common as non-syncopal falls. Annually, falls occur in approximately 33% of community-dwelling older adults and 50% of nursing home residents. The nursing home resident rate, 1.5 falls per bed annually, is probably due to the increased frailty of these residents and the increased reporting in this setting[1]. Depending upon the published series, while up to 2% of falls result in hip fractures, other fractures can occur in up to 5% and other serious injuries (such as head injury) can occur in up to 10%. Over 50% of fallers sustain at least some minor injury (such as a laceration). These and other fallers may develop fear of falling and self-imposed mobility restrictions, which then may lead to loss of independence and institutionalization[2]. Fallers, particularly repeat fallers, tend to have activities of daily living (ADL) and instrumental activities of daily living (IADL) disability, and are at high risk for subsequent hospitalization, further disability, institutionalization, and death[3-5].

## Gait disorders

Determining that a gait is 'disordered' is difficult, because there are generally no clearly accepted standards of 'normal' gait for older adults. Some believe that slowed gait speed suggests a disorder, while others believe that deviations in smoothness, symmetry, and synchrony of movement patterns suggest a disorder. However, a slowed and esthetically abnormal gait may in fact provide the older adult with a safe, independent gait pattern. Self-reports of difficulty walking are common. At least 20% of non-institutionalized older adults admit to walking difficulty or require the assistance of another person or special equipment to walk[6]. Limitations in walking also increase with age. In some samples of non-institutionalized older adults aged 85 and over, the incidence of limitation in walking can be over 54%[6]. While age-related gait changes such as in speed are most apparent past age 75–80, the majority of gait disorders appear in connection with underlying diseases, particularly as disease severity increases. Attributing a gait disorder to a particular disease etiology in older adults is particularly difficult, because similar gait abnormalities are common to many diseases[7].

## Causes, risk factors, and clinical manifestations

Multiple factors frequently contribute to falls, fall-related injury, and gait disorders. In falls,

**Table 1**  Intrinsic factors contributing to risk of falls, fall-related injury, and gait disorders

| Factor | Typical diseases involved |
|---|---|
| Central processing | dementia |
| Neuromotor | Parkinson's disease, stroke, myelopathy (such as from cervical or lumbar spondylosis), cerebellar degeneration, carotid sinus hypersensitivity, peripheral neuropathy, vertebrobasilar insufficiency |
| Vision | cataracts, glaucoma, age-related macular degeneration |
| Vestibular | acute labyrinthitis, Meniere's disease, paroxysmal positional vertigo |
| Proprioception | peripheral neuropathy (such as from diabetes mellitus), vitamin $B_{12}$ deficiency |
| Musculoskeletal | arthritis, foot disorders |
| Systemic | postural hypotension, metabolic disease (e.g. thyroid), cardiopulmonary disease, other acute illness (e.g. sepsis) |

**Table 2**  Medications contributing to risk of falls, fall-related injury, and gait disorders

| Medication function | Typical medications |
|---|---|
| Reduce alertness or retard central processing | analgesics (especially narcotics) |
| | psychotropics (especially tricyclics, long-acting benzodiazepines, phenothiazines) |
| Impair cerebral perfusion | antihypertensives (especially vasodilators) |
| | antiarrythmics |
| | diuretics (especially when dehydration occurs) |
| Direct vestibular toxicity | aminoglycosides |
| | high-dose loop diuretics |
| Extrapyramidal syndromes | phenothiazines |

there is often a complex interaction between intrinsic factors (individual impairments), situational factors (aspects related to the ADL task being performed), and extrinsic factors (environmental demand and hazards). In terms of intrinsic factors, the diseases and impairments implicated in gait disorders are similar to those that place an older adult at risk for falls and fall-related injury. At least seven major intrinsic factors/conditions can be implicated, and while age-related changes may be present (such as in reduction of leg strength), the major contributors to fall risk and gait disorders are the diseases that influence each factor (Table 1). These functions include vestibular, proprioceptive, and visual function, cognition, and musculoskeletal factors. For example, patients with leg arthritis (with associated pain and limited range of motion and strength) and dementia (with associated lack of judgment, inattention, and confusion, are at

risk for falls. Risk of falling increases dramatically with the number of impairments (intrinsic factors)[8] and, accordingly, recurrent fallers have more impairments[9]. Medications are also major risk factors and are categorized according to their major mechanism of effect (Table 2). Extrinsic and situational factors (Table 3) contribute to the risk of falls and fall-related injury when: environmental hazards are present; the environment or tasks performed demand greater postural control and mobility; situations require changing positions (such as transferring and turning). For example, a patient with Parkinson's disease (intrinsic factor) may trip over a rug (extrinsic factor) but only under certain situations, such as walking to the bathroom at night (situational factor). Situational factors are particularly important when an injury results from a fall[10]. For example, major injuries are more likely when falling from an upright position (with greater potential

**Table 3** Extrinsic and situational factors contributing to risk of falls and fall-related injury. From the author's own original work and adapted with permission from King MB, Tinetti ME. Falls in community-dwelling older persons. *J Am Geriatr Soc* 1995;43:1146–54[3]

| Factor | Examples |
|---|---|
| Environmental hazard | slippery or uneven walking surface, poor lighting |
| Increased environmental demand | using stairs, rising from a low chair |
| Situational | changing position, risk-taking behavior, recent relocation to new nursing home |

energy to be dissipated) and when falling laterally, with direct impact on the hip. Other environmental factors (such as hardness of impact surface) contribute to the increased risk of fall-related injury. In general, however, the intrinsic factors noted above, as well as other factors such as low femoral bone mineral density and body mass index, are major contributors to increased risk of fall-related injury[11–13].

The relative contribution of intrinsic, extrinsic and situational factors also depends on the faller and their living environment. Community-dwelling fallers tend to be exposed to greater environmental demand and hazards and tend to be less physically impaired. Therefore, extrinsic factors make larger contributions to fall and fall injury risk[3]. Nursing home fallers are usually more physically impaired and are exposed to fewer environmental hazards and demands. Therefore, intrinsic factors such as weakness and balance disorders make larger contributions to fall and fall injury risk[1].

## Assessment of gait disorders and fall risk

### Diagnoses contributing to falls and gait disorders

Disordered gait may not be an inevitable consequence of aging but rather a reflection of the increased prevalence and severity of age-associated diseases. These underlying diseases, both neurological and non-neurological, are the major contributors to disordered gait. In a primary care setting, patients consider pain, stiffness, dizziness, numbness, weakness, and sensations of abnormal movement to be the most common contributors to their walking difficulties[14]. The most common diagnoses found in a primary care setting thought to contribute to gait disorders include degenerative joint disease, acquired musculoskeletal deformities, intermittent claudication, post-orthopedic surgery and post-stroke impairments, and postural hypotension[14]. Usually, more than one contributing diagnosis is found. Factors such as dementia and fear of falling also contribute to gait disorders. The diagnoses found in a neurological referral population are primarily neurologically oriented[15,16] and include frontal gait disorders (usually related to normal-pressure hydrocephalus (NPH) and cerebrovascular processes), sensory disorders (also involving vestibular and visual function), myelopathy, previously undiagnosed Parkinson's disease or Parkinsonian syndromes, and cerebellar disease. Known conditions causing severe gait impairment, such as hemiplegia and severe hip or knee disease, are frequently not found in these neurological referral populations. Many gait disorders, particularly those that are classical and discrete (such as those related to stroke and osteoarthritis), and those that are mild and/or may relate to irreversible disease (such as multi-infarct dementia), are presumably diagnosed in a primary care setting and treated without a referral to a neurologist. Other less common contributors to gait disorders include metabolic disorders (related to renal or hepatic disease), central nervous system (CNS) tumors or subdural hematoma, depression, and psychotropic medications. Case reports also document reversible gait disorders due to clinically overt hypo- or hyperthyroidism and vitamin $B_{12}$ and folate deficiency (for detailed review, see reference 7).

Other factors that contribute to gait disorders are frequently disease-associated (such as those related to cardiopulmonary disease) but are often assessed separately. These include marked reductions in activity and aerobic fitness, reductions in joint strength and range of motion, and previous falls.

While older adults may maintain a relatively normal gait pattern well into their eighties, some slowing occurs, and decreased stride length thus becomes a common feature described in older adult gait disorders[7]. Some authors have proposed the emergence of an age-related gait disorder without accompanying clinical abnormalities, i.e. an essential 'senile' gait disorder[17]. This gait pattern is described as broad-based with small steps, diminished arm swing, stooped posture, flexion of the hips and knees, uncertainty and stiffness in turning, occasional difficulty in initiating steps, and a tendency towards falling. These and other non-specific findings (such as the inability to perform tandem gait) are similar to gait patterns found in a number of other diseases and yet the clinical abnormalities are insufficient to make a specific diagnosis. This 'disorder' may be a precursor to an as-yet-asymptomatic disease (for example, related to subtle extrapyramidal signs) and is likely to be a manifestation of concurrent progressive cognitive impairment (such as Alzheimer's disease or vascular dementia)[18]. 'Senile' gait disorder thus potentially reflects several potential disease etiologies and is generally not useful in labeling gait disorders in older adults.

## History and physical examination

According to a recent consensus panel, older adults who present for medical attention because of a fall, who report recurrent falls in the past year, or who demonstrate abnormalities of gait and/or balance, should have a fall assessment[8] as follows. The panel also recommended asking every patient annually about falls, and patients who report a single fall should be evaluated for an abnormal 'Get Up and Go' test (see below) prior to embarking on a full fall assessment[8]. Emphasis should be placed on assessing the cardiovascular, visual, vestibular, musculoskeletal, and neurological systems, and assessing medication use. A history of the fall and circumstances surrounding the fall, including associated symptoms and associated movements or activities that may have elicited the fall, is useful. Subject reports of premonitory or associated symptoms such as palpitations, shortness of breath, chest pain, vertigo, light-headedness, and associated activities helps determine contributing medical conditions. Of particular importance is the determination of syncope or near-syncope, which leads to a different differential diagnosis and work-up, including Holter monitor, tilt table, and carotid massage. Recent data from selected populations suggest under-recognition of near-syncope, as caused by carotid sinus hypersensitivity[19,20], but the contribution of carotid sinus hypersensitivity to an actual fall is not completely clear. Symptoms that are postprandial or postmicturition may help better define accompanying risk. The vestibular or cardiovascular origin of dizziness or light-headedness, particularly when positional, is sometimes difficult to differentiate (see examination below). A careful medical history and a review of the factors given in Table 1 will help elucidate the multiple factors contributing to the fall. A brief systemic evaluation for evidence of subacute metabolic disease (such as thyroid disorders), acute cardiopulmonary disorders (such as a myocardial infarction), or other acute illness (such as sepsis) is warranted, because falling may be the presenting feature of acute and subacute systemic decompensation in an older adult. An assessment of mobility is also indicated, to include ADL function and ambulation, for example, wheelchair use, distance ambulated, and the extent of human or device assistance required (see below).

Using the factors given in Table 1, the physical examination should include an attempt to identify motion-related factors, as by provoking both objective and subjective responses to the Hallpike–Dix maneuver and to supine and standing blood pressure and pulse measurement. In the Hallpike–Dix maneuver, while the patient is seated on an examination table, the examiner holds the patient's head, turns the head to one side and lowers the head to the level of the table, classically 30° below the table level. The patients then sits up and the maneuver is repeated again to the other side. Blood pressure should be measured with the patient both supine and standing, to rule out orthostatic hypotension. Vision screening, at least for acuity, is essential. Examining the cardiovascular system helps exclude arrhythmia, valvular heart disease and heart failure. The neck, spine, extremities and feet should be evaluated for deformities and pain/limitations in range of motion. A formal neurological assessment is critical, to include assessment of strength and tone, sensation (including proprioception), co-ordination (including cerebellar function), and station and gait. For the latter, the Romberg test screens for simple postural control and whether the proprioceptive and vestibular systems are functional. Some investigators have proposed one-legged stance time of less than 5 seconds as a risk factor for injurious falls[21], although even relatively healthy older adults aged 70 may have difficulty with one-legged stance[22]. Given the importance of cognition as a risk factor, screening for mental status is also indicated.

## Performance-based functional assessment

Technologically oriented assessments involving formal kinematic and kinetic analyses have not been applied widely in clinical assessments of older adult balance and gait disorders. Using a functional gait and balance battery (which includes aspects such as turning while standing) has been proposed as a means to detect and quantify abnormalities and direct interventions. Fall risk, for example, may be increased with more abnormal gait and balance scale scores[23]. Clinical gait assessments utilize a battery of items either timed or scored semi-quantitatively, usually based upon whether a subject is able to perform the task and, if able, how normal or abnormal the performance was. Batteries that focus primarily on gait include: the Functional Ambulation Classification

scale[24], rating the use of assistive devices, the degree of human assistance (either manual or verbal), the distance the patient can walk, and the types of surfaces the patient can negotiate; the Performance Oriented Balance and Mobility Assessment (POMA) gait subsection[25], i.e. a rating of gait initiation, turning, step length and height, step symmetry and continuity, path deviation, and trunk sway; the Get Up and Go test[26], a timed sequence of rising from a chair, walking 3 m, turning, and returning to the chair; the Dynamic Gait Index[27], a rating of a series of tasks including turning, walking while turning the head, clearing obstacles, and using stairs; the Functional Obstacle Course[28], a timed test of negotiating different floor textures, graded surfaces and stairs, and simultaneous functional activities while walking (such as opening and closing doors); the Gait Abnormality Rating Scale[29], modified to score gait variability, guardedness, staggering, foot contact, hip range of motion, shoulder extension, and arm–heel synchrony; and the Emory Functional Ambulation Profile[30], a battery of timed tasks including walking on a hard floor and on a carpeted surface, stepping over an obstacle, and up and down four stairs. These scales were used reliably in smaller selected published samples, although perhaps less reliably in larger epidemiological settings (for example, see reference 31 for a critique of the Get Up and Go test).

Comfortable gait speed has become a powerful assessment and outcome measure. Gait speed measured as part of a timed short distance (for example, eight foot; 2.5 m) walk or as measured in terms of distance walked over time (such as 6 minutes) predicts disease activity (such as in arthritis), cardiac and pulmonary function (particularly in congestive heart failure), and ultimately mobility (and ADL), disability, institutionalization, and mortality[7].

## Laboratory/diagnostic tests

Depending upon the history and physical examination, further laboratory and diagnostic evaluation may be warranted. Tests such as electrocardiograms, Holter monitors, cardiac enzymes and echocardiograms are not routinely recommended unless a cardiac source is suspected. Similarly, complete blood count, chemistries and stool for occult blood are useful only where acute systemic disease is suspected. Head or spine imaging, including X-ray, computed tomography (CT), or magnetic resonance imaging (MRI) are of unclear use unless there are neurological abnormalities by history and physical examination, either preceding the gait disorder or of recent onset. A possible exception relates to cerebral white matter changes on CT scan, considered to be ischemic in nature (termed leukoaraiosis), which can cause non-specific gait disorders. Recently, periventricular high-signal measurements on MRI as well as increased ventricular volume, even in apparently healthy older adults[32] (see discussion in reference 32 for review of previous studies) are associated with gait slowing. Age-specific guidelines, sensitivity, specificity, and cost-effectiveness of these work-ups remain to be determined.

## Interventions to reduce falls, fall-related injury, and gait disorders

### Falls

These interventions attempt to improve functional capacity, decrease falls, and decrease injuries, but sometimes patterns of independence are altered as well (for example, for safety reasons, ambulating in inclement weather conditions is discouraged).

Interventions can be divided into at least four categories (Table 4). Interventions that deal directly with intrinsic factors focus on decreasing disease-related impairment and providing therapy. Extrinsic factor interventions have thus far focused primarily on decreasing hazards and decreasing environmental demand. Examples of these extrinsic interventions include improving lighting, adding grab bars, raising the toilet seat, finding an appropriate bed height, and providing an appropriately structured environment for those who are cognitively impaired. Since restraint use may

be associated with more falls and injuries[33], reducing active mechanical restraints (such as vests) may not necessarily increase falls or fall-related injury. More passive alternatives such as wheelchair adaptations, removable belts and wedge seating can apparently provide adequate fall protection with less mobility limitation. Few controlled studies have addressed situational factors, although caregiver or nurse surveillance, particularly with those who are considered for restraint, may be useful. Use of motion detectors has a mixed benefit because a member of staff still needs to be present to respond to the triggered alarm. Finally, protective padding worn over the hip may become a useful alternative for fallers at risk for hip injury. A recent randomized community-based study found a reduction in hip fractures (relative hazard 0.4) in those wearing hip protector pads[34]. In that study, the majority of hip fractures in the hip pad group occurred in those who were not wearing the pad at the time of the fall. Note, however, that as in previous hip pad studies, compliance was still a problem; 31% of those randomized to the hip pad group refused to wear the pad. Alternatively, flooring materials exist that will help dissipate the impact force, although a floor that is too compliant may be destabilizing in itself.

Among community-dwelling older adults, a multifactorial approach seems most appropriate, individualizing a combination of medical, rehabilitative, environmental, and intervention strategies for each faller/potential faller[8,35]. In one example of a multifactorial approach[36] for non-syncopal falls, in-home interventions were identified for community-dwelling older adults with at least one of the following risk factors: postural hypotension; use of benzodiazepines or hypnotic sedatives; use of four or more prescription medications; inability to transfer safely to a bathtub or toilet; environmental hazards for falls or tripping; gait impairment; balance impairment; and arm and/or leg strength or range of motion impairment. While 47% of the controls fell during 1-year follow-up, only 35% of the intervention group

**Table 4** Interventions to reduce falls, fall-related injury, and gait disorders

---

*Intrinsic*
Treat the underlying disease
Eliminate drugs and/or reduce dosages
Initiate physical therapy program
   balance and gait training (including training with an assistive device)
   vestibular rehabilitation and habituation training
Initiate exercise program
   tai chi
   resistive (strength) training
   other balance training

*Extrinsic*
Reduce environmental hazards
Reduce active restraints
Improve fall surveillance
   identify those at risk
   increase staff proximity and ratio
   improve motion detection
Decrease/dissipate impact force
   protective pads and flooring

---

fell[36]. Reductions in postural blood pressure changes (and medication use) and in balance, gait, and transfer problems contributed the most to the reduction in falls[36]. The intervention group had a lower incidence of injurious falls and hospitalizations but the difference did not reach statistical significance. However, given the financial costs of the injuries and medical care required, average costs for the controls exceeded that of those in the intervention group[37]. A bi-disciplinary intervention (medical and single occupational therapy home visit) also showed a reduction of falls (odds ratio 0.39 versus controls) in community-dwelling emergency room patients seen for non-syncopal and syncopal falls[38].

In long-term care settings, this multidisciplinary approach includes an emphasis on staff education, gait training and advice on the appropriate use of assistive devices, and review and modifications of medications, especially psychotropic medications[8]. A randomized trial of a fall reduction consultation service in 14 nursing homes showed a decline in the proportion of recurrent fallers (44% in intervention homes versus 54% in control homes) and

a trend toward a lower incidence of injurious falls[39]. The consultation service made a series of recommendations according to domains (in order of most- to least-commonly suggested) related to wheelchairs, the environment, transferring and ambulation, and psychotropic medication use. Notably, multidisciplinary interventions to reduce falls have not been shown to be effective in acute hospital settings[8,40].

Other controlled studies provide more caveats about the effect of interventions on fall reduction. No fall prevention study has had sufficient power to show a reduction in serious fall injuries such as hip fracture[41] (although note the reduction in hip fracture with use of hip pads, see above). Some studies have demonstrated no change in falls but, owing to the multidisciplinary evaluation, other co-morbid conditions are identified, which might lead to improved overall health and decreased hospitalizations[42]. Some studies have suggested that environmental hazards relate poorly to fall occurrence[43] and that even home modification interventions may have reduced falls by mechanisms unrelated to the modifications themselves[44,45]. The success of fall reduction with withdrawal of psychotropic medications (66% reduction in falls) is notable, but by 1 month following study completion, 47% had restarted their psychotropic medications[46]. Studies that focus on low-intensity exercise or behavioral interventions find small and transient, if any, effects on fall reduction, with the greatest effects in targeted high-risk groups who are given individually tailored exercise programs[35]. A recent meta-analysis of seven independent, randomized clinical studies suggested that intervention programs that include exercise, and balance training in particular, may reduce falls by 10%[47]. Moreover, one recent controlled study found that a 15-week program of tai chi reduced the risk of falls by 48%[48].

## Gait disorders

Even if a diagnosable condition is found on evaluation, many conditions causing a gait disorder are only, at best, partially treatable (for a more extensive review of the studies below, see reference 49). The patient is often left with at least some residual disability. However, other functional outcomes such as reduction in weight-bearing pain may be equally important in justifying treatment. Achievement of pre-morbid gait patterns may be unrealistic, and improvement in measures such as gait speed is reasonable as long as gait remains safe. Co-morbidity, disease severity, and overall health status tend to have a strong influence on treatment outcome.

Many of the reports dealing with treatment and rehabilitation of gait disorders in older adults are retrospective chart reviews and case studies. Gait disorders presumably secondary to vitamin $B_{12}$ deficiency, folate deficiency, hypothyroidism, hyperthyroidism, knee osteoarthritis, Parkinson's disease, and inflammatory polyneuropathy show improvement in ambulation as a result of medical therapy. A variety of modes of physical therapy for diseases such as Parkinson's disease, knee osteoarthritis, and stroke also result in modest improvements but continued residual disability. Recent studies suggest the use of special apparatus and techniques for gait rehabilitation of patients with specific diseases and impairments, such as body weight support and a treadmill to enhance post-stroke gait retraining[50].

Modest improvement and residual disability is also the result of surgical treatment for compressive cervical myelopathy, lumbar stenosis, and NPH. Few controlled prospective studies and virtually no randomized studies have addressed the outcome of surgical treatment for these conditions. A number of problems plague the available series: outcomes such as pain and walking disability are not reported separately; the source of the outcome rating is not clearly identified or blinded; the criteria for classifying outcomes differ; the follow-up intervals are variable; the selection factors for conservative versus surgical treatment between studies differ or are unspecified; and there is publication bias (only positive results are published). Many of the surgical series include all ages, although the mean age is usually above 60 years. Many older adults have reduction in pain and improvement in maximal walking distance following laminectomies and lumbar fusion surgery, although they have continued residual disability. A few studies document equivalent surgical outcomes with conservative, non-surgical treatment. Finally, it is unclear how much of the initial postoperative gains are maintained in the long term, particularly in NPH.

Outcomes for hip and knee replacement surgery for osteoarthritis are better, although some of the same study methodological problems exist. Other than pain relief, sizable gains in gait speed and joint motion occur, although residual walking disability continues for several reasons, including residual pathology on the operated side and symptoms on the non-operated side.

# References

1. Rubinstein LZ, Josephson KR, Robins AS. Falls in the nursing home. *Ann Intern Med* 1994; 121:442–51

2. Cumming RG, Salkeld G, Thomas M, *et al*. Prospective study of the impact of fear of falling on activities of daily living, SF-36 scores, and nursing home admission. *J Gerontol* 2000;55: M299–305

3. King MB, Tinetti ME. Falls in community-dwelling older persons. *J Am Geriatr Soc* 1995; 43:1146–54

4. Tinetti ME, Williams CS. Falls, injuries due to falls, and the risk of admission to a nursing home. *N Engl J Med* 1997;337:1279–84

5. Tinetti ME, Williams CS. The effect of falls and fall injuries on functioning in community-dwelling older persons. *J Gerontol* 1998;53A: M112–19

6. Oschiega Y, Harris TB, Hirsch R, *et al*. The prevalence of functional limitations and disability in older persons in the US: data from the National Health and Nutrition Examination Survey III. *J Am Geriatr Soc* 2000; 48:1132–5

7. Alexander NB. Gait disorders in older adults. *J Am Geriatr Soc* 1996;44:434–51

8. American Geriatrics Society. Guideline for prevention of falls in older persons. *J Am Geriatr Soc* 2001;49:664–72

9. Nevitt MC, Cummings SR, Kidd S, *et al*. Risk factors for recurrent nonsyncopal falls. A prospective study. *J Am Med Assoc* 1989;261: 2663–8

10. Tinetti ME, Douchette JT, Claus EB. The contribution of predisposing and situational risk factors to serious fall injuries. *J Am Geriatr Soc* 1995;43:1207–13

11. Cummings SR, Nevitt MC. A hypothesis: the causes of hip fractures. *J Gerontol* 1989;44: M107–11

12. Greenspan SL, Myers ER, Maitland LA, *et al*. Fall severity and bone mineral density as risk factors for hip fracture in ambulatory elderly. *J Am Med Assoc* 1994;271:128–33

13. Graafmans WC, Ooms ME, Hofstee HM, *et al*. Falls in the elderly: a prospective study of risk factors and risk profiles. *Am J Epidemiol* 1996;143:1129–36

14. Hough JC, McHenry MP, Kammer LM. Gait disorders in the elderly. *Am Fam Pract* 1987; 30:191–6

15. Sudarsky L, Rontal M. Gait disorders among elderly patients: a survey study of 50 patients. *Arch Neurol* 1983;40:740–3

16. Fuh JL, Lin KN, Wang SJ, *et al*. Neurologic diseases presenting with gait impairment in the elderly. *J Geriatr Psychiatry Neurol* 1994;7: 89–92

17. Koller WC, Wilson RS, Glatt SL, *et al*. Senile gait: correlation with computed tomographic scans. *Ann Neurol* 1983;13:343–4

18. Elble RJ, Hughes L, Higgins C. The syndrome of senile gait. *J Neurol* 1992;239:71–5

19. Ward CR, McIntosh S, Kenny RA. Carotid sinus hypersensitivity – a modifiable risk factor for fractured neck of the femur. *Age Ageing* 1999;28:127–33

20. Allcock LM, O'Shea D. Diagnostic yield and development of a neurocardiovascular investigation unit for older adults in a district hospital. *J Gerontol* 2000;55A:M458–62

21. Vellas BJ, Wayne SJ, Romero L, *et al*. One-leg balance is an important predictor of injurious falls in older persons. *J Am Geriatr Soc* 1997; 45:735–8

22. Rossiter-Fornoff JE, Wolf SL, Wolfson LI, *et al*. A cross-validation study of the FICSIT common data base static balance measures. *J Gerontol* 1995;50A:M291–7

23. Tinetti ME, Speechley M, Ginter SF. Risk factors for falls among elderly persons living in the community. *N Engl J Med* 1988;319:1701–7

24. Holden MK, Gill KM, Magliozzi MR. Gait assessment for neurologically impaired patients: standards for outcome assessment. *Phys Ther* 1986;66:1530–9

25. Tinetti ME. Performance-oriented assessment of mobility problems in elderly patients. *J Am Geriatr Soc* 1986;34:119–26

26. Posiadlo D, Richardson S. The timed 'Up & Go': a test of basic functional mobility for frail elderly persons. *J Am Geriatr Soc* 1991;39:142–8

27. Shumway-Cook A, Woollacott MH. Assessment and treatment of the patient with mobility disorders. In *Motor Control: Theory and Practical Applications*, 1st edn. Baltimore, MD: Williams and Wilkins, 1995

28. Means KM, Rodell DE, O'Sullivan PS, *et al*. Comparison of a functional obstacle course with an index of clinical gait and balance and postural sway. *J Gerontol* 1998;53A:M331–5

29. Van Swearingen JM, Paschall KA, Bonino P, *et al*. Assessing recurrent fall risk of community-dwelling frail older veterans using specific tests of mobility and the physical performance test of function. *J Gerontol* 1998;53A:M457–64

30. Wolf SL, Catlin PA, Gage K, *et al*. Establishing the reliability and validity of measurements of

walking time using the Emory Functional Ambulation Profile. *Phys Ther* 1999;79: 1122–33

31. Rockwood K, Awalt E, Carver D, *et al*. Feasibility and measurement properties of the functional reach and timed up and go tests in the Canadian Study of Health and Aging. *J Gerontol* 2000;55A:M70–3

32. Camicoli R, Moore MM, Sexton G, *et al*. Age-related changes associated with motor function in healthy older people. *J Am Geriatr Soc* 1999; 47:330–4

33. Capezuti E, Strumpf NE, Evans LK, *et al*. The relationship between physical restraint removal and falls and injuries among nursing home residents. *J Gerontol* 1998;3A:M47–52

34. Kannus P, Parkkari J, Niemi S, *et al*. Prevention of hip fracture in elderly people with use of a hip protector. *N Engl J Med* 2000;343:1506–13

35. Feder G, Cryer C, Donovan S, *et al*. Guidelines for the prevention of falls in people over 65. *Br Med J* 2000;321:1007–11

36. Tinetti ME, Baker DI, McAvay G, *et al*. A multifactorial intervention to reduce the risk of falling among elderly people living in the community. *N Engl J Med* 1994;331:821–7

37. Rizzo JA, Baker DI, McAvay G, *et al*. The cost-effectiveness of a multifactorial targeted prevention program for falls among community elderly persons. *Med Care* 1996;34:954–69

38. Close J, Ellis M, Hooper R, *et al*. Prevention of falls in the elderly (PROFET): a randomized controlled trial. *Lancet* 1999;353:93–7

39. Ray WA, Taylor JA, Meador KG, *et al*. A randomized trial of a consultation service to reduce falls in nursing homes. *J Am Med Assoc* 1997;278:557–62

40. Oliver D, Hopper A, Seed P. Do hospital fall prevention programs work? A systematic review. *J Am Geriatr Soc* 2000;48:1679–89

41. Gardner MM, Robertson MC, Campbell AJ. Exercise in preventing falls and fall related injuries in older people: a review of randomized controlled trials. *Br J Sports Med* 2000;34: 7–17

42. Rubinstein LZ, Ribbins A, Josephson K, *et al*. The value of assessing falls in the elderly population: a randomized clinical trial. *Ann Intern Med* 1990;113:308–16

43. Sattin RW, Rodriguez JG, DeVito CA, *et al*. Home environmental hazards and the risk of fall injury events among community-dwelling older persons. Study to Assess Falls among the Elderly (SAFE) group. *J Am Geriatr Soc* 1998;46:669–76

44. Cumming RG, Thomas M, Szonyi G, *et al*. Home visits by occupational therapists for assessment and modification of environmental hazards: a randomized trial of falls prevention. *J Am Geriatr Soc* 1999;47:1397–402

45. Gill TM. Preventing falls: to modify the environment or the individual? *J Am Geriatr Soc* 1999;47:1471–2

46. Campbell AJ, Robertson MC, Gardner MM, *et al*. Psychotropic medication withdrawal and a home-based exercise program to prevent falls: a randomized controlled trial. *J Am Geriatr Soc* 1999;47:850–3

47. Province MA, Hadley EC, Hornbrook MC, *et al*. The effects of exercise on falls in elderly persons: a population-based randomized trial. *J Am Med Assoc* 1995;273:1341–7

48. Wolf DSL, Barnhart HX, Kutner NG, *et al*. Reducing frailty and falls in older persons: an investigation of Tai Chi and computerized balance training. *J Am Geriatr Soc* 1996;44: 489–97

49. Alexander NB. Differential diagnosis of gait disorders in older adults. *Clin Geriatr Med* 1996;12:697–8

50. Visintin M, Barbeau H, Korner-Bitensky N, *et al*. A new approach to retrain gait in stroke patients through body weight support and treadmill stimulation. *Stroke* 1998;29:1122–8

# 12

# Cardiovascular disease in the geripause

*William P. Castelli*

## Introduction

Women pass through the menopause at about the age of 50 and begin a process that transforms their risk of atherosclerotic vascular diseases such as coronary heart disease, stroke, peripheral vascular disease, and other atherosclerotic vascular problems from a state where only those women who had the familial forms of hyperlipoproteinemia, or had diabetes and smoked, could get these diseases, to where eventually half the women will die from these diseases[1,2]. About 10–15 years later, the real start of the geripause, women have reached the same high rates of these diseases as men; 80% of the vascular disease in women occurs in women who are older than 60, with the highest rate obtained in the geripause. All of these diseases are preventable. Most of the women who live on this Earth will not get these diseases unless they migrate to America and adopt the American diet and exercise practices.

Of the women destined to get these measured diseases, 75% could be identified years in advance by having a simple set of numbers measured on their bodies. These numbers refer to the 'risk factors' such as the different kinds of cholesterol, high blood pressure, smoking, high blood sugar, excess weight, and many other measures described in this chapter[3].

In the geripause, 25% of women die when they have a heart attack; 75% live. Half the women who live have lost their normal ejection fractions and lose their jobs if they are still working, but especially reduce the quality of their lives. Ten per cent of those who have a stroke, die. Of the 90% who live, 75% have a residual neurological deficit. Many of these

chronically ill women populate our nursing homes. Most of this would be preventable.

Women have been involved in many trials to control risks such as their high cholesterol and blood pressure. Their responses have been as great as, if not greater than, those of men. Recent data described later in this chapter will reveal that, if some of these risks are treated, women will live longer, even if they are in their eighties. We can now fashion an algorithm of assessing and treating risk to improve the lives of older women.

## Blood lipids

Total cholesterol was the first lipid to rank women for risk of coronary heart disease (CHD), the most prevalent of the atherosclerotic vascular diseases. As Figure 1 shows, from the Framingham Heart Study, the higher the level of cholesterol, the higher the rate of CHD. The older the woman, the higher the absolute rate of disease, indicating that the more time the woman was exposed to the detrimental characteristics of the American life style, the higher the rate of these diseases. Multivariate adjustments for the major confounding factors do not explain away the impact of total cholesterol on risk[4].

Alas, as useful as the total cholesterol looks, one has to admit that the total cholesterol is not the critical factor. Figure 2 shows two bell-shaped curves: one, showing the total cholesterol of all the men and women of the Framingham Study who did not develop CHD in the first 26 years of the study, and the

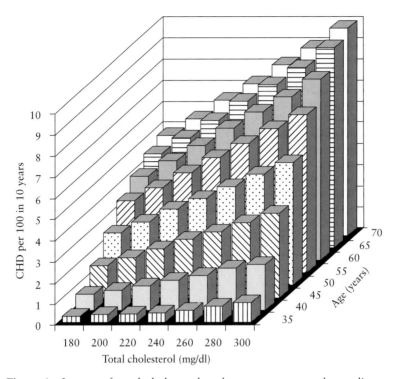

**Figure 1** Impact of total cholesterol and age on coronary heart disease (CHD) in women. From the Framingham Heart Study/National Heart, Lung and Blood Institute, Boston University School of Medicine. Reproduced with permission from Castelli WP. Cholesterol and lipids in the risk of coronary artery disease. The Framingham Heart Study. *Can J Cardiol* 1988;4(Suppl A): 5A–10A[4]

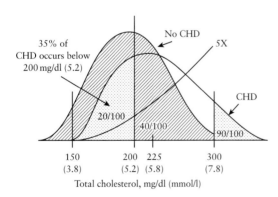

**Figure 2** Relative, absolute, and population-attributable risk fractions of men and women in the Framingham Heart Study who did not develop coronary heart disease (CHD) (leftbell-shaped curve) and those who did (right bell-shaped curve). Values in parentheses and mmol/l. Reproduced with permission from Castelli WP. Cholesterol and lipids in the risk of coronary artery disease. The Framingham Heart Study. *Can J Cardiol* 1988; 4(Suppl A):5A–10A[4]

second, showing the total cholesterol of all the men and women who did. Note that these curves overlap when the total cholesterol is between 150 mg/dl (3.8 mmol/l) and 300 mg/dl (7.8 mmol/l). This is roughly 90% of the total cholesterol in these individuals and it is impossible to tell whether a subject is on the curve to get a heart attack or on the curve to stay free. We understand three kinds of risk in medicine. The first is relative risk, and in Figure 2, it can be appreciated that the higher the cholesterol, the higher the heart attack rate; those at 300 mg/dl run five times the rate of those at 150 mg/dl. We understand absolute risk, the second kind of risk. Take the subjects who had a total cholesterol of 300 mg/dl or above: 90/100 developed CHD in the first 26 years of our study. If one treats people with a 300 mg/dl cholesterol, one knows that the chances of treating someone who did not need treatment is tiny. However, the risk we need to understand in the clinical

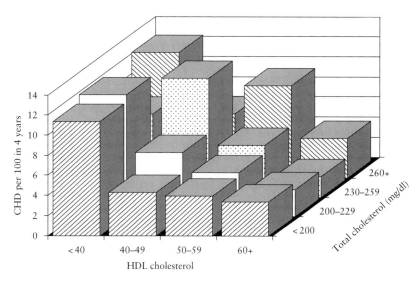

**Figure 3** Coronary heart disease (CHD) in men and women aged 50–59 in the Framingham Study according to total cholesterol and high-density lipoprotein (HDL) cholesterol. Reproduced with permission from Castelli WP, Garrison RJ, Wilson PWF, *et al*. Incidence of coronary heart disease and lipoprotein cholesterol levels. The Framingham Study. *J Am Med Assoc* 1986;256:2835–8[5]

sense has to do with the third kind of risk, that is the attributable fractions. What fraction of the patients who developed CHD had a cholesterol under 200 mg/dl (5.2 mmol/l)? In the Framingham study, 35% – twice as many as those who developed CHD from a cholesterol over 300 mg/dl. Then why have the guidelines suggesting a cholesterol under 200 mg/dl desirable? Because they focused on the absolute risk that was 20/100 but did not realize that it was 20/100 of 45% of the population, which is twice as many cases as 90/100 of 3% of the population. However, the dilemma is: how do you find the 20 out of 100 who will get the disease so you do not treat the 80 out of 100 not destined for such an outcome?

The total cholesterol is about 18 different kinds of cholesterol-containing particles in the blood. Seven of these particles are in the low-density lipoprotein (LDL) class. All are atherogenic as they rise in blood; the smaller, denser ones may be somewhat more atherogenic than the larger particles. Four of the 18 particles have more triglyceride than cholesterol. Two of these, the chylomicrons, which appear in our blood immediately after eating fat, and the large 'fluffy-puffy' very-low-density lipoproteins

(VLDL) that come out of the liver are not very atherogenic. However, the chylomicron remnants and the small dense beta VLDL are among the most atherogenic kinds of particles. About five of the particles fall into the high-density lipoprotein (HDL) class, and these are generally good for us, although there are some small dense HDL particles which are less protective. Figure 3 shows how to find the women with a total cholesterol under 200 mg/dl who are at high risk. They have a low HDL cholesterol. Note that, as one goes up the quartile of cholesterol values in Figure 3, one needs a higher and higher HDL cholesterol for protection[4].

Rather than have one remember a whole series of HDL cholesterols to go with a whole series of total cholesterols, once the total cholesterol reaches 150 mg/dl and goes beyond, make a simple ratio: the total cholesterol divided by the HDL cholesterol. This ratio, given its simplicity, is the best lipid predictor of CHD risk in the Framingham Heart Study[5], the Harvard Nurses Study, the Physicians Health Study, the Lipid Research Clinic Study, the 4S study, and virtually any study which took the time to measure it and compare it to total cholesterol, LDL cholesterol,

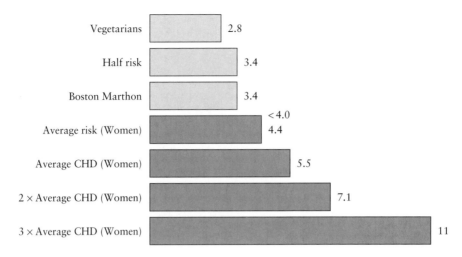

**Figure 4** Ratio of total cholesterol/high-density lipoprotein in women of the Framingham Heart Study. CHD, coronary heart disease. Adapted with permission from Castelli WP. Cholesterol and lipids in the risk of coronary artery disease. The Framingham Heart Study. *Can J Cardiol* 1988;4(Suppl A):5A–10A[4]

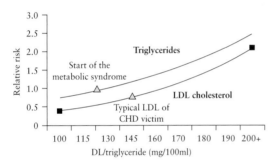

**Figure 5** Low-density lipoprotein (LDL) cholesterol and triglyceride trends in coronary heart disease (CHD)

**Table 1** Low-density lipoprotein (LDL) cholesterol and triglyceride levels for identifying types of hyperlipoproteinemia

| Age (years) | LDL (type II) | Triglycerides (type IV) |
| --- | --- | --- |
| 0–4 | | 96 |
| 5–9 | 125 | 90 |
| 10–14 | 126 | 114 |
| 15–19 | 127 | 107 |
| 20–24 | 136 | 112 |
| 25–29 | 141 | 116 |
| 30–34 | 142 | 123 |
| 35–39 | 161 | 137 |
| 40–44 | 164 | 155 |
| 45–49 | 173 | 171 |
| 50–54 | 192 | 186 |
| 55–59 | 204 | 204 |
| 60–64 | 201 | 202 |
| 65–69 | 208 | 204 |
| 70 | 189 | 204 |

triglyceride, or HDL cholesterol as discriminators of risk.

Figure 4 shows the relationship of the total/HDL ratio to risk in women. No one would want to be at the values of the average woman in America (4.5), since half of them die of this disease process; rather, we need to consider a more ideal ratio, where it would be difficult to get this disease, for example a ratio under 4[3].

The same thing could be said for the LDL cholesterol. The higher the LDL cholesterol rose in the Framingham Study, the higher the heart attack rate, as seen in Figure 5. However, as with the total cholesterol, one cannot interpret an LDL cholesterol unless one knows the patient's HDL cholesterol. When LDL levels reach the numbers by age in Table 1, those women almost always have an autosomal dominant genetic disorder producing premature atherosclerotic risk. These women need to be found at any age. Half of their children (and other first-degree blood relatives) need to be evaluated, since they risk inheriting these genes[6]. Women who develop CHD before they

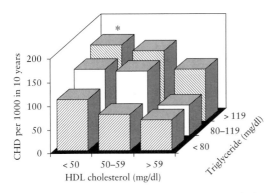

**Figure 6** High-density lipoprotein (HDL) cholesterol and triglyceride trends in coronary heart disease (CHD) in women in the Framingham Study *$p$ = 0.003. Reproduced with permission from Castelli WP. Cholesterol and lipids in the risk of coronary artery disease. The Framingham Heart Study. *Can J Cardiol* 1988;4(Suppl A):5A–10A[4]

**Table 2** Risk factors for coronary heart disease, from the Adult Treatment Program III

| |
| --- |
| Cigarette smoking |
| Hypertension (140/90) consider 120/80 |
| HDL < 40 mg/dl |
| Family history (first-degree relatives): under 55 for men and under 65 for women |
| Age 45 for men, 55 for women |

HDL, high-density lipoprotein

reach the age of 50 generally have one of these disorders; 85% will develop these diseases in the geripause.

As triglycerides rose in the Framingham Study the rate of coronary disease rose also, as seen in Figure 5. In multivariate analyses using the best epidemiological studies, triglyceride is an independent risk factor after adjusting for HDL[7]. Triglycerides cannot be interpreted unless one knows the patient's HDL cholesterol. As Figure 6 shows, it is important to find women who have a triglyceride level that is 120 mg/dl or higher when their HDL cholesterol is under 50 mg/dl. It is now felt that these women belong to a new syndrome called the metabolic syndrome. This begins in most women by adding weight to their abdomen, to where their waist size reaches 35 inches (89 cm) or beyond. They have hypertension defined as 130/85 or greater. They have blood sugars that reach 110 mg/dl because they have started to have insulin resistance. Many of these women have a total cholesterol under 200 and LDL cholesterol in the 120s and so are missed in American medicine. In addition to developing CHD at a high rate they run three times the rate of maturity-onset diabetes mellitus compared to their thinner cohorts[3,8].

The National Cholesterol Education Program has issued new guidelines for evaluating lipid risk in the Adult Treatment Program III[9]. Before one looks at the patient's LDL cholesterol one must calculate how many risk factors the patient has. One risk factor is counted for each defined in Table 2. Then one proceeds to Table 3. For example, if the woman only has one or no risk factors and no vascular disease, she has to have her LDL cholesterol put under 160 mg/dl. Therapeutic lifestyle changes (diet and exercise) are tried first; if they fail to lower the LDL under 160 mg/ml, drugs cannot be used to lower the LDL unless it is still over 190 mg/dl. In the next category, where the person has no disease, but two or more risk factors, the goal of therapy is an LDL under 130. If lifestyle changes do not succeed, one can treat with drugs only after downloading the Framingham Risk Calculator from www. nhlbi.nih.gov. Punch in the requested numbers and if the CHD risk is 10–19% in the next 10 years one can treat with drugs to reduce the LDL to under 130. If the Framingham Risk score is under 10% one should not treat with drugs unless the LDL is still 160 or higher. The third category are people with vascular disease of any sort (coronary, cerebral, peripheral vascular, etc.) or people who have what is now called a CHD Equivalent. There are two: diabetes mellitus or a risk score on the Framingham Risk calculator of 20% in the next 10 years. These patients have to have their LDL cholesterol reduced to under 100 mg/dl. Supposedly, if lifestyle does not succeed, drugs should be used for those at 130 or above. This author does not agree with these strategies, since, if 160, 130 and 100 are the goals, and one fails with diet and exercise, by all means

**Table 3** Adult Treatment Program III treatment guidelines. Adaptad from http://www.nhlbi.nih.gov

| Risk category | LDL goal (mg/dl) | TLC | Drug |
|---|---|---|---|
| CHD, or equivalent: 10-year risk > 20% | < 100 | ≥ 100 | ≥ 130 |
| 2+ risk factors: 10-year risk ≤ 20% | < 130 | ≥ 130 | 10 year ≥ 10–20%, >130; < 10%, ≥ 160 |
| 0–1 risk factors | < 160 | ≥ 160 | ≥ 190 |

LDL, low-density lipoprotein; TLC, therapeutic lifestyle changes; CHD, coronary heart disease
Metabolic syndrome, triglycerides: 150, waist men 40 inches (101 cm), women 35 inches (89 cm); high-density lipoprotein < 40, < 50; blood pressure 130/85; glucose ≥ 110

**Table 4** Goals and strategies, from the Framingham Cardiovascular Institute

| No further progression (mg/dl) | Regression (mg/dl) |
|---|---|
| LDL < 110 (< 130) | LDL < 80 |
| TC/HDL < 4 | triglycerides < 90 |
| Triglycerides < 120 | TC/HDL < 3 |

LDL, low-density lipoprotein; TC, total cholesterol; HDL, high-density lipoprotein

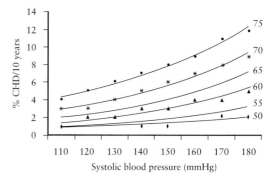

**Figure 7** Systolic blood pressure and the risk of coronary heart disease (CHD) in women. Low risk: no smoking of cigarettes, no diabetes mellitus and average lipids. From the Framingham Heart Study. Adapted from the Framingham Risk Calculator: www.nhlbi.nih.gov

one should go to drug therapy. I am also not in favor of reducing someone's LDL to just under 160 when the average LDL cholesterol of someone who develops CHD is in the 140s, and this number is even lower for women in the geripause.

The Framingham Cardiovascular Institute uses two sets of numbers as goals (Table 4). One set is for primary prevention. These are more ideal values destined to reduce the level of these diseases in most of the people who did not get this disease in the Framingham Study and many of the trials. They are an LDL under 110 mg/dl, a total cholesterol/HDL ratio under 4, and a triglyceride under 120 mg/dl. For people with disease, or diabetes, or the Framingham Risk score of 20%, it is an LDL under 80 mg/dl and a triglyceride under 90 and total/HDL ratio under 3. These are the numbers of the billions of people who cannot get these diseases who live in Asia, Africa, and Latin America, usually outside the big cities, and who are poor.

## Blood pressure

Blood pressure rises with age only in those countries where the inhabitants eat a high-salt diet. Almost half of people in the USA are hypertensive, defined as 140/90 mmHg or higher by the time they reach their fifties. By the time one reaches the geripause it is near 75%. Framingham was one of the first studies to show that the elderly did not tolerate high blood pressure (Figure 7). It was taught, prior to the evidence from the Framingham Study, that the elderly needed a higher pressure because their arteries contained many fat blockages and a higher pressure was needed to maintain perfusion. People were told that their systolic pressure should be 100 plus their age.

**Table 5** 12-year coronary heart disease incidence according to blood pressure category in women ($n$ = 227)

| Blood pressure category | Person years | Events % | Relative odds with 95% CI |
|---|---|---|---|
| Normal 120–129/80–84 mmHg | 20710 | 29% | 1 |
| High normal 130–139/85–89 mmHg | 6043 | 16% | 1.31 (0.86–1.99) |
| Hypertension stage I 140/90 mmHg | 7242 | 32% | 1.78 (1.19–2.51) |
| Hypertension stage II–IV | 4000 | 23% | 2.12 (1.42–3.17) |
| Total | 37995 | | |

This was also the period when one looked only at the diastolic pressure to decide whether the patient had hypertension. Then, they were told that they had a disease only if some organ in their body showed damage from the high pressure, such as a hemorrhage in the fundus of the eye, or left ventricular hypertrophy or a shrinking kidney (target organ damage). The Framingham Study showed that only in the very young did diastolic pressure out-predict the systolic pressure. Furthermore, the older one got, both the absolute and relative risk increased with age. In the geripause, one begins to see a fall in the diastolic pressure such that the difference between the systolic and the diastolic pressures, or what is called the pulse pressure, becomes one of the better predictors of risk. Table 5 shows that half of the coronary risk occurs in people with systolic pressures between 120 and 139 mmHg and diastolic pressures between 80 and 89. Ideal pressure is therefore under 120/80. If the pulse pressure reaches 60 or higher, the patient will require therapy. Genrally this means lowering the systolic pressure, since the diastolic pressure is already low.

## Cigarettes

In the early data from the Framingham Study, cigarettes were a very modest risk in women, because they did not inhale. For example, lung cancer in the 1940s in the USA in women was, of the major cancers, almost dead last. Unfortunately, women learned to inhale in the 1950s and by 1987 lung cancer crossed breast cancer and became the number one cause of cancer death in women as it had been in men since the appropriate data were collected.

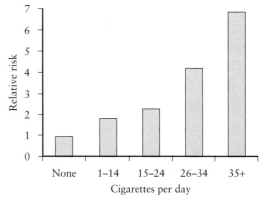

**Figure 8** Cigarette smoking and risk of myocardial infarction in women. Adapted with permission from Rosenberg L, Palmer JR, Shapiro S. Decline in risk of myocardial infarction among women who stop smoking. *N Engl J Med* 1990;322:213–17[10]

Every third woman who smokes dies of lung cancer. Of course, for every woman who dies prematurely of lung cancer there are two women who have developed premature vascular complications. Figure 8 from Rosenberg and colleagues shows that the risk of myocardial infarction is dose-related, rising from a relative risk of 2 for 1–14 cigarettes per day to 7.2 for 35 or more[10]. Add to this all the chronic lung diseases from emphysema to complex chronic bronchitis, and bladder, breast, stomach, and laryngeal cancer and one wonders how anyone could be allowed to see cigarettes at all. More women smoke than men now. Aggressive programs that incorporate behavior modification, nicotine patches, sprays, gums, and nicotine cigarette holder devices can be very successful in reducing the risk in women. Quitting returns the risk in the Rosenberg data

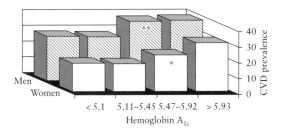

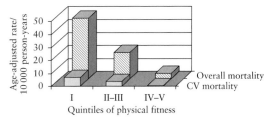

**Figure 9** Hemoglobin $A_{1c}$ and cardiovascular disease in the Framingham Heart Study. *$p < 0.004$; **$p < 0.001$. Reproduced with permission from Singer DE, Nathan DM, Anderson KM, *et al.* Association of HbA1c with prevalent cardiovascular disease in the original cohort of the Framingham Heart Study. *Diabetes* 1992;41:202–8[33]

**Figure 12** Cardiovascular (CV) and overall mortality in women according to exercise, in the Cooper Clinic. Reproduced with permission from Blair SN, Kohl HW III, Paffenbarger RS, *et al.* Physical fitness and all cause mortality. A prospective study of healthy men and women. *J Am Med Assoc* 1989;262:2395–401[15]

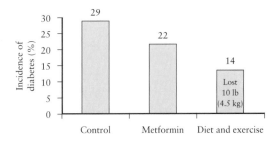

**Figure 10** Development of type 2 diabetes in 3 years, in 3234 obese subjects with impaired glucose tolerance (45% minorities). From the Diabetes Prevention Program of the National Institute of Diabetes, Digestive and Kidney Diseases. Adapted from Diabetes Prevention Program Research Group. Reduction in the incidence of type 2 diabetes with lifestyle intervention of metformin. *N Engl J Med* 2002;346:393–403[13]

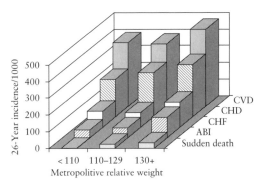

**Figure 11** Metropolitan relative weight and 26-year incidence/1000 of sudden death, atherothrombotic brain infarction (ABI), congestive heart failure (CHF), coronary heart disease (CHD) and cardiovascular disease (CVD). From the Framingham Heart Study

to that of non-smokers in 3 years. In the Framingham Study, where a quit smoker was defined as a person who had quit for an entire year, the risk fell to that of non-smokers in 1 year.

## Diabetes mellitus

As weight has steadily risen since the early 1980s when more systematic surveys were started in the USA, the rate of diabetes has increased with obesity defined as a body mass index (BMI) of 30 or greater to where, in the year 2000, 19.8% of Americans were obese and 7.3% had diabetes mellitus[11]. In 1997 the American Diabetes Association changed the guidelines for diagnosing diabetes. After a glucose tolerance test, impaired glucose intolerance was 140–199 mg/dl and diabetes was 200 or higher. For fasting glucose, impaired fasting glucose is 110–125 mg/dl and diabetes is 126 or higher[12]. Goals of therapy have been given as hemoglobin $A_{1c}$. There are three: under 8, 7 or 6. Consider Figure 9 from the Framingham Study. One starts with a healthy population and sees how they do by measures of hemoglobin $A_{1c}$. Getting to 5.5 is not good. The fasting blood sugar is over 100 mg/dl, where they are running a higher risk of vascular disease and onset of diabetes mellitus. Diabetes is the number-one cause of blindness, renal dialysis and neuritis. The most recently completed trial to prevent diabetes (Figure 10) showed that

(a)

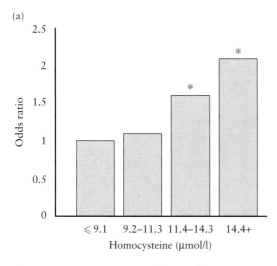

(b)

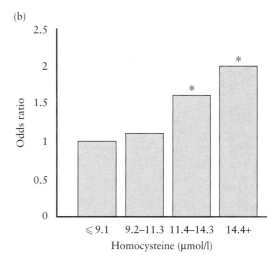

**Figure 13** Homocysteine and carotid artery stenosis: (a) adjusted for age and sex; and (b) adjusted for age, sex, total cholesterol/high-density lipoprotein, cigarette smoking and systolic blood pressure. *significant 95% CI. Adapted with permission from Selhub J, Jacques PF, Bostom AG, *et al.* Association between plasma homocysteine and carotid stenosis. *N Engl J Med* 1995;332:286–91[16]

weight loss actually did better than metformin which did better than nothing, especially in high-risk groups such as Native Americans, African-Americans, Hispanics and Asians[13]. Indeed, a weight loss of over 7 lb (3 kg) resulted in a 14% incidence of diabetes in about 3 years compared to 22% on metformin and 29% in the control group, where those who had lost weight had gained most of it back in the next 3 years.

## Weight

Weight continues to rise in America evey year. In the past decade we went from no states with 20% obesity to more than a quarter of the states. Weight gain from age 25 in the Framingham Study was associated with rises in most of the major risk factors such as unfavourable blood lipids and fall in the favourable HDL. Blood pressure, diabetes, uric acid, left ventricular hypertrophy, all rose. This results in increased rates of all the cardiovascular diseases, especially coronary and cerebral diseases. Sudden death and heart failure have all risen, as seen in Figure 11. Obesity is an independent risk factor[14]. With 7% of the

world's population living in the USA, Americans consume 40% of the food. Sloth and gluttony reign.

## Exercise

All the studies performed so far in America have shown that those who exercise the most develop the lowest rates of vascular disease and die at the slowest rates. The evidence from the Cooper Clinic has demostrated that total and cardiovascular death fell as exercise increased in women (Figure 12)[15]. Cancer deaths also fell. The lowest rates in this figure can be obtained with a 30-minute/day program. The trade-off for calories by exercise is unfair. Walking a mile burns off about 100 cal; an American candy bar takes 2.5 miles. It takes about 35 miles to work off 1 lb (0.45 kg).

## Homocysteine

Homocysteine is an amino acid that may be associated with too high an ingestion of animal protein. It is also higher in people with renal failure. Hyperhomocysteinemia is a recessive

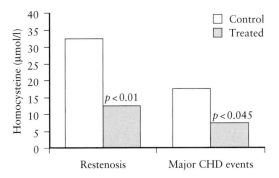

**Figure 14** Restenosis and major coronary heart disease (CHD) events after 6-months' treatment of homocysteine (folic acid 1 mg, vitamin $B_{12}$ 400 µg, pyridoxine 10 mg). Homocysteine fell from 11.1 to 7.2 µmol/l. Adapted with permission from Schnyder G, Roffi M, Pin R, *et al*. Decreased rate of coronary restenosis after lowing of plasma homocysteine levels. *N Engl J Med* 2001;345:1539–1600[17]

**Table 6** Coronary heart disease and electrocardiogram abnormalities in women. From the Framingham Heart Study/National Heart, Lung and Blood Institute, Boston University School of Medicine

| | *Relative odds* |
|---|---|
| Non-specific ST-T wave | 1.92 |
| Left ventricular hypertrophy | 3.22 |
| Atrial fibrillation | 2.7 |
| Right bundle branch block | 3.1 |
| Left bundle branch block | 4.2 |
| +ST segment/+recovery loop | 4.7 |

trait; children who are homozygous with a gene from each parent have values usually over 100 µmol/l, and they develop atherosclerotic disease as teenagers and even as children. Until the discoveries by Dr Kilmer S McCully, lower values of homocysteine were not thought to be important. As Figure 13 shows 40% of the participants in the Framingham Study had elevated homocysteine which was associated with increased carotid artery stenosis. They went on to eventually develop higher stroke rates, heart attack rates and death[16]. These people had low levels of vitamin $B_6$ and folic acid in their blood. The therapy for high homocysteine is eating smaller portions of meat, and taking adequate amounts of folic acid and vitamins $B_{12}$ and $B_6$. Lately, high amounts of a methyl donor such as trimethylglycine have proved effective. As of November 2001 about 17 trials were underway to see whether treating homocysteine could lower vascular disease rates. The first major trial to show this was a co-operative trial to try to prevent coronary restenosis after angioplasty. As shown in Figure 14 they achieved an almost 50% fall in restenosis and vascular disease rates in about 6 months of therapy[17]. The goals of therapy are still under debate. In the Framingham Study it would appear that under 9 µmol/l would be good; there are others who insist that under 7 is better.

## Electrocardiographic and echocardiographic findings

First-degree atrioventricular block, atrial premature beats, and isolated late cycle premature ventricular beats of less than one per hour, were not associated with increased risk in the Framingham Study. As Table 6 shows, non-specific ST-T waves, left ventricular hypertrophy, atrial fibrillation, right and left bundle branch block, +ST segment/+recovery loop all carry significant increased risk of CHD. Echocardiographic left ventricular hypertropy is more common than electrocardiographic hypertrophy and brings significant risk. Mitral valve prolapse was overstated in early studies of the heart, but with better criteria it is present in 2–3% of women.

## C-reactive protein

The Harvard Nurse's Study has supplied us with the best view of C-reactive protein in women. Overall, the women who developed cardiovascular disease had a higher C-reactive protein than the control group, at $p = 0.0001$. The subjects with the highest levels of C-reactive protein had a relative risk of 4.8 (95% CI 2.3–10.1) for any vascular event. For myocardial infarction and stroke the relative risk was 7.3 (95% CI 2.7–19.9)[18]. Aspirin lowers C-reactive protein and in the Physicians Health Study lowered rates of disease. Atorvastatin, simvastatin and pravastatin all lower C-reactive protein.

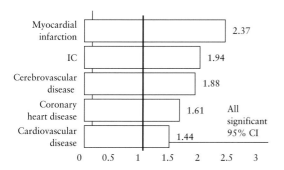

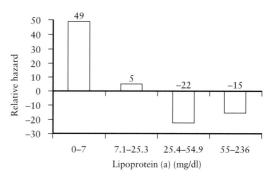

**Figure 15** Reduced pre-β lipoprotein (a) in women in the Framingham Heart Study. Relative odds adjusted for age, body mass index, systolic blood pressure, cigarette smoking, high-density and low-density lipoprotein, glucose and electrocardiographic left ventricular hypertrophy. Reproduced with permission from Bostom AG, Gagnon DR, Cupples LA, *et al.* A prospective investigation of elevated lipoprotein (a) detected by electrophoresis and cardiovascular disease in women. The Framingham Heart Study. *Circulation* 1994;90:1688–95[19]

**Figure 16** Relative hazard of non-fatal myocardial infarction, coronary heart disease or death, when women are treated with estrogen–progestin according to the level of lipoprotein (a). Interaction trend: $p = 0.03$. Adapted from Singer DE, Nathan DM, Anderson KM, *et al.* Association of HbA1c with prevalent cardiovascular disease in the original cohort of the Framingham Heart Study. *Diabetes* 1992;41:202–8[33]

## Lipoprotein (a)

Lipoprotein (a) (Lp(a)) is an LDL particle combined with the little 'a' protein that blocks the conversion of plasminogen to plasmin, which in turn dissolves the fibrin that is deposited on endothelial cells. Apparently we live in this drizzle of platelets clumping and unclumping and fibrinogen being converted to fibrin all day long. When the fibrin hits an endothelial cell it sends tissue-type plasminogen activator to convert plasminogen to plasmin, to dissolve the fibrin. Figure 15 represents one of the first studies in women to show that this is a risk factor for virtually all forms of atherosclerotic cardiovascular disease[19]. So far the only trial to lower Lp(a) and lower cardiac risk is the Heart, Estrogen/progestin Replacement Study (HERS), where, with an Lp(a) of 30 mg/dl or higher, benefit was achieved only from being on estrogen (Figure 16)[34]. The only other drug that has been used with some success to lower Lp(a) is niacin. So far in our clinic it has required doses of 1000–2000 µg for an appropriate effect.

## Clotting factors

In the early 1980s we learned that a blood clot came with virtually every myocardial infarction when we did an angiogram at the very time the heart attack was occuring. Estrogen given at very high doses in early birth control pills led to marked arterial clotting. As the dose of estrogen has come down, there has been less clotting, but good evidence is lacking as to what would be the ideal dose of estrogen, since there is still appreciable clotting occuring on the venous side, even with current birth control pills. Table 7 from Rosendaal gives a short list of clotting factors and their prevalence in the general population and patients with thrombosis[20]. Leiden factor V, high factor VIII and high homocysteine are very prevalent. The question remains unanswered whether any of these and perhaps some of the rarer ones play a role in the early events described in the estrogen trials.

## Other risk factors

No increase in risk has been found for coffee ingestion, hours of sleep, marital status or area of town in the Framingham Study. Number of pregnancies, white blood cell count, fibrinogen, high pulse rate, low pulse rate, low pulse variability, serum amyloid antigen, positive family history, and some forms of stress are all associated with higher risk.

**Table 7** Prevalence of risk factors for thrombosis. Adapted from reference 20

| Risk factor | % General population | % Patients with thrombosis |
|---|---|---|
| Protein C deficiency | 0.2–0.4 | 3 |
| Protein S deficiency | not known | 1–2 |
| Antithrombin deficiency | 0.02 | 1 |
| Factor V Leiden | 5 | 20 |
| Prothrombin 20210A | 2 | 6 |
| High factor VIII (> 1500 IU/l) | 11 | 25 |
| Homocysteine > 18.5 µmol/l | 5 | 10 |

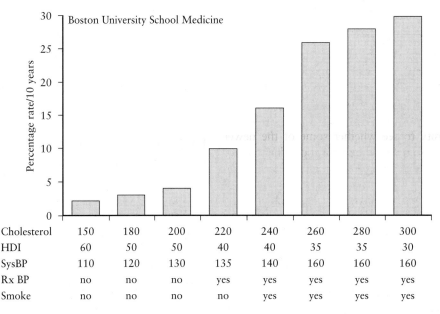

**Figure 17** Risk fo coranary heart disease according to multiple risk factors. HDL, high density lipoprotein cholesterol; Sus BP; systolic blood pressure; Rx BP, treatment for high blood pressure; smoke, smoking cigarettes

## Multiple risk factors

Diabetes has been taken out of the Framingham Risk Calculator because all by itself it represents such a high degree of risk that one must treat the patient as if they have already had a heart attack. The same can now be said for left ventricular hypertrophy. What is left are the remaining risks that need to be added up in the risk calculator. Figure 17 shows a range of factors with women at different levels of risk.

## Estrogen

Estrogen falls at the menopause and women go from a state where they could develop atherosclerotic lesions only with great difficulty and usually with the help of genetic factors to where 10 years later they have caught up with men. In animal studies where controls are tightest, estrogen protects cynomolgus macaques – with 98% of our genome[21] – from atherosclerosis. The use of estrogen is a double-edged sword. At any dose it appears antiatherogenic but at almost all the doses used so far, in some women, it is prothrombotic. At high doses, such as the 2.5 and 3.5 mg of conjugated estrogen taken by the Framingham women at the menopause, it increases the rate of heart attack and stroke[22]. These rates occurred in the Harvard Nurses Study only in women on over

1.25 mg of conjugated estrogen. Men given estrogen at 2.5 mg in the Coronary Drug Project died at such a high rate that the estrogen arm was stopped prematurely[23]. Lower doses have not been fully tested, but 5μg of ethinylestradiol in the Chart study provided the same osteoporosis protection as higher doses[24]. Prospective epidemiology studies show that women on hormone replacement therapy have about half the vascular disease rate as women not treated. In the Harvard Nurse's Study they found the same small increase in vascular disease the first years but then rates fell by half and this has persisted for 20 years[25]. Contrast this with the HERS, where the higher rate of vascular disease occurred in the first year but by years 4 and 5 the rates were 33% lower than the control group, which is better than some of the weaker statin trials. Unfortunately, the HERS trial missed an opportunity to see whether some of the newer clotting factors would explain the higher risk of clotting in the first year. In a similar fashion the Women's Health Initiative has not reported on whether any of the clotting factors were associated with a higher rate of vascular complications. It has stopped the combined use of conjugated estrogen/medroxyprogesterone because of a higher rate of CHD (RR 1.29, 95% CI 1.02–1.63), invasive breast cancer (RR 1–1.59), stroke (RR 1.41, 95%CI 1.07–1.85), and pulmonary embolus (RR 2.13, 95% CI 1.39–3.25)[35]. Colorectal cancer and hip fracture were significantly reduced. In the ERA trial[36], using conjugated estrogen/medroxyprogesterone in women with CHD, no benefit was found in reducing coronary atherosclerosis as viewed by coronary angiography. However, in women without CHD, β-estradiol at 1 mg in the EPAT trial[37] looking at carotid intima-media thickness, estrogen reduced the intimal thickening significantly better than placebo and about the same as statin therapy. Estrogen raises HDL cholesterol and lowers LDL cholesterol. It decreases fibrinogen as shown in the Postmenopausal Estrogen/ Progestin Intervention (PEPI) study[26].

The advantages of estrogen, at appropriate doses, continue to be elucidated by new research. Eskin and colleagues have recently proposed a series of new mechanisms by which estrogen provides benefit. In addition to the aforementioned effects on lipids, there are antioxidant effects, including: cardiac estrogen α and β receptors in mice, which could prevent vascular injury and necorosis; stabilization of the norepinephrine release mechanism in the heart; an increase in endothelium-mediated blood flow through enhancement of nitric oxide and improved coronary vasodilatation; a reduction in coronary artery vasoconstriction via a reduction in endothelin-1; and inhibition of platelet aggregation and stimulation of vasodiliatation by an increase in prostacylin production[27]. For now, women with high Lp(a) definitely need to be on estrogen; non-smokers and possibly women without any of the major new clotting factors could benefit.

## Know your numbers!

Life is a game of numbers. By following one generation of Framingham subjects for over 50 years and a second for over 30 years, we have come to appreciate what some of the numbers should be to be ideal. If your total cholesterol is over 150 mg/dl you need to have your total cholestorel/HDL ratio under 4 and your LDL cholestorel under 110; your triglycerides need to be under 120 mg/dl; blood pressure is best under 120/80; blood sugar needs to be under 100 and the hemoglobin $A_{1c}$ under 5.5; cigarettes need to be at zero; homocysteine under 9; waist/hip ratio needs to be under 0.8; Lp(a) needs to be under 20 mg/dl; you need to walk 2 miles per day; eat less than 15 g of saturated fat and less than 200 mg of cholesterol; eat small portions of low-fat meat laced with at least five servings of vegetables and two of fruits; eliminate white flour for whole grains; and keep calories in line with your exercise program.

For people with disease trying for reversibility, the LDL must be under 80 and the triglycerides under 90. Total fat should be under 40 g and saturated fat under 10 g a day. Cholesterol intake should be under 100 mg.

## Treatment

Taking all the diet trials to date, the better one lowers the serum cholesterol the better one lowers the heart attack rate. One new issue in the diet is the intake of ω-3 fatty acids. Two fish and two α-linolenic trials have lowered total death and vascular disease rates dramatically. The drug trials have now shown that with the arrival of the statin drugs many more people can achieve the goal of therapy, and for people with high triglycerides the use of combinations of statins with niacin and fibrates allow excellent control of the elevated triglyceride. Over 10 000 women have participated in these trials and they generally do better than the men. For a given 1% fall in cholesterol they sometimes show as much as a 4% fall in vascular disease. Discharge from a hospital in Salt Lake City on a statin versus nothing in 7220 persons after a vascular event lowered the total death rate to one-third that of the control group[28], and this occurred even in people over 80 years of age, and it all happened within 3.3 years! The British Heart Protection Study showed that people treated with a statin who are over 75 get just as much benefit as people treated at a younger age[29].

By the late 1970s in the USA the Hypertension Detection and Follow-up Program (HDFP)[30] showed that lowering blood pressure in women improved their outcomes; this was followed by similar benefit in England in the Medical Research Council trial[31]. More recently, for the geripause group the Systolic Hypertension in the Elderly (SHEP) study, treating isolated systolic hypertension, has lowered their stroke rate by 38%[32].

## Conclusion

The average man or woman, at any age, destined to develop a cardiovascular disease, should not be a mystery to them or their physician. Had someone measured a few simple numbers on their bodies they could have been identified many years in advance of their developing disease. Those numbers could be treated starting with diet and exercise and followed by drugs where necessary. About 20–25% of women in the geripause will die when they get a heart attack and about 10% will die from their stroke. Of the people who live after a heart attack, half will lose their normal ejection fraction and, with reduced pumping ability of their heart, many will end up in a nursing home for the rest of their lives. Of the people who live after a stroke, 75% have a neurological residual that damages the quality of their lives. Now we know that therapy not only prolongs their life but preserves the quality of their lives, which in many respects is just as important.

# References

1. Gordon T, Kannel WB, Hortland MC, McNamara PM. Menopause and coronary heart disease. *Ann Intern Med* 1978;89:157–61
2. Lloyd-Jones DM, Larson MG, Beiser A, Levy D. Lifetime risk of developing coronary heart disease. *Lancet* 1999;335:89–92
3. Wilson PWF. Coronary heart disease prediction. *Am J Hypertens* 1994;7:75–125
4. Castelli WP. Cholesterol and lipids in the risk of coronary artery disease. The Framingham Heart Study. *Can J Cardiol* 1988;4(Suppl A):5A–10A
5. Castelli WP, Garrison RJ, Wilson PWF, *et al.* Incidence of coronary heart disease and lipoprotein cholesterol levels. The Framingham Study. *J Am Med Assoc* 1986;256:2835–8
6. Schaefer EJ, Levy RI. Pathogenesis and management of lipoprotein disorders. *N Engl J Med* 1985;312:1300
7. Hokanson JE, Austin MA. Plasma triglyceride level is a risk factor for cardiovascular disease independent of high-density lipoprotein cholesterol level: a meta-analysis of population-based prospective studies. *J Cardiovasc Risk* 1996;3: 213–19
8. Grundy SM. Hypertriglyceridemia, atherogenic dyslipidemia and the metabolic syndrome. *Am J Cardiol* 1998;81:18–25B
9. Executive Summary of the Third Report of the National Cholesterol Education Program (NCEP) Expert Panel on Detection, Evaluation, and Treatment of High Blood cholesterol in Adults (Adult Treatment panel III). *J Am Med Assoc* 2001;285:2486–97
10. Rosenberg L, Palmer JR, Shapiro S. Decline in risk of myocardial infarction among women who stop smoking. *N Engl J Med* 1990;322:213–17
11. Mokdad AH, Bowman BA, Ford ES, *et al.* The continuing epidemics of obesity and diabetes in the United States. *J Am Med Assoc* 2001;286: 1195–200

12. Report of the Expert Committee on the Diagnosis and Classification of Diabetes Mellitus. *Diabetes Care* 1997;20:1183–97

13. Diabetes Prevention Program Research Group. Reduction in the incidence of type 2 diabetes with lifestyle intervention of metformin. *N Engl J Med* 2002;346:393–403

14. Hubert HB, Feinleib M, McNamara P, Castelli WP. Obesity as an independent risk factor for cardiovascular disease; a 26 year follow-up of participants in the Framingham Heart Study. *Circulation* 1983;67:768–77

15. Blair SN, Kohl HW III, Paffenbarger RS, *et al.* Physical fitness and all cause mortality. A prospective study of healthy men and women. *J Am Med Assoc* 1989;262:2395–401

16. Selhub J, Jacques PF, Bostom AG, *et al.* Association between plasma homocysteine and carotid stenosis. *N Engl J Med* 1995;332:286–91

17. Schnyder G, Roffi M, Pin R, *et al.* Decreased rate of coronary restenosis after lowing of plasma homocysteine levels. *N Engl J Med* 2001;345:1539–1600

18. Ridker PM, *et al.* Prospective study of C-reactive protein and risk of future cardiovascular events among apparently healthy women. *Circulation* 1998;98:731–3

19. Bostom AG, Gagnon DR, Cupples LA, *et al.* A prospective investigation of elevated lipoprotein (a) detected by electrophoresis and cardiovascular disease in women. The Framingham Heart Study. *Circulation* 1994;90:1688–95

20. Rosendaal FR. Venous thrombosis: a multicausal disease. *Lancet* 1999;353:1167–73

21. Clarkson TB, Adams MR, Kaplan JR, *et al.* From menarche to menopause: coronary artery atherosclerosis and protection in cynomolgus monkeys. *Am J Obstet Gynecol* 1989;160:1280–5

22. Wilson PWF, Garrison RJ, Castelli WP. Postmenopausal estrogen use, cigarette smoking and cariovascular morbidity in women over 50. The Framingham Study. *N Engl J Med* 1985;313:1038–43

23. Canner PL, Berge KG, Wenger NK, *et al.* Fifteen year mortality in Conronary Drug Project patients: long-term benefit with niacin. *J Am Coll Cardiol* 1986;8:1245–55

24. Speroff L, *et al.*, for the CHART group. The comparative effect of bone density, endometrium and lipids of continuous hormones as replacement therapy (CHART study). A randomized control trial. *J Am Med Assoc* 1996;276:1397–408

25. Grodstein F, Stampfer MJ, Colditz GA, *et al.* Postmenopausal hormone therapy and mortality. *N Engl J Med* 1997;336:1769–75

26. The Writing Group of the PEPI Trial. Effects of estrogen or estrogen/progestin regimens on heart disease risk factors in postmenopausal women. *J Am Med Assoc* 1995;273:199–208

27. Eskin BA, Synder DL, Gayheart P, Roberts J. The protective effect of estrogen on the cardiac adrenergic nervous system. In *Cardiovascular Disease in Women*. Dallas, TX: American Heart Association, 1997:23–30

28. Muhlestein JB, Horne BD, Bair TL, *et al.* Very elderly individuals with severe coronary artery disease also benefit from statin therapy. *Circulation* 2001;194:abstract 2841

29. Heart Protection Study Collaborative Group. MRC/BHF Heart Protection Study of Cholesterol lowering with simvastatin in 20,536 high-risk individuals: a randomized placebo-controlled trial. *Lancet* 2002;360:7–22

30. Hypertension Detection and Follow-Up Program Cooperative Group. Five-year findings of the hypertension detection and follow-up program. I. Reduction in mortality of persons with high blood pressure, including mild hypertension. *J Am Med Assoc* 1979;242:2562

31. Medical Research Council Working Party. MRC trial of treatment of mild hypertension; principal results. *Br Med J* 1985;219:97

32. SHEP Cooperative Research Group. Prevention of stroke by antihypertensive drug treatment in older persons with isolated systolic hypertension; final results of the Systolic Hypertension in the Elderly Program (SHEP). *J Am Med Assoc* 1991;265:3255

33. Singer DE, Nathan DM, Anderson KM, *et al.* Association of $HbA_{1c}$ with prevalent cardiovascular disease in the original cohort of the Framingham Heart Study. *Diabetes* 1992;41:202–8

34. Shlipak MG, Simon JA, Vittinghoff F, *et al.* Estrogen and progestin, lipoprotein(a), and the risk of recurrent coronary heart disease events after menopause. *J Am Med Assoc* 2000;283:1845–52

35. Writing Group for the Women's Health Initiative Investigators. Risks and benefits of estrogen plus progestin in healthy post-menopausal women. *J Am Med Assoc* 2002;288:321–33

36. Herrinton DM, Rebousian DM, Brosnekan KB, *et al.* Effects of estrogen replacement on the progression of coronary-artery atherosclerosis. *N Engl J Med* 2000;313:522–9

37. Hodis HN, Mack WJ, Lobo RA, *et al.* Estrogen in the prevention of atherosclerosis. A randomized, double-blind, placebo-controlled trial. *Ann Intern Med* 2001;735:939–53

# 13

# Osteoporosis

*Bruce R. Troen, Angela M. Inzerillo and Mone Zaidi*

## Introduction

Osteoporosis, one of the leading causes of serious morbidity and functional loss in old age, was once thought to be a natural part of the aging process. Although, at times, it is difficult to distinguish between the disease and normal skeletal aging *per se* in the clinical approach to osteoporosis management, progress in the scientific understanding of the underlying disease process has made it largely a preventable disease. Defining the point at which these age-related skeletal changes require intervention presents a major challenge to researchers and clinicians alike, since there is a long latent period of bone loss before the onset of clinically apparent disease. While current diagnostic procedures have been shown to distinguish those at risk of fracture from those not at risk, there is a large overlap in bone density between persons who fracture and persons who do not. Fortunately, the demographic revolution resulting in increasing numbers of elderly at high risk for osteoporosis has impelled the recent rapid development in better diagnostic tools and therapeutic modalities to treat this disorder.

Osteoporosis is a skeletal disorder where bone strength is compromised due to loss of bone density and a decline in the quality of bone. Osteoporosis is due, in large part, to an uncoupling of bone formation and resorption. There is an absolute osteoclast overactivity (possibly with increased numbers of cells) in *high-turnover* osteoporosis, including type I primary osteoporosis, also known as postmenopausal osteoporosis. In contrast, in *low-turnover* osteoporosis, as occurs with type II primary osteoporosis seen with aging (also known as involutional or senile osteoporosis), bone formation lags behind resorption; hence, the rate of resorption is relatively higher than that of formation, with net bone loss. Osteoporosis is characterized not only by low bone mass, but also by microarchitectural deterioration of bone tissue with a consequent increase in bone fragility and susceptibility to fractures[1]. The bone mass of an individual depends not only on the amount lost as a function of hormonal status and age, but also upon the peak bone mass attained during growth and development. Thus, osteoporosis and attendant fractures can occur either when there is a failure to reach peak bone mass or when resorption exceeds formation after peak bone mass is achieved (Figure 1). Other factors could contribute to osteoporosis. Aging is associated with a number of disorders of vitamin D metabolism as well as with diminished intestinal calcium absorption. Dietary calcium also decreases with age, further exacerbating this calcium-deficient state. It is important to clarify the difference between osteoporosis and osteomalacia. Osteoporosis results from abnormalities in bone remodelling, whereas osteomalacia results from defects in bone mineralization due to calcium deficiency.

Secondary osteoporosis due to conditions other than aging or menopause arises from a variety of causes (Table 1). The most common of these is hypercortisolism, endogenous as in Cushing's syndrome, or more commonly iatrogenic secondary to chronic glucocorticoid administration. Osteoporosis induced by

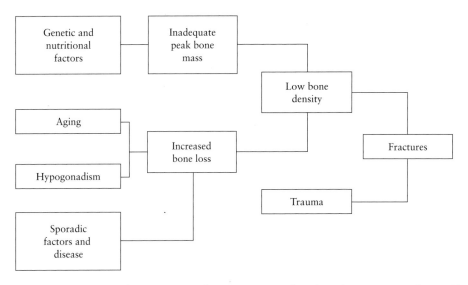

**Figure 1** Pathophysiology of osteoporotic fractures. Reproduced with permission from Olson RE. Osteoporosis and vitamin K intake. *Am J Clin Nutr* 2000;71:1031–2, © *Am J Clin Nutr*. American Society for Clinical Nutrition

glucocorticoid excess is characterized by decreased bone formation, causing an increase in resorption and bone loss. Trabecular bone (which is most predominant in the lumbar spine) is more affected than cortical bone. Decreased bone formation results from reduced osteoblast proliferation, reduced bone matrix protein secretion, and increased apoptosis. In addition, there is often a negative calcium balance due to decreased gastrointestinal calcium absorption and increased urinary calcium loss. Secondary hyperparathyroidism can ensue with a further increase in net bone resorption. Steroids may also induce hypogonadotropic hypogonadism, further aggravating bone loss. Another common cause of secondary osteoporosis is hyperthyroidism. In hyperthyroidism, similar to postmenopausal osteoporosis, there is increased bone remodelling with resorption exceeding formation and hence, net bone loss. This is mostly reversible with treatment of the hyperthyroid state. Postmenopausal women with significant hyperthyroidism are at the greatest risk, because they have increased bone loss and fracture risk. This category also includes women on suppressive doses of levothyroxine for the treatment of thyroid diseases. Additional common causes of secondary osteoporosis

include hyperparathyroidism, hypogonadism, immobilization (commonly due to stroke), nutritional deficiency, alcoholism, and immunosuppressive treatment.

## Epidemiology

Osteoporosis is the most common bone disease. The prevalence of low bone mass is dependent on a number of variables, including the study population examined, diagnostic thresholds, densitometric techniques, and the skeletal sites measured. The prevalence of low bone mass increases with increasing age in both men and women, reflecting age-associated bone loss. It is higher for women (approximately 80% of all cases) than men, because accelerated bone loss occurs in the immediate postmenopausal period[2]. The differences between men and women are partially related to the achievement of higher peak bone mass and absence of an accelerated phase of bone loss in men. Low bone mass is also more prevalent in Caucasians than in African-Americans[2].

Based on data from the National Health and Nutrition Examination Survey III (NHANES), 10 million people in the USA have osteoporosis at the hip and nearly 18 million

**Table 1** Secondary causes of systemic osteoporosis

*Endocrine*
Hypogonadism
Cushing's syndrome
Hyperthyroidism
Type 1 diabetes
Hyperparathyroidism

*Malignancy*
Multiple myeloma
Lymphoma
Leukemia
Malignancy-induced PTHrP secretion
Mastocytosis

*Gastrointestinal*
Alcohol
Malabsorption
Celiac disease
Crohn's disease
Lactase deficiency
Hepatic failure
Low vitamin D intake
Anorexia nervosa
Gastrectomy
Small bowel resection

*Lifestyle*
Smoking

*Drugs*
Anticonvulsants
Heparin
Glucocorticoids
FK 506
Thyroid suppression
Vitamin A excess
Methotrexate
Cyclosporin A
Alcohol

*Immobilization*
Hip fracture
Paralysis

*Genetic and Other*
Osteogenesis imperfecta
Homocystinuria
Marfan's syndrome
Rheumatoid arthritis
Ehlers–Danlos syndrome

*Renal*
Renal failure
Renal tubular acidosis
Idiopathic hypercalciuria

PTHrP, parathyroid hormone related protein

more have low bone mass at the hip, placing them at risk for future hip fractures. The prevalence of osteoporosis will probably increase as the population ages. The occurrence of osteoporotic fractures is even more striking. In the USA alone, these approximate 1.5 million per year. This includes 700 000 spine fractures, 300 000 hip fractures, 250 000 wrist fractures and 300 000 other fractures. One in two women and one in eight men over the age of 50 will have an osteoporotic fracture in her or his lifetime. Of those who reach the age of 90, one-third of women and one-sixth of men will suffer a hip fracture. The risk for African-Americans is about half of that for Caucasians[3]. As of 1995, 28 million women were affected with osteopenia and osteoporosis[4]. After the age of 65, the incidence of hip fracture in Caucasian women is greater than the incidence of stroke, breast cancer, and diabetes[5]. Osteoporotic fractures entail a significant economic burden, costing between $10 and 15 billion per year. Hip fractures alone total between $4 and 6 billion per year[6]. Health costs due to osteoporosis are predicted to reach $64 billion in 2025[7].

## Risk factors

Family history, age, history of fracture, smoking, female sex, Caucasian race, estrogen deficiency, and low body weight are risk factors for the development of osteoporosis[8] (Table 2). Smoking poses a major risk for the development of osteoporosis; it increases the relative incidence of hip fracture by 1.5–2[9]. Low calcium intake below the recommended daily allowance (RDA) of 800 mg/day has been observed in about 75% of US women[10]. Other risk factors associated with hip fracture are maternal history of hip fracture, past fracture particularly after age 50, anticonvulsants, hyperthyroidism and others. Low bone mass accurately predicts fracture risk[11]. For every standard deviation decrease in bone density measured at any site, the odds ratio for a fracture at any site is 1.6–2.4[12–14]. This relationship holds for both men and women. Other factors clearly predictive of risk are the type of fall

**Table 2**  Risk factors for osteoporotic fractures

Age
Female sex
Caucasian
Low bone density
Prior fracture after age 50
Hypogonadism
Smoking
Falls
Anticonvulsant therapy
Hyperthyroidism
Alcoholism
Excess dietary protein
Family history
Inactivity

(falls directly on the hip or wrist increase fracture risk at that site)[15] and history of prior fractures at any site[12,14]. A combination of low bone density plus one or more prior vertebral fractures increases relative risk of fracture 2.5-fold[12,14]. Fracture risk increases progressively and exponentially with decreasing bone density. A family history of osteoporosis (particularly a maternal one) is a risk factor for osteoporosis[8] and suggests a hereditary component to the disease. However, since bone mass is a complex trait with multiple external influences, it has become difficult to separate external from genetic influences. Despite this, positive correlations have been noted between polymorphisms of several candidate genes and bone mass. These include the vitamin D receptor, collagen type I, estrogen receptor, transforming growth factor β (TGFβ), and interleukin-6[16]. Although the potential implications for treatment and diagnosis are vast, since bone mass is a complex trait, it is unlikely that a monogenetic cause of osteoporosis will be found. More linkage studies are needed to unravel the genetic predisposition to this trait.

## Clinical presentation

The clinical presentation of osteoporosis can vary from a symptomatic vertebral compression fracture to the observation of low bone mineral density on baseline dual-energy X-ray absorptiometry (DEXA), screening ultrasound or even a plain radiograph. Vertebral fractures are the most common type of osteoporotic fracture, and their prevalence increases with increasing age. Vertebral fractures are often asymptomatic and are detected on routine chest radiography. The most common sites for fractures are the lower thoracic and upper lumbar spine. Fractures occurring in the cervical and upper thoracic (above T6) vertebrae suggest a secondary or pathological cause, such as tumor or infection (Table 1). An acute vertebral compression fracture may present with sudden onset of pain at the site of the fracture with associated radiation of pain laterally, paravertebral muscle spasm, and signs and symptoms of spinal cord compression. Vertebral fractures may occur in clusters of five or six over short time periods. New crush fractures may result in substantial short-term pain and disability, but many patients with vertebral osteoporosis can experience chronic back discomfort, height loss and postural changes[17,18]. In the absence of radiographic evidence of fracture or bone scan evidence of microfracture, back pain should not be attributed to a diagnosis of osteoporosis. Sufficient numbers of wedge or crush fractures may lead to height loss and kyphosis with attendant back pain and impaired functional capacity. Associated abdominal distention, discomfort, and pulmonary restriction may also occur in severe cases of thoracic kyphosis. Hip fractures are second in frequency, are associated with substantial morbidity and mortality, and occur primarily in persons over the age of 75. Morbidity is between 30 and 50%, as most of those affected are unable to return to their previous level of function. As many as one-third of patients with hip fracture are discharged to a nursing home[3]. Mortality is estimated between 10 and 20% and increases with age and co-morbid conditions[3,19]. Hip fractures are almost always associated with a fall, but whether the fracture precedes or follows the fall is not always clear. Occasionally, a patient with an impacted hip fracture retains the ability to walk, but most hip fracture patients are unable to stand. The involved limb may appear shorter and externally rotated. Patients with osteoporosis generally suffer one of two types of hip fracture: intracapsular or intertrochanteric. In the former, fracture occurs within the joint capsule and frequently results in interruption of the vascular supply to the femoral head. There is thus a high rate of non-union and avascular necrosis. Intertrochanteric fractures are extra-capsular and the fracture occurs between the greater and lesser trochanter. In contrast to intracapsular fracture, these are not associated with non-union or avascular necrosis. Distal radial fractures (Colles fracture) are the third most common osteoporotic fracture and usually occur in middle-aged women who attempt to break a fall with outstretched arms and hands (parachute reflex). Some elderly patients experiencing this type of fracture with concomitant medical problems may require hospitalization. Presentation with pain and deformity is usually straightforward. Rehabilitation exercises of the hand and forearm may be necessary.

## Diagnosis

Fracture risk assessment requires a history and physical examination, including assessment for loss of height and change in posture and a falls and mobility assessment (see Chapter 9). All patients with unexplained bone loss should be considered candidates for laboratory evaluation for secondary causes that may also be superimposed upon primary bone loss. To exclude common secondary causes, basic laboratory tests, thyroid function tests, immunoprotein electrophoresis, $1,25\text{-}(OH)_2$ vitamin $D_3$, 24-hour urine free cortisol, testosterone and/or estrogen, 24-hour urinary calcium and intact parathyroid hormone (PTH) should be obtained. Alkaline phosphatase is normal in postmenopausal and age-related osteoporosis; if it is elevated a diagnosis of Paget's disease should be entertained. Bone mass measurements have now been shown in multiple prospective studies to predict fracture risk accurately[11,13]. The World Health Organization has defined osteoporosis in terms of bone mineral density in postmenopausal Caucasian women (Table 3). A bone density

**Table 3** World Health Organization diagnostic criteria for osteoporosis

| Diagnosis | Bone mineral density |
|---|---|
| Normal | T score ≤ – 1 |
| Osteopenia | T score between –1 and –2.5 |
| Osteoporosis | T score ≥ – 2.5 without fractures |
| Severe osteoporosis | T score ≥ – 2.5 with a history of fragility fracture |

T score, the number of standard deviations above or below the average bone mineral density value for young healthy Caucasian women

measurement of more than 2.5 standard deviations below the mean for young adult women, without fractures, is osteoporosis[20]. Note that these criteria identify approximately 30% of postmenopausal women as having osteoporosis, using DEXA of spine, hip or forearm. It predicts equivalent life-time risk for spine, hip, and forearm fracture as approximately 17% and life-time fracture risk for any of the three fractures as approximately 40%[20]. The World Health Organization (WHO) diagnostic criteria are not appropriate for groups other than postmenopausal Caucasian women or sites other than spine, hip, or forearm, or modalities other than DEXA. This is in part due to the different normative databases utilized. Diagnostic criteria for osteoporosis in groups other than postmenopausal women are controversial and ambiguous at the least. The National Osteoporosis Foundation has recommended bone mineral density (BMD) tests for all post-menopausal women under the age of 65 who have additional risk factors and for all women over the age of 65. However, there is not yet evidence-based medicine to support universal BMD screening, especially in peri-menopausal women[3]. BMD should be considered in patients receiving glucocorticoids for 2 months or more, in patients with fractures in the absence of trauma, in those with unexpected or unexplained osteopenia on X-ray, and in cases with unexpected hypogonadism (particularly in males). BMD testing may also be useful

**Table 4** National Osteoporosis Foundation treatment recommendations

Postmenopausal women with T score $\leq -2$
Postmenopausal women with T score $\leq -1.5$ with additional risk factors:
    previous fracture
    current smoking
    body weight $\leq 127$ lb (57 kg)
    family history of osteoporosis

**Table 5** Monitoring treatment

Total or bone-specific alkaline phosphatase before initiating treatment; repeat 3–6 months later
Estradiol levels in women receiving replacement therapy
Testosterone in men receiving replacement
Vitamin D before initiating treatment; repeat in 1–2 months
Bone densitometry infrequently needed; requires minimum 1-year interval

in helping a patient to accept treatment for osteoporosis[21]. The National Osteoporosis Foundation has issued treatment recommendations for those patients in whom the BMD is known (Table 4). Peripheral measurements of bone density (such as heel ultrasound) are being increasingly utilized because of their low cost, lack of radiation exposure, and portability. However, results are difficult to determine, because different normative databases are utilized and T scores do not correspond to the WHO criteria applicable to central DEXA measurements. Although BMD testing has been used to follow bone mass changes over time in response to disease or anti-resorptive treatments[22], biochemical markers may be more useful and cost effective (see below).

Biochemical markers of bone turnover are a useful adjunct in the management of osteoporosis. Although serial BMD measurements have been useful in research to monitor clinical response to treatment, most anti-resorptive therapies require long-term administration with little-to-modest increases in BMD necessitating intervals of 2 or more years before repeat determinations are obtained. High bone turnover, which can be measured by biochemical markers, is an independent predictor of increased fracture risk[23–25]. Biochemical markers are useful in assessing rapid bone loss, risk of fracture and monitoring therapy[26]. Common markers of bone formation available for clinical use include alkaline phosphatase, bone-specific alkaline phosphatase and osteocalcin. Resorption markers include pyridinoline, deoxypyridinoline, and N- and C-telopeptides. The latter

are collagen breakdown products that enter the circulation following bone resorption. Total alkaline phosphatase, which is readily available in routine laboratory testing, can be used to assess the efficacy of alendronate therapy within 3 months of initiation of therapy[27] (Table 5). Telopeptide testing, while more expensive, can be used to assess anti-resorptive efficacy as soon as 6 weeks after therapy begins. BMD testing is more expensive than both and requires a minimum interval of 1 year between assessments to give clinically useful information.

## Prevention and treatment

Osteoporosis therapy should ideally be aimed at the underlying type of osteoporosis, i.e. involutional, postmenopausal or secondary causes. The majority of agents available today are anti-resorptive and exert the most beneficial effect in osteoporosis with a high rate of bone turnover (Table 6). They include estrogen, selective estrogen receptor modulators (SERMs), bisphosphonates and calcitonin. Investigational agents that increase formation include PTH, vitamin D analogs, fluoride and new osteoblastic stimulatory agents.

### Calcium

The physiological role of calcium in the body is two-fold. First, calcium provides structural integrity of the skeleton. In the extracellular fluids and in the cytosol, the $Ca^{2+}$ concentration is critical to a number of biochemical

**Table 6** Treatment/prevention of osteoporosis

*Habits*
Discontinue smoking and excess alcohol

*Exercise*
All age groups, weight-bearing 30 minutes three times a week

*Calcium*
Men: 800 mg/day
Premenopausal women: 1000 mg/day
Women taking estrogen: 1000 mg/day
Postmenopausal women: 1500 mg/day

*Vitamin D*
400–800 IU/day with calcium

*Estrogen*
Conjugated estrogen: 0.3–0.625 mg/day for 25 days
Transdermal patch: 50–100 μg/day
Uterus: add progestin 10 mg/day on days 16–25
Consider 2.5 mg/day continiously with daily estrogen

*Raloxifene*
60 mg/day

*Alendronate*
10 mg/day at least 30 minutes before breakfast with 8 oz (225 ml) of water; must not lie down
70 mg once a week

*Risedronate*
5 mg/day (taken similarly to alendronate)
35 mg once a week

*Calcitonin*
200 IU nasal salmon calcitonin everyday

processes, and its levels are tightly regulated. In states of high bone turnover, as with estrogen deficiency, there is an elevation in PTH levels. Administration of calcium in this setting, in part, inhibits PTH secretion and further bone loss. Multiple placebo-controlled studies[28,29] have demonstrated the importance of adequate calcium intake for both primary and secondary prevention of osteoporosis. Chronic deficiency inevitably leads to skeletal demineralization and enhanced fracture risk[28]. The effects of calcium supplementation are maximized in patients in whom baseline intake is low, especially in the elderly. Premenopausal women[28,29], postmenopausal women[30,31], middle-aged men and older men[28], and frail female nursing home residents[32] respond to calcium supplementation with increases in BMD. Women in early menopause, presumably because of the dominant effect of gonadal hormone loss, do not show such an effect[28,29]. Calcium and vitamin D administration reduced non-vertebral and hip fractures over an 18-month period in frail female nursing home residents[32]. Since calcium and vitamin D deficiencies are common in the elderly, calcium and vitamin D supplementation in institutionalized elderly should be routine, particularly in those who have subclinical secondary hyperparathyroidism. How much calcium is enough? The 1994 Consensus Development Conference on optimal calcium intake recommended increases in the RDA for calcium in most age groups, particularly during childhood and adolescence, when 40% of total adult bone mineral is formed. There is little evidence that one form of calcium supplementation is superior to another. Older persons have a high prevalence of gastric achlorhydria and should take their supplements with meals. Calcium supplementation alone is not sufficient to prevent either menopausal or age-related bone loss. Risks of calcium supplementation are minimal, but persons with a personal or family history of nephrolithiasis must be screened with 24-hour urinary calcium determination. In addition, some older patients may suffer from constipation and/or rebound gastric hyperacidity. Calcium citrate or calcium glubionate may be better tolerated in persons unable to tolerate other forms of calcium supplementation. A 24-hour urinary calcium corrected for creatinine is a useful and inexpensive tool for evaluation of the adequacy of dietary calcium intake. With the recommended intake, the 24-hour urinary calcium should remain in the 150–250-mg range. Calcium supplements should be prescribed with care in patients with end-stage renal disease, mainly for phosphate control. Calcium citrate should be avoided, as it enhances the absorption of aluminum, the excessive absorption of which could worsen the bone disease secondary to renal failure.

**Table 7** Fall prevention checklist

Check glasses: correct prescription and worn correctly

Check for factors that impair walking and balance: peripheral neuropathy, arthropathy

Check for postural hypotension, arrhyrthmias

Check for excessive use of transquilizers, sedatives, hypnotics, and anti-depresents

Pay attention to home environments: non-slip floors, good lighting, hand rails, no obstacles, beds/seating – easy in and out

## Exercise and fall prevention

It is evident from multiple studies that immobility and disuse leads to accelerated bone loss. Active individuals have higher bone mass than inactive individuals[33]. Correlations have been shown between muscle mass and bone density. For example, athletes have higher bone mass in skeletal regions of greatest exertion, and some prospective controlled studies in menopausal women have demonstrated increases in bone mass, total body calcium and improved calcium balance in the exercising groups[33,34]. However, only a small percentage of the variability in bone density over a broad range of ages can be accounted for by differences in physical activity[33,35]. In addition, compliance with exercise recommendations is difficult to achieve in clinical practice, and there is some evidence that exercise-induced gains in bone mass are lost within months of discontinuation of the regimen[34]. Questions regarding timing, age at onset, frequency, duration, and type of exercise most beneficial to bone remain to be answered. Many have proposed that the principal benefit of exercise in reducing fracture is its enhancement of muscle strength, balance and co-ordination, and associated reduction in falls risk[35]. General recommendations include exercise that loads the axial skeleton (such as walking) for 30 minutes/day, 3–5 days/week, maintenance of a high level of activities of daily living and adaptation according to the individual's age, lifestyle, strength, and agility. Osteoporotic fractures, particularly hip and wrist fractures, are commonly due to falls.

Many elderly patients are at high risks for falls (see Chapter 11). Consequently it is important to lower the chances of falling by avoiding adverse drug reactions, optimizing treatment for co-morbidities and eliminating environmental hazards (Table 7).

## Estrogen

Evidence for the role of estrogen loss in osteoporosis is several-fold: bone loss is accelerated as ovarian function ceases[36]; such loss is inhibited with initiation of estrogen replacement therapy[37,38]; and loss of bone resumes when estrogen replacement is terminated[39]. Estrogen treatment begun early in menopause (i.e. within the first 5 years) and continued for at least 10 years reduces hip fracture by 50% and significantly reduces distal radial and vertebral fractures[40,41]. However, to date, no prospective randomized controlled trials have demonstrated that estrogen reduces hip fracture. Optimally, hormone therapy should begin as soon after menopause as possible in order to inhibit the accelerated loss of bone that rapidly ensues. Thereafter, bone mass is stabilized or the rate of loss is slowed until treatment is discontinued, whereupon rapid loss once again begins. Thus, while estrogens theoretically should be given indefinitely, every year of use delays the onset of clinically important osteopenia as demonstrated by the reduced hip fracture incidence seen in elderly women treated in the distant past with several years of hormone replacement[38,42–44]. Studies of estrogen replacement in the elderly or in women with established osteoporosis have yielded conflicting results. Several have shown stabilization or improved bone density in estrogen-treated women after more than 10 years following menopause[45–47]. Estrogen treatment of frail elderly women (aged 75 or older) significantly increased bone mineral density in the lumbar spine and the hip[48]. The initiation of hormone replacement even in women well beyond the menopause may result in a substantial decrease in fracture risk and suggests that osteopenic elderly women are, contrary to widespread assumption, good candidates for estrogen treatment for fracture risk reduction.

There are a number of dosing regimens of estrogen currently utilized, including continuous and cyclic progestins. The most commonly used combination is Premarin® 0.625 mg plus medroxyprogesterone 2.5 mg daily. Alternatively, estrogen is administered on days 1–30 plus medroxyprogesterone 5 or 10 mg on days 1–12. The former minimizes the risk of bleeding. Estrogen alone is utilized in women without a uterus. Previously, several studies concluded that the minimum effective daily dose of oral conjugated estrogens is 0.625 mg or its equivalent. A recent randomized, double-blind placebo-controlled study evaluated the efficacy of low-dose estrogen 0.3 mg/day plus medroxyprogesterone 2.5 mg/day and revealed an increase in spinal bone mineral density of 3.5%, but without a significant change at the hip after 3.5 years[49]. Additionally, the availability of transdermal estrogen formulations (which avoid the first-pass effect of oral estrogens on hepatic protein synthesis) may prove useful in patients with hepatic disease, coagulopathies, hypertension, or congestive heart failure. The minimum transdermal estrogen dose necessary to inhibit bone loss has not yet been determined, although one study showed fracture reduction at a daily dose of 0.1 mg estradiol[46]. For a discussion of the other beneficial and potential adverse effects of estrogen therapy, refer to Chapter 10.

An important addition to our armamentarium of osteoporosis treatment is the development of selective estrogen receptor modulators (SERMs). By binding differently than parent estrogens to the same receptor, SERMs can act as an agonist in bone and with respect to lipoproteins, but, in contrast to estradiol, act as an antagonist at the breast and uterus. The SERMs currently include tamoxifen, raloxifene and draloxifene. Raloxifene (60 mg/day) is approved by the Food and Drug Administration (FDA) for the prevention and treatment of osteoporosis. The clinical effects of raloxifene on BMD and anti-fracture efficacy have been shown by a number of prospective placebo-controlled trials. Raloxifene can increase BMD by 2.4% at the spine and the hip after 3 years of treatment[50]. In one large

trial, raloxifene significantly reduced vertebral fractures by approximately 30–50%, but treatment did not alter the incidence of non-vertebral fractures[51]. Additional benefits of raloxifene include its favorable lipoprotein profile and a 76% reduction in invasive breast cancer[52]. Its side-effects include venous thromboembolism and lack of relief of postmenopausal vasomotor symptoms. More long-term studies are needed to evaluate hip fracture efficacy as well as possible side-effects on the uterus and breast.

## Calcitonin

Prospective controlled trials have documented stabilization of, and in some cases modest short-term increases in, bone mass in osteoporotic patients treated for 5 years or less with calcitonin[53–55]. Much of this benefit has been observed in trabecular bone; the benefit of calcitonin in reducing cortical bone loss has not been clearly demonstrated[55,56]. Similar effects have been demonstrated utilizing calcitonin as a preventive treatment for menopausal trabecular bone loss[55,57]. Three studies directly evaluating the impact of calcitonin on fracture reduction in both postmenopausal and elderly women have all shown significant reduction in hip fractures, vertebral compression fractures and peripheral limb fractures[56,58,59]. Data from the PROOF trial (Prevent Recurrence Of Osteoporotic Fractures), a 5-year double-blind, randomized, placebo-controlled study of 1255 postmenopausal women with osteoporosis demonstrated that 200 IU salmon calcitonin nasal spray reduced the relative risk of vertebral fractures by 36% versus placebo. The major drawbacks of calcitonin therapy include its high cost and the need for parenteral, nasal, or rectal administration. Analgesic effects of calcitonin have also been documented in multiple studies of patients with vertebral fracture, but these results have been compromised by failure to utilize appropriate control groups[55]. The major side-effect of parenteral calcitonin therapy, the use of which is now generally restricted to acute vertebral compression syndrome, is transient nausea and vomiting, which are both self-limited. Nasal calcitonin is generally well tolerated; its use may be associated with local irritation and rhinitis, which usually subsides with continued therapy. There is no evidence of any serious or long-term side-effects in studies of up to 5 years' duration[60].

## Bisphosphonates

Bisphosphonates are stable analogs of pyrophosphate that inhibit bone resorption. Their main effects include decreased osteoclast progenitor development, decreased osteoclast recruitment and induction of osteoclast apoptosis leading to inhibition of bone resorption. Bisphosphonates are tightly bound to the hydroxyapatite crystal and can be retained in bone for many years. Only a small percentage of an oral dose is absorbed, mandating avoidance of food and other medications for several hours before a dose and at least 30 min after ingestion. Alendronate sodium, a second-generation aminobisphosphonate, has been used for the prevention and treatment of post-menopausal osteoporosis as well as the treatment of glucocorticoid-induced osteoporosis and Paget's disease. The recommended dose of alendronate for treatment of osteoporosis is 10 mg and that for prevention of osteoporosis is 5 mg. It is to be taken daily in the morning on an empty stomach with 8 oz (225 ml) of plain water. Patients need to remain upright and delay eating or taking other medications for a minimum of 30 minutes. These measures reduce the risk of esophagitis and help to maximize absorption. Calcium supplements, at a different time of day, of at least 1500 mg/day must be given with bisphosphonates to reduce the risk of mineralization defects. Randomized controlled trial data using alendronate in post-menopausal women demonstrated significant reductions in both vertebral and non-vertebral fractures in association with significant gains in bone mineral density[27]. The 10-mg dose of alendronate resulted in bone mineral density increases of 8.8% in the spine and 5.9% in the femoral neck in postmenopausal women over 3 years and decreased vertebral fracture by

48%[61]. Over a 3-year period, alendronate reduced new vertebral fractures by 47% and hip fractures by 51% in women aged 55–81, who were postmenopausal and had at least one vertebral fracture and low femoral neck bone mineral density[62]. A 7-year study in 350 post-menopausal osteoporotic women revealed that 10 mg of alendronate increased spine bone mineral density by 11.4%, and 5 mg of alendronate increased spine bone mineral density by 8.4%[63]. Although tolerability profiles of alendronate are similar to those of placebo in the literature, there is a rare association of alendronate with erosive esophagitis. More commonly patients experience nausea, dyspepsia and other non-specific gastrointestinal side-effects prompting their discontinuation. Recent short-term studies reveal that once and twice weekly dosing of alendronate increases bone mineral density similarly to daily administration[64,65]. Hopefully, the intermittent dosing of alendronate will minimize gastrointestinal side-effects and maximize compliance. A newer bisphosphonate, risedronate sodium, which is a potent third-generation bisphosphonate, is also effective for the prevention and treatment of postmenopausal osteoporosis[66] and treatment of glucocorticoid-induced osteoporosis in men and women[67]. The current dose is 5 mg by oral administration daily. Clinical trials are currently assessing whether the intravenous administration of newer and more potent bisphosphonates as infrequently as once or twice a year will be effective in preventing and treating osteoporosis[68].

## Combination therapy

The effects of combination therapy and efficacy in the treatment of osteoporosis have been studied. One study evaluated 72 post-menopausal women in a 4-year study evaluating the efficacy of etidronate plus hormone replacement therapy, hormone replacement alone, etidronate alone and placebo[69]. Patients on combination therapy experienced a significant increase in hip bone mineral density compared with monotherapy with etidronate or

**Table 8**  Corticosteroid-induced osteoporosis

Consider bone mineral densitometry
Ensure adequate calcium/vitamin D intake
Consider thiazide diuretic in calciuric patients
Women: estrogen replacement therapy; then consider bisphosphonate or calcitonin
Men: bisphosphonate or calcitonin

estrogen. There was no statistically significant decrease in fracture rates among groups. Another study found that combination therapy with alendronate 10 mg and continued hormone replacement therapy in postmenopausal women significantly increased bone mineral density at the lumbar spine compared with control groups (3.6 vs. 1%, $p < 0.001$) and trochanter (2.7 vs. 0.5%, $p < 0.001$)[70].

## Treatment of secondary osteoporosis

Wherever possible, the underlying primary disease process leading to bone loss in secondary osteoporosis should be treated. When this is not possible, routine calcium and vitamin D supplementation, as well as treating hypogonadism in women and men, may be of benefit. Similarly, it is reasonable to utilize other antiresorptive agents (such as calcitonin or bisphosphonates) in an effort to minimize bone loss. Osteoporosis is among the most serious consequences of long-term glucocorticoid treatment, leading to a 50% increase in risk of hip and other fractures (Table 8). Glucocorticoids inhibit osteoblastic bone formation, increase osteoclastic bone resorption and inhibit intestinal calcium absorption. Alendronate has been shown to increase BMD while on oral glucocorticoid at a daily dose of prednisone 7.5 mg or greater[71]. Doses of 5 and 10 mg significantly increased both lumbar spine BMD and BMD at the femoral neck compared with control groups. The dosage of alendronate for the prevention of glucocorticoid-induced osteoporosis is 5 mg, except in postmenopausal women not receiving estrogen, where the dosage is 10 mg once daily. There were no data on fracture efficacy,

owing to an insufficient number of patients. Risedronate (5 mg daily) also significantly increased bone mineral density at the lumbar spine, the femoral neck and the trochanter during 12 months of glucocorticoid treatment[72].

## Other treatments

### Sodium fluoride

Sodium fluoride is an agent capable of stimulating new bone formation by increasing osteoblastic activity. Prospective controlled clinical trials have demonstrated linear increases in spine and hip bone mass but decreased radial cortical bone mass[73,74]. Vertebral fractures were not reduced and non-vertebral fractures at sites high in cortical bone were actually increased[73,74]. Slow-release sodium fluoride at lower doses appears to reduce vertebral and total fracture rates[75] but is not commercially available in the USA. Substantial side-effects accompany fluoride use, including lower extremity pain, nausea, vomiting, peptic ulcers, and gastrointestinal bleeding[75]. Fluoride remains an experimental drug and is not approved for treatment of osteoporosis by the FDA.

### Parathyroid hormone

Recent trials have indicated that intermittent PTH is anabolic for bone. Daily subcutaneous PTH administration to men with idiopathic osteoporosis for 18 months increased bone mineral density in the lumbar spine by 13.5% and in the hip by 2.9%[76]. PTH also significantly reduces vertebral and non-vertebral fractures in postmenopausal women, while increasing vertebral, femoral and total body BMD[77]. A major drawback to using PTH is the requirement, at present, for parenteral administration. While still investigational, PTH treatment appears to hold great promise and may be approved for use in the near future. Eventually therapies for osteoporosis may include a combination of agents used sequentially and cyclically first to stimulate bone formation and then to prevent resorption.

## Vitamin D

Gastrointestinal calcium absorption diminishes with age and is abnormally low in patients with osteoporosis, in association with diminished calcitriol levels and decreased responsiveness of the 1-α-hydroxylase enzyme to parathyroid hormone stimulation[78,79]. While vitamin D may indirectly stimulate bone resorption, it also enhances gastrointestinal calcium absorption, promotes mineralization, and inhibits PTH-induced bone resorption[79]. One clinical trial utilizing cholecalciferol (800 IU daily) in combination with calcium supplements (1200 mg daily) significantly reduced hip and other fractures in a nursing home population[32]. Another controlled trial of annual injection of 150 000 IU of vitamin D alone also demonstrated a significant reduction in fracture rate in an elderly population[80]. However, results from multiple trials of calcitriol (1,25-dihydroxyvitamin D) have been contradictory, with four showing increased bone mass and/or fewer fractures, three showing lower bone mass or more fractures, and three showing no effect[79]. Because of the risk of hypercalcemia and hypercalciuria with calcitriol, regular monitoring of calcium intake and serum and 24-hour urinary calcium is required. Given the risks and the contradictory findings of available clinical trials, pharmacological doses of vitamin D metabolites must be considered experimental. However, physiological replacement of vitamin D (800 IU/day) has demonstrated efficacy in reducing fractures in the elderly, and should now be considered routine treatment.

## Acute management of fractures

Acute vertebral compression fractures can cause debilitating pain and muscle spasm. Treatment including bed rest and use of a brace may be helpful, but should be minimized because of the potential for worsening bone loss due to immobility (Table 9). Potent analgesics and muscle relaxants are often needed until the acute pain syndrome resolves. It is necessary to be alert for side-effects, particularly those involving alterations in cognition.

**Table 9** Acute management of osteoporotic fractures

Strong analgesics
Immobilization (temporary!)
Physical therapy for muscle spasm
Pool therapy (builds confidence and mobility)
Improve muscle strength; resume activities of daily living
Prompt surgery for hip fracture if needed

Parenteral calcitonin has been an effective analgesic in this clinical context[81]. The pain usually resolves within several months. Physical therapy can reduce muscle spasm and improve strength. Pool therapy can accelerate the restoration of mobility and the confidence to resume normal activities without discomfort. Persistent pain mandates re-evaluation for possible pathological causes of fracture or other sources of pain. Additionally, acute compression fracture in a patient with a pre-existing malignancy or receiving chronic immunosuppression mandates exclusion of metastases or infection. The treatment options for intracapsular hip fractures are reduction and internal fixation or hemiarthroplasty. The choice depends on the degree of fracture displacement. Aseptic necrosis and poor healing, due to fracture-related disruption of the blood supply, may complicate displaced femoral head and neck fractures within intracapsular fractures. Intertrochanteric fractures are usually unstable and may be associated with substantial blood loss and hemodynamic compromise in the elderly. Depending on the type of fracture, the surgical approach may require internal fixation with nail and plate, placement of a prosthetic femoral head and neck, or total hip replacement. Prompt surgical stabilization and fixation of the fracture are critical to the prevention of the complications of immobility in the elderly, including altered mental status, pneumonia, fat embolism, venous thrombosis, deconditioning, pressure ulcers, and pulmonary embolism. The overall goal is to maximize the patient's ability to resume activities of daily living.

## Male osteoporosis

Osteoporosis is a significant but understated problem in men; approximately 2 million American men have osteoporosis. Although men are less likely to fracture, the lifetime risk of fracture is 13–25%[82]. The prevalence of osteoporosis in men will increase as the population ages. Recent studies suggest a higher prevalence of secondary causes of osteoporosis in men than in women. Over one-third of men presenting with osteoporotic vertebral fractures have a secondary cause such as glucocorticoid administration, hypogonadism, gastrectomy, and hypercalciuria with nephrolithiasis; there is also a high incidence of cigarette smoking, alcoholism, and low body weight[83]. Careful evaluation for secondary and potentially remediable causes of osteoporosis is mandatory in male patients[84]. There is some controversy in the diagnosis of osteoporosis in men. Currently there are no established guidelines for the use of BMD in male patients. Males facing long-term glucocorticoid administration, those with hypogonadism and those with unexplained fragility fractures or osteopenia on X-ray are candidates for BMD measurement. Therapeutic intervention in male osteoporosis has been poorly studied. Controlled trials utilizing available treatment modalities are few. One controlled trial of calcium (1000 mg/day) with vitamin D (1000 IU/day) failed to reduce radial or spinal bone loss in men[85]. Replacement of testosterone in hypogonadal patients has led to increased bone mass, but there is no experimental basis for such therapy in eugonadal osteoporotic men. Routine calcium, low-dose vitamin D supplementation and weight-bearing exercise are reasonable and safe measures, but are not yet supported by controlled studies. Bisphosphonates have been shown to increase BMD and decrease fracture rates in males on chronic glucocorticoid treatment[71,72]. A recent 2-year clinical trial of alendronate in osteoporotic men revealed increases at the lumbar spine (7.1%), femoral neck (2.5%), and total body (2%)[86]. More prospective long-term controlled trials are required to establish the efficacy of these therapeutic options in osteoporotic men[87].

# References

1. NIH conferences. Diagnosis and management of asymptomatic primary hyperparathyroidism: consensus development conference statement. *Ann Intern Med* 1991;114:593–7
2. Looker AC, Orwoll ES, Johnston CC, *et al*. Prevalence of low femoral bone density in older U.S. adults from NHANES III. *J Bone Miner Res* 1997;12:1761–8
3. Osteoporosis prevention, diagnosis, and therapy. *J Am Med Assoc* 2001;285:785–95
4. Melton LJ. How many women have osteoporosis now? *J Bone Miner Res* 1995;10:175–7
5. Melton LJ 3rd. Epidemiology of hip fractures: implications of the exponential increase with age. *Bone* 1996;18:121S–125S
6. Ray NF, Chan KJ, Thamer M, Melton LJ. Medical expenditures for the treatment of osteoporotic fractures in the United States in 1995: report from the National Osteoporosis Foundation. *J Bone Miner Res* 1997;12:24–35
7. Cooper C, Campion G, Melton LJ 3rd. Hip fractures in the elderly: a world-wide projection. *Osteoporos Int* 1992;2:285–9
8. Fulton JP. New guidelines for the prevention and treatment of osteoporosis. National Osteoporosis Foundation. *Med Health R I* 1999;82:110–1
9. Williams AR, Weiss NS, Ure CL, *et al*. Effect of weight, smoking, and estrogen use on the risk of hip and forearm fractures in postmenopausal women. *Obstet Gynecol* 1982;60: 695–9
10. Heaney RP, Gallagher JC, Johnston CC, *et al*. Calcium nutrition and bone health in the elderly. *Am J Clin Nutr* 1982;36:986–1013
11. Cummings SR, Black DM, Nevitt MC, *et al*. Bone density at various sites for prediction of hip fractures. The Study of Osteoporotic Fractures Research Group [see comments]. *Lancet* 1993;341:72–5
12. Ross PD, Davis JW, Epstein RS, Wasnich RD. Pre-existing fractures and bone mass predict vertebral fracture incidence in women. *Ann Intern Med* 1991;114:919–23
13. Faulkner KG, Cummings SR, Black D, *et al*. Simple measurement of femoral geometry

predicts hip fracture: the study of osteoporotic fractures. *J Bone Miner Res* 1993;8:1211–17

14. Wasnich R. Bone mass measurement: prediction of risk. *Am J Med* 1993;95:6S–10S

15. Nevitt MC, Cummings SR. Type of fall and risk of hip and wrist fractures: the study of osteoporotic fractures. The Study of Osteoporotic Fractures Research Group. *J Am Geriatr Soc* 1993;41:1226–34

16. Nguyen TV, Blangero J, Eisman JA. Genetic epidemiological approaches to the search for osteoporosis genes. *J Bone Miner Res* 2000;15: 392–401

17. Ryan PJ, Blake G, Herd R, Fogelman I. A clinical profile of back pain and disability in patients with spinal osteoporosis. *Bone* 1994; 15:27–30

18. Kanis JA, Pitt FA. Epidemiology of osteoporosis. *Bone* 1992;13:S7–15

19. Cooper C, Atkinson EJ, Jacobsen SJ, *et al.* Population-based study of survival after osteoporotic fractures. *Am J Epidemiol* 1993;137: 1001–5

20. Kanis JA, Melton LJ, Christiansen C, *et al.* The diagnosis of osteoporosis. *J Bone Miner Res* 1994;9:1137–41

21. Chestnut C. The imaging and quantitation of bone by radiographic and scanning methodologies. In *Disorder of Bone and Mineral Metabolism*. New York: Raven Press, 1992: 447–8

22. Riggs BL, Wahner HW. Bone densitometry and clinical decision-making in osteoporosis. *Ann Intern Med* 1988;108:293–5

23. Riggs BL, Melton LJ 3rd, O'Fallon WM. Drug therapy for vertebral fractures in osteoporosis: evidence that decreases in bone turnover and increases in bone mass both determine antifracture efficacy. *Bone* 1996;18:197S–201S

24. Garnero P, Dargent-Molina P, Hans D, *et al.* Do markers of bone resorption add to bone mineral density and ultrasonographic heel measurement for the prediction of hip fracture in elderly women? The EPIDOS prospective study. *Osteoporos Int* 1998;8:563–9

25. Melton LJ 3rd, Khosla S, Atkinson EJ, *et al.* Relationship of bone turnover to bone density and fractures. *J Bone Miner Res* 1997;12: 1083–91

26. Miller PD, Baran DT, Bilesikian JP, *et al.* practical clinical application of biochemical markers of bone turnover: consensus of an expert panel. *J Clin Densitom* 1999;2:323–42

27. Liberman UA, Weiss SR, Broll J, *et al.* Effect of oral alendronate on bone mineral density and the incidence of fractures in postmenopausal osteoporosis. The Alendronate Phase III Osteoporosis Treatment Study Group [see comments]. *N Engl J Med* 1995;333:1437–43

28. Heaney RP. Nutritional factors in osteoporosis. *Annu Rev Nutr* 1993;13:287–316

29. Dawson-Hughes B. Calcium supplementation and bone loss: a review of controlled clinical trials. *Am J Clin Nutr* 1991;54:274S–280S

30. Reid IR, Ames RW, Evans MC, *et al.* Effect of calcium supplemetation on bone loss in postmenopausal women [see comments]. *N Engl J Med* 1993;328:460–4

31. Aloia JF, Vaswani A, Yeh JK, *et al.* Calcium supplementation with and without hormone replacment therapy to prevent postmenopausal bone loss. *Ann Intern Med* 1994;120:97–103

32. Chapuy MC, Arlot ME, Duboeuf F, *et al.* Vitamin $D_3$ and calcium to prevent hip fractures in the elderly women. *N Engl J Med* 1992; 327:1637–42

33. Chesnut CD. Bone mass and exercise. *Am J Med* 1993;95:34S–36S

34. Dalsky GP, Stroke KS, Ehsani AA, *et al.* Weight-bearing exercise training and lumbar bone mineral content in postmenopausal women. *Ann Intern Med* 1988;108:824–8

35. Drinkwater BL. Exercise in the prevention of osteoporosis. *Osteoporos Int* 1993;3:169–71

36. Heaney RP, Recker RR, Saville PD. Menopausal changes in bone remodelling. *J Lab Clin Med* 1978;92:964–70

37. Nachtigall LE, Nachtigall RH, Nachtigall RD, Beckman EM. Estrogen replacement therapy I: a 10-year prospective study in the relationship to osteoporosis. *Obstet Gynecol* 1979;53: 277–81

38. Lindsay R. Osteoporosis. *Clin Geriatr Med* 1988;4:411–30

39. Lindsay R, Hart DM, Maclean A, *et al.* Bone response to termination of oestrogen treatment. *Lancet* 1978;1:1325–7

40. Kiel DP, Felson DT, Anderson JJ, *et al.* Hip fracture and the use of estrogens in postmenopausal women. The Framingham Study. *N Engl J Med* 1987;317:1169–74

41. Maxim P, Ettinger B, Spitalny GM. Fracture protection provided by long-term estrogen treatment. *Osteoporos Int* 1995;5:23–9

42. Kreiger N, Kelsey JL, Holford TR, O'Connor T. An epidemiologic study of hip fracture in postmenopausal women. *Am J Epidemiol* 1982;116:141–8

43. Smith DM, Khairi MR, Johnston CC. The loss of bone mineral with aging and its relationship to risk of fracture. *J Clin Invest* 1975;56:311–18

44. Ettinger B, Genant HK, Cann CE. Long-term estrogen replacement therapy prevents bone loss and fractures. *Ann Intern Med* 1985;102: 319–24

45. Lindsay R, Tohme JF. Estrogen treatment of patients with established postmenopausal osteoporosis. *Obstet Gynecol* 1990;76:290–5

46. Lufkin EG, Wahner HW, O'Fallon WM, *et al.* Treatment of postmenopausal osteoporosis with transdermal estrogen [see comments]. *Ann Intern Med* 1992;117:1–9

47. Marx CW, Dailey GE 3rd, Cheney C, *et al.* Do estrogens improve bone mineral density in osteoporotic women over age 65? *J Bone Miner Res* 1992;7:1275–9

48. Villareal DT, Binder EF, Williams DB, *et al.* Bone mineral density response to estrogen replacement in frain elderly women: a randomized controlled trial. *J Am Med Assoc* 2001; 286:815–20

49. Reckar RR, Davies KM, Dowd RM, Heaney RP. The effect of low-dose continuous estrogen and progesterone therapy with calcium and vitamin D on bone in elderly women. A randomized, controlled trial. *Ann Intern Med* 1999;130:897–904

50. Delmas PD, Bjarnason NH, Mitlak BH, *et al.* Effects of raloxifene on bone mineral density, serum cholesterol concentrations, and uterine endometrium in postmenopausal women. *N Engl J Med* 1997;337:1641–7

51. Ettinger B, Pressman A, Silver P. Effect of age on reasons for initiation and discontinuation of hormone replacement therapy. *Menopause* 1999;6:282–9

52. Cummings SR, Eckert S, Krueger KA, *et al.* The effect of raloxifene on risk of breast cancer in postmenopausal women: results from the MORE randomized trial. Multiple Outcomes of Raloxifene Evaluation. *J Am Med Assoc* 1999;281:2189–97

53. Gruber HE, Ivey JL, Baylink DJ, *et al.* Long-term calcitonin therapy in postmenopausal osteoporosis. *Metabolism* 1984;33:295–303

54. Mazzuoli GF, Passeri M, Gennari C, *et al.* Effects of salmon calcitonin in postmenopausal osteoporosis: a controlled double-blind clinical study. *Calcif Tissue Int* 1986;38:3–8

55. Reginster JY. Calcitonin for prevention and treatment of osteoporosis. *Am J Med* 1993;95: 44S–47S

56. Overgaard K, Hansen MA, Jensen SB, Christiansen C. Effect of salcitonin given intranasally on bone mass and fracture rates in established osteoporosis: a dose-response study. *Br Med J* 1992;305:556–61

57. McDermott MT, Kidd GS. The role of calcitonin in the development and treatment of osteoporosis. *Endocr Rev* 1987;8:377–90

58. Kanis JA, Johnell O, Gullberg B, *et al.* Evidence for efficacy of drugs affecting bone metabolism in preventing hip fracture. *Br Med J* 1992;305: 1124–8

59. Rico H, Hernandez ER, Revilla M, Gomez-Castresana F. Salmon calcitonin reduces vertebral fracture rate in postmenopausal crush fracture syndrome. *Bone Miner* 1992;16: 131–8

60. Wimalawansa SJ. Long- and short-term side effects and safety of calcitonin in man: a prospective study. *Calcif Tissue Int* 1993;52: 90–3

61. Eastell R. Treatment of postmenopausal osteoporosis. *N Engl J Med* 1998;338:736–46

62. Black DM, Cummings SR, Karpf DB, *et al.* Randomised trial of effect of alendronate on risk of fracture in women with existing vertebral fractures. Fracture Intervention Trial Research Group. *Lancet* 1996;348:1535–41

63. Tonino RP, Meunier PJ, Emkey R, *et al.* Skeletal benefits of alendronate: 7-year treatment of postmenopausal osteoporotic women. Phase III Osteoporosis Treatment Study Group. *J Clin Endocrinol Metab* 2000;85:3109–15

64. Schnitzer T, Bone HG, Crepaldi G, *et al.* Therapeutic equivalence of alendronate 70 mg once-weekly and alendronate 10 mg daily in the treatment of osteoporosis. Alendronate Once-Weekly Study Group. *Aging (Milano)* 2000;12:1–12

65. Rossini M, Gatti D, Girardello S, *et al.* Effects of two intermittent alendronate regiments in the prevention or treatment of postmenopausal osteoporosis. *Bone* 2000;27:119–22

66. McClung MR, Geusens P, Miller PD, *et al.* Effect of risedronate on the risk of hip fracture in elderly women. Hip Intervention Program Study Group. *N Engl J Med* 2001;344:333–40

67. Chapurlat RD, Delmas PD. Risedronate: clinical usage. *Int J Clin Pract* 2001;55:275–8

68. Reid IR, Brown JP, Burckhardt P, *et al.* Intravenous zoledronic acid in postmenopausal women with low bone mineral density. *N Engl J Med* 2002;346:653–61

69. Wimalawansa SJ. A four-year randomized controlled trial of hormone replacement and bisphosphonate, alone or in combination, in women with postmenopausal osteoporosis. *Am J Med* 1998;104:219–26

70. Lindsay R, Cosman F, Lobo RA, *et al.* Addition of alendronate to ongoing hormone replacement therapy in the treatment of osteoporosis: a randomized, controlled clinical trial. *J Clin Endocrinol Metab* 1999;84:3076–81

71. Saag KG, Emkey R, Schnitzer TJ, *et al.* Alendronate for the prevention and treatment of glucocorticoid-induced osteoporosis. Glucocorticoid-Induced Osteoporosis Intervention Study Group. *N Engl J Med* 1998;339:292–9

72. Reid DM, Hughes RA, Laan RF, *et al.* Efficacy and safety of daily risedronate in the treatment of corticosteroid-induced osteoporosis in men and women: a randomized trial. European Corticosteroid-Induced Osteoporosis Treatment Study. *J Bone Miner Res* 2000;15:1006–13

73. Riggs BL, Hodgson SF, O'Fallon WM, *et al.* Effect of fluoride treatment on the fracture rate in postmenopausal women with osteoporosis. *N Engl J Med* 1990;322:802–9

74. Kleerekoper M, Peterson EL, Nelson DA, *et al.* A randomized trial of sodium fluoride as a treatment for postmenopausal osteoporosis. *Osteoporos Int* 1991;1:155–61

75. Pak CY, Sakhaee K, Adams-Huet B, *et al.* Treatment of postmenopausal osteoporosis with slow-release sodium fluoride. Final report of a randomized controlled trial [see comments]. *Ann Intern Med* 1995;123:401–8

76. Kurland ES, Cosman F, McMahon DJ, *et al.* Parathyroid hormone as a therapy for idiopathic osteoporosis in men: effects on bone mineral density and bone markers. *J Clin Endocrinol Metab* 2000;85:3069–76

77. Neer RM, Arnaud CD, Zanchetta JR, *et al.* Effect of parathyroid hormone (1–34) on fractures and bone mineral density in postmenopausal women with osteoporosis. *N Engl J Med* 2001;344:1434–41

78. Slovik DM, Adams JS, Neer RM, *et al.* Deficient production of 1,25-dihydroxyvitamin D in elderly osteoporotic patients. *N Engl J Med* 1981;305:372–4

79. Brandi ML. New Treatment strategies: ipriflavone, strontium, vitamin D metabolities and analogs. *Am J Med* 1993;95:69S–74S

80. Heikinheimo RJ, Inkovaara JA, Harju EJ, *et al.* Annual injection of vitamin D and fractures of aged bones. *Calcif Tissue Int* 1992;51:105–10

81. Lyritis GP, Tsakalakos N, Magiasis B, *et al.* Analgesic effect of salmon calcitonin in osteoporotic vertebral fractures: a double-blind placebo-controlled clinical study. *Calcif Tissue Int* 1991;49:369–72

82. Bilezikian JP. Osteoporosis in men. *J Clin Endocrinol Metab* 1999;84:3431–4

83. Seeman E, Melton LJ 3rd, O'Fallon WM, Riggs BL. Risk factors for spinal osteoporosis in men. *Am J Med* 1983;75:977–83

84. Kelepouris N, Harper KD, Gannon F, *et al.* Severe osteoporosis in men. *Ann Intern Med* 1995;123:452–60

85. Orwoll ES, Oviatt SK, McClung MR, *et al.* The rate of bone mineral loss in normal men and the effects of calcium and cholecalciferol supplementation. *Ann Intern Med* 1990;112:29–34

86. Orwoll E, Ettinger M, Weiss S, *et al.* Alendronate for the treatment of osteoporosis in men. *N Engl J Med* 2000;343:604–10

87. Seeman E. Osteoporosis in men: epidemiology, pathophysiology, and treatment possibilities. *Am J Med* 1993;95:22S–28S

88. Olson RE. Osteoporosis and vitamin K intake. *Am J Clin Nutr* 2000;71:1031–2

# 14

# Urological issues in the aging woman

*Nina S. Davis and Tamara G. Bavendam*

## Introduction

A complete understanding of urinary tract issues in older women is impossible, as they are continually evolving as the life expectancy of women increases. This evolution occurs in women who are living into old age with excellent health and those living longer with multiple serious medical conditions. It also depends on numerous medications that can ultimately affect the function of the lower urinary tract. Treating lower urinary tract conditions in elderly women is often less about the urinary tract and more about mobility, cardiovascular status, mental status, and their medications.

Currently we are seeing women at both extremes of the hormone replacement continuum: those who went through menopause on long-term estrogens and those who were never on hormone replacement therapy (HRT). Aside from vaginal dryness, the symptoms of estrogen deprivation in urogenital tissues are often not considered in the discussion of starting or withdrawing HRT. While the issues of urinary incontinence, pelvic organ prolapse, and urinary tract irritation are not typically life threatening, they do have tremendous quality of life implications for older women struggling to maintain their independence. The issues discussed in this chapter are not to be overlooked.

## Urinary incontinence

Millions of women face the involuntary loss of urine every day. While urinary incontinence is thought to occur primarily in older women,

50% of 4211 healthy, nulliparous women 18–25 years of age were recently reported as having experienced involuntary loss of urine with activity, 16% on a daily basis[1]. The prevalence of all types of urinary incontinence in adult women ranges from 40 to 45%[2]. In a study of women 60 years and older, mixed stress and urge incontinence was the most prevalent (55.3%), followed by pure stress incontinence (26.7%), urge incontinence (9.1%) and other forms of incontinence (8.9%)[3]. An estimated $16 billion is spent yearly as a result of urinary incontinence[4]. One-third of feminine sanitary pads sold are used for urinary incontinence[5] rather than for the management of menses.

Public and professional education campaigns are vitally important to raise the level of recognition that urinary incontinence is a common and treatable condition. We need to identify the condition early and work towards solutions before the vicious downhill cycle of isolation, depression and loss of self-esteem results. Urinary incontinence should be discussed as easily as shortness of breath. Questions such as 'What have you done to minimize your episodes of urinary incontinence?' and 'What physical and social activities are you no longer comfortable doing because of your bladder?' help women understand the impact of incontinence on their lives. Urinary incontinence is multifactorial in etiology and rarely is one treatment strategy good for all patients, so treatment needs to be individualized to each woman.

## Evaluation

The history begins with eliciting a description of the circumstances of the incontinence: what provokes it, how often it occurs and the impact of the incontinence on the woman's life. Clinical descriptions of the types of urinary incontinence are as follows. *Stress urinary incontinence* is defined as urine leakage secondary to sudden increases in intra-abdominal pressure resulting from such acts as coughing, laughing, lifting, and sneezing. In *urge incontinence*, the patient perceives the sudden onset of the sensation to void and is unable to suppress it, so leakage of a variable amount of urine results. With *total or continuous incontinence*, the patient is constantly wet, both at rest and during stress maneuvers. *Spontaneous or 'unaware' incontinence* is associated with episodes of urinary leakage that occur without a perceived urge or stress-related activity. *Overflow incontinence* occurs when the bladder is at maximal capacity and the intravesical pressure exceeds bladder outlet pressure. *Nocturnal enuresis* (bedwetting) is urinary incontinence occurring while asleep and suggests an underlying neurogenic etiology. *Mixed urinary incontinence* occurs when more than one type of incontinence is present in the same patient. It commonly combines stress and urge incontinence.

The most important risk factors for the development of urinary incontinence in women include vaginal childbirth, age, estrogen deficiency, constipation, and obesity. Vaginal delivery can cause neuromuscular damage to the pelvic floor with stretching and compression of the pelvic nerves. Stretching of the pudendal nerves can also affect the innervation of the bladder neck and proximal urethra[5]. Aging and estrogen deficiency appear to worsen neuromuscular injury, since incontinence is often not clinically evident until decades after the childbirth injury. Conditions commonly associated with chronic increases in intra-abdominal pressure include constipation, obesity, chronic coughing from smoking or pulmonary disease, and occupational or recreational heavy lifting.

## Bladder diary

A bladder diary is the record of daily fluid intake, number and volume of voids and the number of incontinent episodes in a 24-hour period. Incontinent episodes are recorded along with any associated activity or sensation of urge. Daily fluid intake including the type of fluids is also noted. A voiding diary provides insight into the pattern of the incontinence and allows the initiation of conservative therapies such as fluid restriction and behavioral modification.

## Physical examination

The physical assessment for urinary incontinence consists of a pelvic examination and a screening neurological survey. The neurological examination assesses the sensation, motor strength and deep tendon reflexes of the lower extremities as well as the bulbocavernosus (BC) reflex. The absence of the BC reflex suggests a neurological deficit at the S2–S4 level. The pelvic examination begins with inspection of the external genitalia for lesions, discharge, and evidence of hypoestrogenism.

Pelvic floor support is evaluated with the speculum examination. Mild relaxation or prolapse is present when the bladder base is partially visible high in the upper half of the vagina, moderate relaxation when the bladder base is in the lower half of the vagina and severe relaxation when the bladder is through the introitus. The woman is asked to cough and 'bear down' to assess the maximum extent of movement of the anterior vaginal wall in response to increased intra-abdominal pressure. Assessment of pelvic muscle function is a key part of the examination. The woman is asked to 'tighten' the muscles she would use to 'stop the flow of urine' and/or to do a 'Kegel' exercise. The ability to isolate the pelvic floor muscles without activating the gluteal, inner thigh and lower abdominal muscles is important. A woman who cannot voluntarily isolate and contract the pelvic floor muscles would be a poor candidate for a self-directed program of pelvic muscle exercises.

## Urinalysis

A urinalysis can reveal evidence of conditions that cause or contribute to urinary incontinence including tumors, urinary tract infection (UTI), and diabetes. Microscopic examination may detect hematuria (> 3 red blood cells/high-power field) and pyuria (> 10 white blood cells/high-power field). A urine culture should be carried out to rule out infection in women with pyuria. A positive culture should be treated with 3–5 days of an appropriate antibiotic with immediate follow-up to determine whether there was any improvement in the urinary incontinence during or immediately after the antibiotics.

## Post-void residual

Assessment of the post-void residual urine is a simple and invaluable part of the incontinence evaluation. This can be approximated on bimanual examination by directly palpating immediately above the pubic symphysis. Suprapubic ultrasound examination or urethral catheterization provide more accurate measurements and the catheterized urine can be submitted for urinalysis and culture if indicated.

## Treatment

The treatment of incontinence is based upon an accurate assessment of all of the factors contributing to the involuntary urine loss determined from a complete history and physical examination (Table 1). In most elderly women, at least half a dozen of these contributing factors are present. Successful treatment plans must take into account the type(s) of incontinence present as well as any mitigating factors. Medical problems and social or environmental factors that may exacerbate incontinence must be addressed. Once identified, non-genitourinary causes of incontinence are often easily treated. Treatment choices for incontinence may be divided into non-surgical and surgical categories.

**Table 1** Causes and contributing factors to urinary incontinence

Behavioral factors
Environmental factors
Medications
Chronic illness
Decreased mobility
Hormonal deficiency
Bowel dysfunction
Psychosocial factors
Pelvic muscle function
Pelvic muscle support
Bladder dysfunction
Urethral dysfunction

## Non-surgical treatment

### Behavioral therapy

Behavioral therapy consists of modification of fluid intake, bladder training, and pelvic muscle rehabilitation. Through unclear mechanisms, dietary substances that are spicy, acidic or carbonated can irritate the bladder and contribute to urinary incontinence. The practice of limiting fluid intake to decrease the risk of urinary incontinence is usually not helpful. Dehydration potentiates constipation, concentrates the urine and increases the effect of irritants on the bladder. A more appropriate measure would be to decrease or eliminate the intake of dietary irritants and maintain a water intake of 6–8 glasses per day.

### Bladder training

The goal of bladder training or bladder drill is to manage urinary incontinence with a timed voiding schedule. The woman is instructed to void at certain predetermined times of the day rather than by urinary urge alone. The voiding schedule is based upon a review of the voiding diary. The goal is for the patient to be able to regain control of continence and increase voiding intervals by trying to suppress urinary urges and by maintaining gradually increasing bladder volumes. Bladder training is effective for treating both urge and stress incontinence.

## Pelvic muscle rehabilitation

Several options are available to help women with pelvic muscle rehabilitation including pelvic floor exercises, vaginal weights, biofeedback and electrical stimulation. Self-directed pelvic muscle exercises, commonly referred to as Kegel exercises, utilize techniques that allow the patient to identify, contract and relax the pelvic floor muscles. When properly performed on a consistent basis, they can strengthen the pelvic floor musculature. All women with incontinence should be offered pelvic muscle rehabilitation. There are no adverse effects and they can supplement all forms of incontinence treatment.

When women are unable to localize their pelvic floor muscles adequately, biofeedback may be added to a pelvic muscle exercise regimen to ensure that the proper muscles are being utilized. Feedback to the patient is provided with either an auditory, visual or tactile signal. For patients who are compliant, pelvic floor exercises can cure 30–70% of women with incontinence[6]. Fifty per cent of patients followed-up 1 year after beginning pelvic floor exercises avoided surgery. Pelvic floor exercises may be performed with vaginal cones weighing 20–90 g. Heavier cones are used as strength is improved. Electrical stimulation is a more passive way of strengthening the pelvic floor muscles and is performed via an electrode-containing probe placed into the vagina. Variable results have been documented with short follow-up.

Intravaginal support devices (pessaries) and the contraceptive diaphragm are *barrier* options for the treatment of urinary incontinence. These devices support the bladder neck/proximal urethra and prevent their downward movement in response to increased intra-abdominal pressure. Success of this form of treatment is defined by resolution of the incontinence, comfort with the device in place and no interference with normal voiding or defecation. The newest non-surgical treatment is a disposable intraurethral insert (Femsoft®) from Rochester Medical Corporation, Rochester MN[7]. Women place the device into their urethra and remove it for urination. It is an immediately effective treatment that eliminates the need for external protection and is covered by Medicare.

## Pharmacological treatment

Pharmacological options begin with *estrogen*. This increases blood flow to the submucosal plexus of the urethra and the epithelium of the urethra. Topical estrogen should be considered in the management of urinary incontinence in all women, taking into account the overall risk/benefit of estrogen replacement in each individual patient. Women taking oral replacement may benefit from adding regular topical vaginal application if vaginal tissues remain atrophic. In addition to estrogen, other pharmacological agents may be prescribed either alone or in combination with behavioral interventions.

Anticholinergic/antispasmodic agents are useful to treat detrusor instability and urgency. They produce detrusor relaxation, thereby improving bladder storage. α-adrenergic agonists increase urethral pressure and may be used to treat mild cases of stress incontinence. In contrast, α-adrenergic antagonists decrease bladder outlet resistance. They can precipitate stress incontinence but relieve urinary retention. Imipramine has both anticholinergic and α-adrenergic properties and is useful in treating both urge and activity-related urinary incontinence by suppressing involuntary bladder contractions while increasing urethral tone (Table 2). More than one drug may be needed to increase efficacy and/or to minimize side-effects, and more than one mode of treatment may be required to achieve continence. A timed voiding schedule is useful for many patients on medical therapy. With anticholinergic agents, it is important to monitor bowel function, as constipation may develop. A stool-bulking agent should be given in anyone with baseline constipation.

## Surgical treatment

Surgical treatment of incontinence is reserved for those patients who fail or who are not

**Table 2** Medications for urge incontinence (overactive bladder)

| Drug | Dosage |
| --- | --- |
| Oxybutinin | 2.5–5 mg orally 2–3 times a day |
| Tolterodine | 1–2 mg orally twice a day |
| Hyoscyamine | 0.125 mg every 4 hours, as circumstances may require |
| | 0.375 mg twice a day |
| Imipramine | 10–25 mg 1–3 times a day |
| Detrol LA® | 2–4 mg daily |
| Ditropan XL® | 5–15 mg daily |

candidates for non-surgical therapy. Surgery is used to treat symptomatic pelvic floor defects and intrinsic urethral deficiency. The risks of anti-incontinence surgery include urinary retention, new onset frequency and urgency of urination, and persistent incontinence. Since urinary incontinence has multiple causes and contributing factors, it is unrealistic to expect that surgery alone will lead to a lifetime 'cure'.

Procedures for stress incontinence are classified as retropubic suspensions, repairs, needle suspensions, pubovaginal slings, and periurethral injections with bulking agents. Retropubic suspensions anchor the pubocervical fascia to ligaments located on the bony pelvis. They are performed either laparoscopically or via a laparotomy. Needle suspensions utilize a combined suprapubic and transvaginal approach. Sutures are placed on both sides of the urethra, incorporating the endopelvic fascia, and then secured to the rectus fascia or ligaments attached to the pubic bone. Pubovaginal sling procedures utilize a transabdominal and/or a transvaginal approach. A strip of autologous fascia, cadaveric dermis or fascia, or man-made material is placed between the bladder neck and anterior vaginal wall and secured in the suprapubic or retropubic area. Periurethral injection of bovine collagen, Contigen®[8], or a slurry of polymer microspheres, Durasphere®[9], is performed under cystoscopic guidance with local anesthesia or intravenous sedation. These substances will eventually be degraded to some degree, and repeated injections are usually required to maintain continence.

## Pelvic organ prolapse

Pelvic organ prolapse is commonly seen in conjunction with urinary tract complaints including urinary incontinence, obstructive voiding, and recurrent UTI. The underlying causes are the same as those discussed for urinary incontinence. As women continue to live longer and remain more active into old age, the risk of prolapse will increase with the chronic 'wear and tear' on the pelvic floor support produced by normal increases in intra-abdominal pressure. Evolution from a quadriped to a biped was not favorable to the female pelvic floor. The ability to safely deliver infants of larger birth weight through the vagina will have long-term implications on the mother's pelvic floor integrity.

Prolapse can occur from the anterior vaginal wall, the vaginal apex, and the posterior vaginal wall. Anterior vaginal wall prolapse involves descent of the bladder (cystocele) or urethra (urethrocele). A cystocele and urethrocele often occur together. Prolapse from the apex may include uterine descent, vaginal vault prolapse and enterocele; a rectocele occurs through the posterior vaginal wall. Vaginal vault prolapse and an enterocele usually occur after a vaginal hysterectomy.

Treatments for prolapse include observation for minimally symptomatic prolapse, pelvic floor muscle rehabilitation, pessaries and surgical pelvic floor reconstruction. Mild-to-moderate prolapse is often identified on routine yearly pelvic examination and may be associated with urinary or fecal incontinence or constipation. Women often become aware of the anatomic changes when they feel something different while wiping themselves after urination. As the prolapse progresses, they feel a bulge protruding from the introitus, especially when they are standing or walking.

A pessary occupies space in the vagina to reduce the prolapse. Pessaries come in many sizes and shapes. Choosing the best pessary is based on experience and trial and error. A pessary that works well is comfortable for the patient, cannot be expelled spontaneously or with activities that increase intra-abdominal pressure, does not provoke urinary incontinence or difficulty with rectal evacuation and does not cause bleeding, discharge, or irritation of the vaginal tissues. When vaginal tissues are atrophic, topical estrogen should be used for 2–3 weeks before placing a pessary.

Transvaginal pelvic floor reconstruction can be performed safely in women well into their eighties and even nineties when they present a reasonable operative risk. When quality of life is significantly compromised by the prolapse and non-surgical management is unsuccessful, surgery can be offered to elderly women. Most women are discharged on the second postoperative day with minimal pain and minimal spontaneous voiding. The only restrictions are to avoid lifting more than 10 lb (4.5 kg) and to avoid sexual intercourse for 6 weeks. Eighty women have undergone pelvic floor reconstruction at MCP Hospital over the past 4 years. Ten women were 50 years of age or younger; 44 women were between 51 and 64 years old; and 28 were 65 years of age or beyond. Of 28 geripausal women, seven were older than 80, and all of these women had unremarkable postoperative courses (unpublished data).

Although urinary incontinence and the pelvic organ prolapse often associated with it are among the most prevalent genitourinary disorders affecting aging women, there are a number of signs and symptoms that may occur concurrently or independently and that may be harbingers of serious genitourinary pathology or adversely affect quality of life. These include hematuria, frequency, urgency, nocturia, and urinary retention. The significance of each of these will be individually considered.

## Hematuria

Asymptomatic hematuria, either microscopic or visible (gross), is one of the most common reasons for referral to a urologist, as it is the sign most frequently associated with genitourinary tract pathology[10]. Even a single episode of gross hematuria is reason for concern and demands investigation; however, what constitutes significant microscopic hematuria is controversial. That the American Urological Association recently appointed a Best Practice Policy Panel on Asymptomatic Microscopic Hematuria attests to the importance of this issue. The panel's mission was to draft best practice guidelines for the detection and evaluation of microscopic hematuria. The resultant consensus recommendations[11-13] defined clinically significant microscopic hematuria as 'three or more red blood cells/high-power field on microscopic evaluation of the urinary sediment from two or three properly collected urinalysis specimens'. Nevertheless, if a patient is a smoker or is otherwise at risk for genitourinary disease, any degree of hematuria should be considered significant and should be evaluated. This is particularly applicable to the elderly population, as it has been shown that the incidence of malignancy in this group is 7.5% overall and 34.5% in those with gross blood in their urine[14].

The conventional work-up of microscopic hematuria consists of intravenous pyelography followed by cystourethroscopy. However, for patients with painful hematuria, a history of urolithiasis or other indicator of a renal or ureteral calculus, unenhanced helical computed tomography (CT urography) has supplanted intravenous pyelography as the radiographic study of choice in most centers. CT urography comprises a spiral CT scan of the abdomen and pelvis without intravenous contrast. Often a plain radiograph of the abdomen (kidney, ureter and bladder) is included in the study for correlation in the sagittal plane. The advantages of CT urography are that it is faster than intravenous pyelography and will demonstrate non-opaque stones.

Because bladder lesions may be small and poorly seen on radiographic images, cystoscopy must be performed even if the preceding radiographic study demonstrates genitourinary pathology that might be responsible for the hematuria. For those individuals with a serum creatinine above 1.4 ng/dl, which precludes administration of intravenous contrast, a renal ultrasound examination followed by cystoscopy with bilateral retrograde pyelography can provide information equivalent to that of intravenous pyelography. Cystoscopy is particularly beneficial when it is performed during an episode of bleeding, as this allows localization and identification of the source[15].

The most common etiologies of hematuria in women aged 40–60 are acute UTI, stones, and bladder cancer, primarily transitional cell carcinoma. In women 60 years of age or older, bladder cancer and UTI are the most common reasons for hematuria. Although a rare disease, urethral carcinoma should be included in the differential diagnosis of microscopic hematuria in the mature woman, because it is most prevalent in this age group. Affected patients more commonly present with a urethral mass and symptoms of urethral obstruction including urinary retention (see below). Renal cell carcinoma, although less common than bladder cancer, must also be ruled out in the patient with microhematuria.

Postmenopausal hematuria may be caused by non-malignant lesions. Caruncles are polypoid lesions of the urethral meatus that may bleed or, less frequently, produce discomfort. They are inflammatory in nature and do not appear to undergo malignant transformation. Intervention is rarely indicated, but if the caruncle is bothersome to the patient or actively bleeding, it is easily removed under local anesthesia in the office. Other inflammatory disorders may affect the bladder and mimic cancer. Chronic cystitis, which resembles carcinoma *in situ* (CIS) of the bladder, may not have an apparent microbial etiology. It can be distinguished from CIS only by biopsy. Tuberculosis can affect any portion of the genitourinary tract, causing asymptomatic pyuria and hematuria.

In the diabetic patient or one who abuses non-steroidal anti-inflammatory drugs, intravenous pyelography may demonstrate calyceal blunting characteristic of papillary necrosis. During the acute phase of the disorder, sloughed papillae may appear as polypoid intrarenal or ureteral masses. At such times, affected patients will not only report gross hematuria and perhaps some flank pain, but they will often note the passage of tissue fragments in the urine as well.

Painful hematuria, gross or microscopic, is most commonly associated with renal or ureteral calculi. Irritative voiding symptoms occur when a stone lies in the distal ureter near the bladder. Such symptoms often indicate that stone passage is imminent.

Finally, conditions unique to the postmenopausal woman may produce microscopic hematuria. Women taking HRT, particularly the estrogen–progesterone combinations, can experience overt or occult vaginal bleeding. Contamination of the urine with vaginal secretions then results in small quantities of blood in the urine. Conversely, in women who are not being treated with systemic or local HRT, atrophy alone, because of the associated tissue fragility, may give rise to microscopic hematuria.

## Urinary frequency and urgency

Urinary frequency is diurnal or daytime voiding episodes that are excessive in number and out of proportion to the patient's fluid intake. Definitions vary somewhat, but urinating every 2 hours or more than seven times a day should be considered abnormal[16]. Urgency, a sudden, strong desire to void, is commonly associated with frequency. Hence, current terminology combines frequency and urgency with or without urge incontinence into a syndrome designated the 'overactive bladder' (OAB)[17]. Strictly speaking, OAB refers to detrusor dysfunction, either detrusor hyperreflexia or detrusor instability, that results in involuntary detrusor contractions on urodynamic testing[18]. It is thought to represent motor impairment of bladder function as opposed to 'sensory instability', in which bladder capacity is reduced on urodynamic testing, but there is no corresponding involuntary detrusor activity[19]. In keeping with their differing mechanisms of dysfunction, patients with OAB are more likely to respond to anticholinergic therapy when appropriate; whereas those with 'sensory urgency' or 'bladder hypersensitivity' tend not to benefit from such treatment. Because OAB is common among the elderly, and bladder hypersensitivity occurs infrequently in this population[20], subsequent discussion will focus on the OAB, frequency, and urgency as manifestations of intrinsic or extrinsic pathology of the aging bladder and urethra.

In evaluating the patient with urinary frequency and urgency, details of the history should include prior genitourinary disorders and treatments, especially UTI; the presence or absence of diabetes; use of hormonal therapy; prior pelvic surgery or radiation; neurological disorders, particularly stroke (cerebrovascular accident, CVA); and hematuria. The patient's daily fluid intake should be determined. Often, a formal voiding diary is helpful in assessing patients and choosing therapy for their voiding dysfunction as well as for monitoring their response to therapy. On physical examination, abdominal scars or masses, vulvovaginal lesions and discharges, and pelvic masses/prolapse should be noted. A general neurological survey should include assessment of the bulbocavernosus and anocutaneous reflexes, gait appraisal, and coarse evaluation of extremity strength and sensation. A complete urinalysis is necessary to rule out UTI, a common and easily treatable cause of OAB. Each patient needs to be scanned or catheterized to determine whether an elevated post-void residual urine volume is present. Further work-up is dependent on the causative pathology and may include urodynamics, cystoscopy, or imaging studies.

Treatment of the OAB may involve behavioral, medical or surgical interventions or combinations of these. Bladder retraining and urge inhibition techniques may be beneficial for patients with detrusor instability. For those patients who drink excessive quantities of fluid, particularly beverages that irritate the bladder such as colas and coffee, fluid restriction with increased relative intake of water produces immediate normalization of voiding frequency and resolution of urgency.

Loss of the beneficial effects of estrogen on the genitourinary tissues of postmenopausal women can alone cause frequency and urgency. Either local or systemic estrogen therapy can produce dramatic improvement in these symptoms and should be employed alone or in conjunction with other treatments.

Elderly diabetic women often suffer frequency and urgency of urination that resolves with anticholinergical therapy. Patients with neurological disorders affecting the bladder also experience significant improvement or resolution of their symptoms with anticholinergics. After a CVA, detrusor hyperreflexia producing frequency, urgency and, often, urge incontinence is the most prevalent form of vesical dysfunction, occurring in approximately 40–80% of affected individuals[21,22]. For these patients, anticholinergics are the mainstay of therapy. Additionally, anticholinergic medications are indicated for idiopathic OAB and OAB due to surgical damage or interruption of the pelvic nerves. If a patient does not respond to a therapeutic trial of medication, urodynamic testing is indicated. Further, if a patient's symptoms are exacerbated on anticholinergic drugs, this usually means that they are retaining excessive urine volumes such that they reach maximum bladder capacity sooner and have to void even more frequently. Such patients may require clean intermittent catheterization in addition to the anticholinergic medication.

Pelvic organ prolapse produces anatomic effects that both directly and indirectly affect bladder function. Prolapse alters the urethrovesical angle and can produce bladder outlet obstruction. Urinary retention develops and predisposes to infection, which in turn causes irritative voiding symptoms. Alternatively, obstruction by itself can cause bladder instability. Detrusor function may be impaired via a number of mechanisms including peripheral denervation[23]. Surgical repair of the prolapse, in most cases, restores normal detrusor function.

Various masses, both benign and malignant, may produce symptoms of OAB. Uterine leiomyomas, when large, can compress the bladder. Other extrinsic masses may also affect bladder function via compression or invasion of the bladder wall or urethra.

Frequency and urgency that occur in conjunction with hematuria suggest a neoplasm of the bladder or urethra. Cystoscopy and imaging studies establish the diagnosis and provide staging information. Subsequent endoscopic resection of the tumor establishes its histological identity and may also be therapeutic, depending on the type and extent of the neoplasm.

Although bacterial cystitis is the most common inflammatory disorder that causes urinary frequency and urgency, any inflammatory process can induce detrusor instability. Pelvic irradiation, particularly during and just after completion of the treatment course, can cause severe irritative voiding symptoms. These generally resolve over time, but may persist in some individuals. Foreign bodies in the bladder and bladder calculi also produce inflammation. Avoiding bladder irritants and anticholinergic medications are effective therapies for radiation cystitis. Bladder stones or foreign bodies should be removed via endoscopy or open surgery, but the cause of the bladder calculi must also be identified and treated to avoid recurrence.

Iatrogenic causes of frequency and urgency include various medications, particularly diuretics, and pelvic surgery. The timing or dosage of medication can be adjusted to reduce bladder symptoms or, if this is not possible, anticholinergics may be tried. With regard to surgery, it is not unusual to have transient irritative voiding symptoms following procedures to repair prolapse and treat incontinence. However, if over-correction of the urethrovesical angle or obstruction of the urethra occur after a suspension or sling procedure, extended problems with OAB may occur. In some cases, it may be necessary to take down or revise the repair in order to restore more normal bladder function. Interim management may require use of anticholinergic medication, self-catheterization or both.

Common causes of urinary frequency and urgency in the elderly are summarized in Table 3.

**Table 3** Causes of an overactive bladder in the elderly

*Behavioral*
Polydipsia
Large intake of bladder irritants
Anxiety

*Anatomic*
Urogenital atrophy
Pelvic organ prolapse

*Inflammatory*
Urinary tract infection
Bladder calculi
Radiation cystitis
Foreign bodies in the bladder

*Neurogenic*
Diabetes mellitus
Cerebrovascular accidents
Parkinson's disease

*Neoplastic*
Uterine leiomyomas
Bladder cancers
Urethral carcinoma
Metastatic lesions to the pelvis, bladder, or urethra
Brain tumor

*Medical*
Diuretics
Anticholinergics (via urinary retention)

*Surgical*
Pelvic procedures for gastrointestinal,
    gynecological, or genitourinary disorders
Vascular procedures

*Idiopathic*

## Nocturia

Nocturia is a condition that is restricted largely to the elderly. It affects women and men equally and increases with advancing age. The term refers to an excessive number of episodes of urination at night, i.e. nocturnal frequency. It is generally agreed that awakening to void more than twice in a given period of sleep is excessive. Implicit in this definition is the element of bother. The frequent interruption of sleep to urinate can result in sleep deprivation whose effects include diminished mental acuity, reduced coordination, mood alterations, muscle stiffness, and impaired immune function[24]. Nocturia is distinguished from enuresis (incontinence during sleep) in that micturition is voluntary in patients with nocturia. Nocturia may exist alone or may be part of the complex dubbed 'irritative voiding symptoms' by urologists: a triad of frequency, urgency, and nocturia with or without urge incontinence.

The prevalence of nocturia in women is quite high. In one community-based sample, 51% of women ≥ 80 years of age reported having nocturia[25]. In an earlier study, 61% of women 65 or older were affected[26]. Nevertheless, patients may not volunteer this information in the normal course of history gathering, so it is important to question them specifically about the symptom. It is also necessary to distinguish those patients with insomnia or other sleep disturbances who merely void because they happen to be awake. In such individuals, treatment is directed toward the sleep disorder, not the night-time urination. The evaluation of the patient with nocturia parallels that for urinary frequency and urgency detailed above.

The marked prevalence of nocturia among the elderly is based, in large part, on age-related changes in renal and vesical physiology. Older individuals tend to produce greater volumes of urine in the supine position. This 'nocturia of recumbency' occurs as a result of the diminished renal concentrating ability that accompanies aging: when patients are supine, renal blood flow increases, producing a corresponding increase in urine volume. Additionally, as people age, they experience an increase in the secretion of atrial natriuretic peptide, a decrease in the activity of the renin–angiotensin–aldosterone system and a loss of the circadian secretion of antidiuretic hormone (ADH)[27]. All of these contribute further to night-time polyuria. In turn, the bladder, which is on the receiving end of this increased urine volume, undergoes age-related diminution in functional capacity and an increase in instability. Greater volumes of urine therefore translate into more frequent voids. It is then easy to understand how any concomitant genitourinary pathology or dysfunction can exacerbate this 'physiological nocturia', creating a potentially debilitating problem for the affected individuals.

Patients who have nocturia but no diurnal frequency or urgency generally have cardiac disease or other source of fluid retention. Fluid mobilization occurs on assuming the recumbent position, producing isolated nocturia. The administration of diuretics later in the day may be the only treatment necessary. Indeed, changing the timing of diuretic administration is a principle that can be applied to any patient with nocturia[28,29]. When a patient routinely takes a diuretic in the morning, she should switch to late afternoon or early evening so diuresis of accumulated fluid will occur prior to going to bed. This should result in decreased fluid mobilization and a corresponding decrease in urine volume produced during the night.

Sometimes nocturia results either from increased fluid intake at night or from significant intake of liquids such as coffee, tea, and alcohol, all of which act as diuretics. Merely diminishing fluid intake after dinner or restricting diuretic beverages at night can improve nocturia without the need for further intervention. In many cases, however, the nocturia is a symptom of genitourinary pathology that affects anatomy or voiding function. In this regard, the causes of nocturia are identical to the causes of OAB and treatments are similarly focused on the underlying disorder.

For a majority of patients with nocturia, regardless of etiology, temporary or extended medical therapy is indicated for mitigation of night-time voiding. Anticholinergic medications may be beneficial in increasing bladder capacity and reducing instability. In recalcitrant cases, a tricyclic antidepressant such as imipramine may be added to the anticholinergic to enhance retention of urine[30]. Recently, intranasal or oral desmopressin (DDAVP) has been used successfully in adults to treat nocturia[29–32]. The caveat in treating patients with DDAVP is that it can cause the rapid onset of profound hyponatremia or fluid retention[33,34]. Hyponatremia is manifested by altered mental status and seizures. To avoid this, particularly in the initial phases of therapy, it is recommended that electrolytes be monitored closely. Further, total medication administered should not exceed 0.4 mg/dose.

## Urinary retention

Urinary retention is the inability to empty the bladder completely. In acute cases, when the patient cannot pass urine at all, suprapubic pain and lower abdominal distention are usually present and the diagnosis is apparent. Such cases are more prevalent in younger populations and generally follow parturition or surgery. In most instances, brief periods of catheterization resolve the problem.

In contrast, urinary retention in older women tends to be subtle and is often indicative of significant genitourinary pathology. Generally, patients are able to void to some degree, maintaining variable post-void residuals. Bladder sensation is often impaired, so patients are unaware that they are not emptying their bladders adequately. The diagnosis of urinary retention, in many cases, must therefore be based on secondary signs and symptoms such as a diminished urinary stream or dribbling urination; straining to void; frequency; urge, overflow or spontaneous incontinence; or UTI[35]. As with other voiding dysfunctions, it is useful to remember that urinary retention may derive from disorders of either the bladder or the urethra. The various etiologies of retention therefore produce either detrusor dysfunction or urethral (outlet) obstruction. This principle guides patient assessment and serves as the point of departure for the differential diagnosis.

In evaluating a patient for urinary retention, an in-depth medical history is critical to determine the etiology. Chronic constipation, endemic in the elderly, may be associated with difficulties passing urine as well. Neurological disorders, specifically CVA, are common causes of retention in the elderly. The mechanism of retention in these cases is detrusor hyporeflexia or areflexia. The estimates of persistent retention after CVA vary. Arunabh and Badlani cited an incidence of 20%[36]. In a recent series of 80 patients, 29% ($n = 23$) entering rehabilitation after ischemic stroke exhibited urinary retention[37]. Of this group, 17% ($n = 4$) of the patients continued to demonstrate retention upon discharge from rehabilitation.

Since detrusor areflexia is characteristic of lower motor neuron lesions, it would be expected that patients with sacral spinal cord injuries, lower cord tumors or disk disease below T12 would be at risk for urinary retention. Neuropathic vesical dysfunction related to diabetes mellitus is also common and may consist of either detrusor hyperreflexia or areflexia. In the latter case, both sensory and motor impairment contribute to the bladder dysfunction. Interestingly, in patients with tabes dorsalis or pernicious anemia, loss of bladder sensation may lead to overdistention with subsequent detrusor decompensation and retention[38]. Iatrogenic causes must also be considered in cases of neuropathic retention. Medications with anticholinergic effects can impair detrusor contractility, and pelvic surgery may damage or interrupt the nerve supply to the bladder, resulting in the inability to empty. Consequently, it is important to determine the proximity of the onset of dysfunction to medical or surgical intervention.

On physical examination, both evidence of retention and its anatomic causes may be found. Lower abdominal palpation and percussion may reveal a distended bladder. Sometimes suprapubic pressure in such patients will provoke a sense of needing to void. On pelvic examination, an absence of the anocutaneous and bulbocavernosus reflexes is consistent with a lower motor neuron lesion. Urethral scarring or a urethral mass, both potential causes of outlet obstruction, may be noted. A urethral mass is ominous, as it raises the suspicion of urethral carcinoma. Carcinoma of the urethra, though rare, is the only genitourinary neoplasm that is more common in women than in men. It occurs primarily in postmenopausal women[39] and often presents with urinary retention. Severe pelvic organ prolapse suggests the possibility of retention due to distortion of the urethrovesical angle. A large fibroid uterus or other pelvic mass may produce similar kinking or compression of the urethra. Fixation of the bladder or palpable bladder mass is characteristic of invasive transitional cell carcinoma of the bladder which, in an advanced form, may restrict detrusor function.

Unless the patient is completely unable to void, an elevated post-void residual urine establishes the diagnosis of urinary retention. The post-void residual is obtained by either sterile catheterization or bladder ultrasound scanning immediately after voiding. Unfortunately, there is no general consensus as to the residual volume that defines the lower limit of abnormality. Certainly, if an individual retains as much as or more than she voided, this is clearly abnormal. Suggested definitions of a significant residual volume range from 50 ml to an amount equal to the bladder capacity[35]. However, most practitioners would accept a post-void residual of > 100 ml as pathological[36,40], especially when associated with UTI, incontinence or a peak urinary flow of less than 15 ml/s on urodynamic testing.

As with all genitourinary disease, the urinalysis, consisting of dipstick and microscopic examination, is always part of the initial evaluation. The presence of pyuria and bacteriuria with or without hematuria suggests UTI which, in the case of retention, is secondary to urinary stasis. Infection may also be seen when a bladder tumor is present. Conversely, 'dirty' urine (pyuria and hematuria without bacteriuria) with a negative urine culture may occur in conjunction with a malignancy of either the bladder or the urethra. Mucin, a secretory product of urethral carcinoma, may be noted in the urine specimen as well.

Further evaluation of the patient with retention is dependent on the historical findings, physical examination and urinalysis. If a tumor is suspected, staging radiographic work-up is indicated. However, most patients who are not in frank retention, particularly those with neuropathic dysfunction, will need to undergo videourodynamic studies to define the nature of their voiding dysfunction more precisely[40,41]. Cystourethroscopy is a valuable adjunct to urodynamics in defining the anatomic correlates of a patient's retention and in planning treatment.

Though rare, psychogenic retention must be considered when a thorough evaluation has been completed and all other potential etiologies of a patient's voiding dysfunction have been ruled out. Often the onset of the problem can be traced to a major life trauma such as loss of a family member.

The treatment of urinary retention is governed by its etiology and, in some instances, by patient preference. When retention is relatively minor and there are no sequelae such as UTI, it may be appropriate to provide no intervention. If retention can be traced to a specific medication, this should be discontinued or changed. Some patients with low-pressure bladders in whom vesicoureteral reflux has been ruled out may empty sufficiently with Valsalva voiding or the Crede maneuver. Unfortunately, there are no medications that reliably facilitate bladder emptying. Although bethanechol chloride remains available, it is not believed to be effective in the treatment of retention, owing to its inability to stimulate a coordinated bladder contraction. Neuropathic lesions of any etiology that are not amenable to surgical correction are generally treated with clean intermittent catheterization (CIC). This may be performed by the patient herself or by a caretaker[42]. When recurrent UTI becomes problematic, antibiotic suppression or bladder irrigation with antibiotics may be considered. Chronic indwelling catheterization is fraught with complications such as urethral erosion and formation of urethrovaginal fistula, therefore it is to be avoided if possible. A good alternative is chronic suprapubic catheterization.

In cases of benign urethral obstruction, periodic urethral dilatation may be sufficient to ensure adequate bladder emptying. The patient may even be taught to perform self-dilation with a catheter or sound at home. When there is significant prolapse producing obstruction, a pessary may be used to restore more normal anatomy, but incontinence may result. Surgical repair remains the optimal treatment for prolapse.

When urinary retention is believed to be psychogenic in origin, psychotherapy in conjunction with CIC is appropriate. When psychotherapy is successful, the retention will usually resolve and CIC can be discontinued.

# References

1. Wolin LH. Stress incontinence in young, healthy nulliparous females. *J Urol* 1969;101: 545–51

2. Yarnell JWG, Voyle GJ, Richards CJ, *et al*. The prevalence and severity of urinary incontinence in women. *J Epidemiol Commun Health* 1981; 35:71–6

3. Diokno AC, Brock BM, Brown MB, *et al*. Prevalence of urinary incontinence and other urologic symptoms in the non-institutionalized elderly. *J Urol* 1986;136:1022–8

4. Fantl JA, Newman DK, Colling J. *Urinary Incontinence in Adults: Acute and Chronic Management: Clinical Practice Guideline No. 2, 1996 Update*. AHCPR Publication 96-0682. Washington, DC: US Public Health Service, Agency for Health Care Policy and Research: 1996

5. Snooks SJ, Swash M, Henry MM, *et al*. Risk factors in childbirth causing damage to pelvic floor innervation. *Int J Colorect Dis* 1986;1: 20–4

6. Kegel A. Progressive resisting exercises in the functional restoration of the perineal muscles. *Am J Obstet Gynecol* 1949;56:238–46

7. Nygaard I, Brandt D, FemSoft Working Group. FemSoft® urethral insert: a multicenter interventional trial. American Urogynecologic Society. *Proceedings of the 19th Annual Scientific Meeting*, 12–15 November 1998:29

8. Stanton SL, Monga AK. Incontinence in elderly women: is periurethral collagen an advance? *Br J Obstet Gynaecol* 1997;104:154–7

9. Lightner D, Calvosa C, Andersen R, *et al*. A new injectable bulking agent for treatment of stress urinary incontinence: results of a multicenter, randomized, controlled, double-blind study of Durasphere. *Urology* 2001;58: 12–15

10. Grossfeld GD, Carroll PR. Evaluation of asymptomatic microscopic hematuria. *Urol Clin North Am* 1998;25:661–76

11. Grossfeld GD, Wolf JS, Litwin MS, *et al*. Asymptomatic microscopic hematuria in adults: summary of the AUA best practice policy recommendations. *Am Fam Physician* 2001;63:1145–54

12. Grossfeld GD, Litwin MS, Wolf JS, *et al*. Evaluation of asymptomatic microscopic hematuria in adults: the American Urological Association best practice policy – part I: definition, detection, prevalence, and etiology. *Urology* 2001; 57:599–603

13. Grossfeld GD, Litwin MS, Wolf JS, *et al*. Evaluation of asymptomatic microscopic hematuria in adults: the American Urological Association best practice policy – part II: patient evaluation, cytology, voided markers, imaging, cystoscopy, nephrology evaluation, and follow-up. *Urology* 2001;57:604–10

14. Sultana SR, Goodman CM, Byrne DJ, *et al*. Microscopic hematuria: urological investigation using a standard protocol. *Br J Urol* 1996;78:691–6

15. Davis NS. Urological problems. In Eskin BA, ed. *The Menopause: Comprehensive Management*, 4th edn. Carnforth, UK: Parthenon Publishing, 2000:171–84

16. Cardozo LD. Urinary frequency and urgency. In Stanton SL, Monga AK, eds. *Clinical Urogynaecology*, 2nd edn. London: Churchill Livingstone, 2000:309–20

17. Weber AM, Abrams P, Brubaker L, *et al*. The standardization of terminology for researchers in pelvic floor disorders. *Int Urogynecol J Pelvic Floor Dysfunct* 2001;12:178–86

18. Milsom I, Abrams P, Cardozo L, *et al*. How widespread are the symptoms of OAB and how are they managed? A population-based prevalence study. *Br J Urol Int* 2001;87:760–6

19. Karram MM. Detrusor instability and hyperreflexia. In Walters MD, Karram MM, eds. *Urogynecology and Reconstructive Pelvic Surgery*, 2nd edn. St Louis: Mosby, 1999: 297–314

20. Bavendam TG. Urinary frequency and urgency. In Lentz GM, ed. *Urogynecology*. London: Arnold, 2000:251–79

21. Badlani GH. Incontinence associated with cerebrovascular accidents. In O'Donnell PA, ed. *Geriatric Urology*. Boston: Little Brown, 1994: 309–17

22. Marinkovic SP, Badlani G. Voiding and sexual dysfunction after cerebrovascular accidents. *J Urol* 2001;165:359–70

23. Couillard DR, Webster GD. Detrusor instability. *Urol Clin North Am* 1995;22:593–612

24. Hette J. The impact of sleep deprivation caused by nocturia. *Br J Urol Int* 1999;84(Suppl):27–8

25. Swithinbank LV, Donovan J, James MC, *et al*. Female urinary symptoms: age prevalence in a community dwelling population using a validated questionnaire. *Neurourol Urodyn* 1998;16:432–4

26. Milne JS, Williamson J, Maule MM, *et al*. Urinary symptoms in older people. *Mod Geriatr* 1972;2:198–213

27. Miller M. Nocturnal polyuria in older people: pathophysiology and clinical implications. *J Am Geriatr Soc* 2000;48:1321–9

28. Kallas HE, Chintanadilok J, Marcienda J, *et al.* Treatment of nocturia in the elderly. *Drugs Aging* 1999;15:429–37

29. Reynard J. Fluid balance therapy of nocturia in women. *Int Urogynecol J Pelvic Floor Dysfunct* 1999;10:43–8

30. Asplund R, Sundberg B, Bergtsson P. Oral desmopressin for nocturnal polyuria in elderly subjects: a double-blind, placebo-controlled randomized exploratory study. *Br J Urol Int* 1999;83:591–5

31. Suchowersky O, Furtado S, Rohs G. Beneficial effect of intranasal desmopressin for nocturnal polyuria in Parkinson's disease. *Mov Disord* 1995;10:337–40

32. van Kerrebroeck P, Backstrom T, Blaivas JG, *et al.* Oral desmopressin (Minirin®, DDAVP®) in the treatment of nocturia in women. *J Urol* 2001;165(Suppl):250

33. Williford SL, Bernstein SA. Intranasal desmospressin-induced hyponatremia. *Pharmacotherapy* 1996;16:969–70

34. Bernstein SA, Williford SL. Intranasal desmospressin – associated hyponatremia: a case report and literature review. *J Fam Pract* 1997;44:203–8

35. Shah PJR, Dasgupta P. Voiding difficulties and retention. In Stanton SL, Monga AK, eds. *Clinical Urogynaecology,* 2nd edn. London: Churchill Livingstone, 2000:259–72

36. Arunabh MB, Badlani G. Urologic problems in cerebrovascular accidents. *Prob Urol* 1993;7:41–53

37. Kong KH, Young S. Incidence and outcome of poststroke urinary retention. A prospective study. *Arch Phys Med Rehab* 2000;81:1464–7

38. Wein AJ. Neuromuscular dysfunction of the lower urinary tract and its treatment. In Walsh PC, Retik AB, Vaughan ED, *et al.*, eds. *Campbells Urology,* 7th edn. Philadelphia: WB Saunders, 1998:953–1006

39. Schelhammer PF. Urethral carcinoma. *Semin Urol* 1983;1:82–9

40. Dwyer PL, Desmedt E. Impaired bladder emptying in women. *Aust NZ J Obstet Gynecol* 1994;34:73–8

41. Blaivas J, Labib KB. Acute urinary retention in women: complete urodynamic evaluation. *Urology* 1977;10:383–9

42. Lieu PK, Chia HH, Heng LC, *et al.* Carer-associated intermittent urethral catheterization in the management of persistent retention of urine in elderly women. *Ann Acad Med Singapore* 1996;25:562–5

# 15

# Surgery in the postmenopausal and geripausal patient

*Hugh R.K. Barber*

The 21st century is designated by the National Institute of Aging as 'the century of the older woman'. By the year 2030, it is estimated that women will outlive men by 8.5 years. More than 34 million Americans – 12% of the population – are aged 65 years and over. This number will almost triple to 93 million within the next 40–50 years. Most will be women. The graying 'baby boomers' will be included in this 93 million. The trends will dramatically increase health-care delivery costs, which already represent 13% of the gross domestic product of the USA. By the year 2031, one in five Americans will be eligible for Medicare. The fastest growing segment of the population will be between 65 and 85 years and there will be a great deal of surgery among the elderly – and most will be women. The geriatric patient and the geripause patient can have any non-pregnancy-related surgical problem that occurs in premenopausal women, in addition to the usual gynecological problems that require surgery. However, often the presenting clinical picture in these two groups of patients is slightly different from that in the premenopausal patient. Eskin has divided the geripause into the early geripause, which start at about age 65 and ends at about age 85, and the late geripause on up to over 100.

Those who reach age 65 or more are subject to a wide range of disorders, many or which are best treated by surgery. In the past three decades, the indication for surgery in this group has expanded, because of the advance in technology and pharmacology, and an understanding of the physiological changes in the aging woman.

The most important therapeutic advances are related to anesthesia, water and electrolyte balance, method of measuring impaired function of vital organs to determine the individual's capacity to withstand the surgical procedure (particularly of the cardiovascular, respiratory, and kidney functions), and the expanded use of monitoring devices such as the Swann–Ganz catheter.

Although age alone should not be a contraindication to elective surgery, there are increased risks for the geripausal woman undergoing surgery. The patient must be evaluated completely. The geripausal woman may present many different types of systemic aging; some have impairment of heart function or kidney function, or impairment of respiratory function with a fairly good endocrine system reserve. The amount of surgical stress the patient can tolerate is limited by the functional reserve capacity of her organ system. This capacity diminishes with age and can deteriorate further because of chronic or endocrine disease. The distinction must be made between emergency and elective surgery. In emergency surgery, a greater risk may be taken than is permissible with elective and corrective surgery.

## When outside the norm is normal: interpreting laboratory data in the aged

Tables 1–3 summarize laboratory values that do not, and those that do, change with age, and provide useful formulas for calculating laboratory values in the elderly.

**Table 1** Laboratory values that do not change with age

Hepatic function tests
    serum bilirubin
    aspartate aminotransferase
    alanine aminotransferase
Coagulation tests
Biochemical tests
    serum electrolytes
    total protein
    calcium
    phosphorus
    serum folate
Arterial blood tests
    pH
    $PaCO_2$
Renal function tests
    serum creatinine
Thyroid function tests
    thyroxine
Complete blood count
    hematocrit
    hemoglobin
    red blood cell indices
    platelet count

## Cardiovascular function

There are certain changes that occur in the aging woman that must be appreciated. These changes include: more prominent arteries in the head, neck and extremities; decrease in cardiac output up to 40%; increase in blood pressure to compensate for the increased peripheral resistance; less elasticity of the cardiovascular vessels; less sufficient oxygen utilization; and thickening and increased rigidity of the valves.

The most important changes are a reduction of peripheral tissue perfusion, a decreased velocity of blood flow, redistribution and reduced cardiac output, and reduction of cardiac reserves. A myocardial infarction within 3 months preceding surgery is associated with either another myocardial infarction or cardiac death in 30% of these patients. As the interval from the time of infarction increases, the percentage of heart attacks and risks drop. The risks can be kept to an acceptable minimum, owing to advances in anesthesia, preoperative assessment, and perioperative monitoring, and to treatment of arrythmias and hemodynamic problems. The cardiologist is an important member of the team preparing the geripausal patient for surgery.

## Pulmonary function

There are certain changes that alter pulmonary function in the geripausal patient. These respiratory changes include: weaker respiratory muscles; 50% increase in residual capacity; alveoli fewer in number and larger in size; more rigid thoracic muscles; reduced maximum breathing capacity; decreased ciliary action; lungs that appear larger, owing to loss of elasticity; and $PO_2$ reduced as much as 15%.

Superimposed disease, and the effects of heavy smoking, compound the problem. There is increased ventilation of dead space, diminished alveolar ventilation, decreased oxygen uptake, decreased arterial oxygen pressure and reduced ventilatory reserve. Since the patient's pulmonary function is compromised, it is important that controlled respiration be performed in any surgical procedure that takes more than 1 hour. Assisted ventilation during anesthesia and a generous oxygen supply postoperatively for a prolonged period are prerequisites for the maintenance of undisturbed aerobic metabolism. Many elderly patients have emphysema or chronic bronchitis and this should be very carefully evaluated.

Lower abdominal surgery is followed by clinically detectable pulmonary mechanical malfunction in nearly 30% of patients, which contributes significantly to postoperative morbidity. Unlike the internist, who is interested in only diagnosis and treatment, the anesthesiologist is primarily concerned with the pulmonary reserve of the patient and whether or not this reserve, if low, can be improved prior to the administration of anesthesia.

Screening tests are mandatory in all patients suspected of having pulmonary abnormalities, because effective preoperative treatment in airway disease reduces the frequency of postoperative complications. It has been shown that 70% of patients with chronic obstruction pulmonary

**Table 2** Laboratory values that change with age

| Value | Degree of change |
|---|---|
| Alkaline phosphatase | increases by 20% between third and eighth decade |
| Biochemical tests | |
|   serum albumin | slight decline |
|   uric acid | slight increase |
|   total cholesterol | increases by 30–40 mg/dl by ages 55 in women and 60 in men |
|   high-density lipoprotein cholesterol | increases by 30% in men; decreases by 30% in women |
|   triglycerides | increases by 30% in men and by 50% in women |
|   serum vitamin $B_{12}$ | slight decrease |
|   serum magnesium | decreases by 15% between third and eighth decade |
| $PaO_2$ | decreases by 25% between third and eight decade |
| Creatinine clearance | decreases by 10 ml/min per 1.73 $m^2$ per decade |
| Thyroid function tests | |
|   tri-iodothyronine | possible slight decrease |
|   thyroid stimulating hormone | possible slight increase |
| Glucose tolerance tests | |
|   fasting blood sugar | minimal increase (within normal range) |
|   1-hour postprandial blood sugar | increases by 10 mg/dl per decade after age 30 |
|   2-hour postprandial blood sugar | increases up to 100-plus-age after age 40 |
| White blood cell count | decreases |

**Table 3** Useful formulas for calculating laboratory values in the elderly

*Arterial oxygen*
$PaO_2$ (mmHg) = 100.1 − 0.325 × age

*Creatinine clearance*
Creatinine clearance = $\dfrac{(140 - age)\ (weight\ in\ kg)}{72\ (serum\ creatinine)}$
(In women, multiply by 0.85)

*Two-hour postprandial blood sugar (2-hour PPBS) (Over 40 years)*
2-hour PPBS = 100 + age

disease, which is not uncommon in the geripausal patient, develop postoperative pulmonary complications, whereas 3% of patients who had no symptoms will have a normal pulmonary function test.

Evaluating the pulmonary status of patients prior to surgery does not require a battery of expensive time-consuming tests. A careful history will identify those patients with a possible problem and simple preoperative tests may be employed to see whether the patient needs a more sophisticated work-up. These will be covered later in the chapter.

## Renal function

Renal function is altered after the age of 60. The glomerular filtration rate drops, and changes in tubular function occur. Since renal function after the age of 70 is decreased considerably, it is important to regulate the doses of drugs and metabolites that given to the patient. Although these patients have decreased sensitivity to antidiuretic hormone, there is concern that they may develop water retention. The elderly patient often suffers water dehydration due to reduced water intake. Measuring the output and specific gravity, as well as the pH of the urine, is a most important postoperative consideration.

The changes that occur in the urinary tract in the aged woman include: decreased size of renal mass; loss of nephrons; a renal blood flow that is decreased by up to 50% of glomerular filtration rate that also decreases by about the same amount; weaker bladder muscles; and decreased tubular function.

It is important to evaluate the operative risk. The surgeon and anesthesiologist must institute proper and appropriate corrective measures in the preoperative period to establish optimal conditions before the surgical procedure is started. Cardiovascular and renal consults must be requested as the gynecologist feels is indicated. In patients with suspected malignancy, the diagnostic work-up and preoperative care can be carried out simultaneously.

## History

A careful history is most important when caring for the geripausal patient. Knowledge of the patient's past histories and exposures to contagious diseases, type of work, tolerance of physical activity, and smoking habits are essential in helping to determine the patient's ventilatory reserve. It is important to question the patient about cough and sputum characteristics. Because exercise leads to increased oxygen consumption, $CO_2$ production, and lactic acid output, ventilatory reserve can be roughly estimated by having the geripausal patient walk fairly briskly up one or two flights of stairs. If this can be accomplished without marked dyspnea, the respiratory reserve is obviously not seriously compromised. The so-called match test establishes the ability to blow out a match held 3 inches (8 cm) from the patient's widely opened mouth (without pursing the lips) and correlates well with the maximum breathing capacity of more than 40 l/minute and a mid-expiratory flow rate of more than 0.6 l/second. Another test is one that measures how long the patient can hold her breath. If she is unable to do this for more than 10 seconds, she is considered to have a markedly reduced respiratory reserve. However, blood gases provide the best evaluation of pulmonary function.

## Physical examination

On the routine physical examination, pelvic and rectal examination should be carried out and recorded. The Pap smear must be obtained and a clear biopsy of the endometrium should be secured. In addition to the hemoglobin, white blood count differential, red blood cell count and routine urinalysis, the following blood chemistries should be ordered: prothrombin time, partial thromboplastin time, prothrombin consumption time, clot retraction time, and platelet count. An electrocardiogram and chest X-ray, as well as an intravenous pyelogram, should be obtained.

Special preoperative orders should be written as required. Thorough preoperative bowel preparation is important in preparing the patient suspected of having any malignancy that would necessitate working near the bowel or requiring bowel surgery. Mechanical bowel preparation is best, but this can be supplemented with antibiotics if the gynecological surgeon feels it is necessary.

The evening before surgery, an infusion of Ringer's lactate with 1000 units of heparin for each 1000 ml of infusion should be started. This is run through the night, during surgery and throughout the first few days postoperatively. An enema the night before surgery and the morning of surgery is often helpful in having the bowel flattened out and, therefore, less distended.

## Care of the patient during the surgery

In certain geripausal patients who have ascites fluid present, it is important to remove the fluid very slowly. If there is any vascular instability during the removal of the fluid, it is best of replace fluid with plasma or Ringer's lactate solution.

There are certain patients who develop bleeding during an operation that is obviously not from a large vessel. The plan of treatment is based upon three features: clinical judgment, rapid blood tests, and selective therapy. Clinical judgment is based upon careful work-up before the operation. Pre-existing disorders must be evaluated and will usually be revealed by a thorough history, careful physical examination and the necessary preoperative tests. There are a great number of rapid blood tests that can be obtained within 10–15 minutes so that appropriate treatment can be started.

## Postoperative orders

Immediately after operation, the vital signs, including blood pressure, pulse, and respiration, should be noted every 15 minutes until sensoria are fully recovered.

Urinary output is recorded at hourly intervals and the normal rate should be about

50 ml/minute. The specific gravity of the urine should be noted. This is a simple guide for the administration of fluids and it is also a rough indicator of the rate of tissue perfusion.

Sedation for pain is gauged to maintain comfort and to avoid respiratory distress.

Nothing by mouth until continued bowel sounds are normal, for at least 24 hours.

Antibiotics should be used at a gynecologist's discretion and of the type that the gynecologist chooses.

Nasogastric suction should be used as needed. Fluids and electrolytes, plasma and blood should be given at the discretion of the responsible gynecologist. A markedly distended abdomen in the geripausal patient may press on the diaphragm and interfere with proper respiration. This may lead to respiratory acidosis, which is often accompanied by arrythmias, which are so dangerous at this time of life.

Hemoglobin and hematocrit should be recorded twice a day for 2 days and then as judged necessary.

## Postoperative complications

Following surgery for gynecological problems, any of the complications that are associated with major surgery may occur. A few of the more common ones include ileus, intestinal obstruction, peritonitis, and fistula formation, either vesical vaginal or rectal vaginal fistula. Infections, particularly in the wound, may also occur. Dehiscence is more common among cancer patients than among those operated on for benign disease and, for these patients, retention sutures often help cut down on the incidence of this complication. Thromboembolic disease and pulmonary embolism occur more frequently in the geripausal patient.

When ventilation is inadequate, as evidenced by cyanosis, 4–5 l of oxygen per minute may be administered through a nasal catheter or mask. The oropharyngeal passage should be cleared and the state of consciousness monitored. Chest X-rays should be ordered as needed. There are a variety of drugs that are given during the postoperative period that may cause respiratory depression in the geripausal

patient. Attention must be directed carefully to prevent this complication.

## Indications for gynecological surgery

The steps in each operation will not be outlined. A great majority of preoperative diagnoses in the geripausal patient include breast cancer, genital prolapse with or without urinary incontinence, and genital cancer. Gynecologists should be prepared to handle these gynecological problems and take care of the complications that arise from them. Many of the surgical conditions that arise in the geripausal patient are secondary to pelvic relaxation. Most of the cases are cystourethroceles, incontinence, anterior vaginal prolapse, enteroceles, and gynecological malignant diseases. The gynecologist should be prepared to handle these problems and any arising complications. The patient judged to have a very short life expectancy can be followed or given palliative treatment.

## Non-gynecological surgery

The geripausal patient is subject to a wide range of disorders, many of them best treated by surgery. Biliary tract problems and colon cancer are probably among the most frequently encountered, non-gynecological problems. The great progress that has been made in technology and in the training of surgeons has changed the view about operating on the geripausal patient.

The surgical principles to be applied to the geripausal patient are not unlike those applied to patients in all other age groups, including the many ramifications that require recognition, consideration, and meticulous management. While these may primarily involve diseases accompanying the aging process, which are often well defined, the patient's background, environment, and circumstances after surgery must be carefully analyzed.

Different problems are imposed by emergency and elective operations. The decision is usually quite easy under emergency conditions, which may arise from trauma or any procedure to maintain life at the time. This applies more to the non-gynecological patient.

## Conclusion

In general, the geripausal patient is able to tolerate operations that in the past would have been impossible. The support team in intensive care units, hyperalimentation teams, metabolic teams, better anesthesia, and improved technology have added a new dimension to the lives of the geripausal patient who needs surgery.

# References

1. Adkins RB Jr, Scott HW, eds. *Surgical Care for the Elderly*. Baltimore: Williams & Wilkins, 1988
2. Barber HRK. *Perimenopausal and Geriatric Gynecology*. New York: Macmillan, 1988
3. Bygny RL, Speroff L, eds. *A Clinical Guide for the Care of Older Women*. Baltimore: Williams & Wilkins, 1990
4. Cavalieri TA, Chopra A, Bryman, PN. When outside the norm is normal: interpreting lab data in the aged. *Geriatrics* 1992;47:66
5. Eliopoulos E. *Gerontological* Nursing 2nd edn. London: JB Lippincott, 1979
6. Gambert SR, Tsitouras PD, Duthie EH. Interpretation of laboratory results in the elderly. *Pastgrad Med* 1982;72:251
7. Lebow MA. A look at older Americans. In Breen JL, ed. *The Gynecologist and the Older Patient*. Rockville, MD: Aspen, 1988
8. Panagioyes G, Ellenbagen A, Grunstein S. Major gynecologic procedures in the aged. *J Am Geriatr Soc* 1978;26:459
9. Ferre FF, Fretwell MD, Wachtel, TJ, eds. *Practical Guide to The Care of the Geriatric Patient*, 2nd edn. St Louis: Mosby, 1997
10. Rowe JW, Grossman E, Bond E, *et al*. Special report, academic geriatrics for the year 2000. *N Engl J Med* 1987;316:1425
11. Wingate MB. Geriatric gynecology. *Geriatr Med* 1982;9:53
12. Zeig NG. Anesthesia for the aging gynecologic patient. In Breen JL, ed. *The Gynecologist and the Older Patient*. Rockville, MD: Aspen, 1988

# 16

# Gastrointestinal disease in the geripause

*Karen E. Hall*

## Introduction

There are more than 30 million people over the age of 65 in the USA today, and their numbers are steadily increasing. Current predictions estimate that, during the next 20 years, the percentage of people older than 65 in the USA will increase from 12 to 18%. Diagnosis and treatment of disease in patients over 65 account for one-third of the total medical expenditures in the USA. The situation is similar in Canada, Europe and other so-called 'developed' countries, in which life expectancies have increased from 65 to over 80 years. Women will make up an increasingly larger percentage of that population, due to their increased longevity compared with men. As the 'baby boom' generation has aged, new questions are being raised about the process of aging. Is decline in function inexorable, or can function be maintained throughout one's life? Is the loss of function related to 'normal aging', or is superimposed disease the culprit? Finally, what is 'normal aging'? There has been a dramatic increase in research funding available for aging research, primarily owing to the fact that the answers to these questions are likely to have a major impact on the well-being and healthy aging of the world's population for decades to come'.

Physiological changes in gastrointestinal function do occur with age. Current research suggests that this process may accelerate dramatically after the age of 70. Women experience a rapid change in physiological function surrounding the involution of ovarian function that defines the menopause. Although there is no comparable event during aging, there is considerable evidence that a threshold exists in the geriatric age range, beyond which there is significantly increased likelihood of impairment and disease. The actual age varies between individuals; however, most people experience this 'geripause' somewhere between the ages of 60 and 75. Thus, the term 'geripause' can be thought of as a description of the crossing of a threshold during aging that results in significant changes in physiology, leading to potentially impaired function.

## General principles

Physiological changes in gastrointestinal function occur with age[2]. However, many areas of the gastrointestinal tract maintain their youthful properties well into the eighth and ninth decades of life. There is little quantitative difference between a 20-year-old and an 80-year-old in the quantity and quality of biliary, pancreatic, and intestinal secretions, in the absorptive capacity of the small intestine, and in overall nutritional requirements for height and weight (although percentage of body fat increases with age). There does not appear to be a significant change in laboratory values with age, and significant adjustments for age are not required. There are, however, some areas of the gastrointestinal tract that are affected by aging, and these tend to be the same areas involved in clinical disease. The areas of the gastrointestinal tract at greatest risk of developing age-related dysfunction are the upper gastrointestinal tract, particularly the oropharynx and esophagus, and the distal tract (colon and rectum). In practical terms, swallowing and defecation are the two most likely functions to be affected by aging. This is even more likely to be the case if superimposed neurological diseases, such as Parkinson's disease or dementia, are present.

Another point worth stressing is that the signs and symptoms of gastrointestinal disease in older patients may be more subtle than in younger patients. Studies of emergency room visits indicate that up to two-thirds of initial diagnoses of abdominal pain in geriatric-aged patients turn out to be incorrect. However, older individuals are also at risk of acquiring the same diseases that affect younger patients, such as infectious diarrhea. The following sections give an outline of gastrointestinal disorders of particular importance in patients over the age of 65, including practical suggestions for diagnosis and treatment[3].

## Dysphagia

Dysphagia, or difficulty swallowing, is a very common problem with aging. One factor that may contribute to the increased prevalence of dysphagia in geriatric patients is the age-related impairment that occurs in the co-ordination of oropharyngeal motility. Several independent abnormalities have been documented, including slow food bolus transit to the posterior oropharynx, delayed closure of the larynx, delayed relaxation of the upper esophageal sphincter with food reflux into the larynx, and impaired transit of food through the esophagus. This results in increased likelihood that food may be propelled into the larynx instead of the pharynx, and that food may pass through the vocal cords into the lungs. When superimposed neuromuscular disease is present, then dysphagia is almost inevitable. Parkinson's disease, amyotrophic lateral sclerosis, bulbar and pseudobulbar palsies, strokes, and dementia are all significant causes of severe dysphagia.

Although primary neurodegenerative disease is often irreversible, significant benefit can be obtained by training patients to perform maneuvers to protect the airway, such as chin tuck during swallowing. Thickening foods, or using special utensils, may also help. Inserting a feeding tube directly into the stomach can speed up the process of eating considerably, and may assist patients with severe dysphagia to take in adequate calories. Feeding tubes are often inserted for ease of nursing; however, it should be pointed out that a feeding tube does not decrease the risk of aspiration, and several studies have indicated that patients still experience a high rate of pneumonia. This is probably due to aspiration of saliva containing bacteria. Hand-feeding, while time-consuming, can also decrease the risk of aspiration and result in the intake of adequate calories.

In patients with a slow onset of dysphagia in the setting of neurodegenerative disease, the diagnosis is usually made fairly easily by the characteristic history, and by demonstrating impaired swallowing of water in the office. However, because older patients are also at higher risk for malignant causes of dysphagia, it is prudent to visualize the esophagus and stomach in all patients presenting with dysphagia to rule out malignant obstruction. Upper endoscopy provides a more definitive diagnosis of esophageal infection (*Candida*), ulceration and intramural malignancy than barium studies. The addition of endoscopic ultrasound assists in the diagnosis of serosal esophageal tumors, but is not required for initial investigation.

Achalasia is a much more likely cause of dysphagia in geriatric patients than in younger patients. The average patient with achalasia is female (ratio 4 Female : 1 male), aged 65–85 and presents with progressive dysphagia to both solids and liquids. Barium X-rays of the esophagus and upper stomach are usually diagnostic, demonstrating a smooth narrowing of the lower esophageal sphincter (LES) to a 'bird's beak'. This is due to uninhibited contraction of the LES, rather than a fixed stricture. Irregularity of the LES region should raise suspicions of ulceration or malignancy as a cause of the obstruction, rather than achalasia. Endoscopic examination of the esophagus should be performed to rule out malignancy, but requires advance planning to decrease the risk of aspiration and perforation. Forcible balloon dilatation is much more likely to give long-term relief of obstruction than passive dilatation using Mallory bougies, but has a higher risk of perforation. Botulinum toxin injection during endoscopy has also been used successfully in geriatric-aged patients; however, the duration of improvement is usually shorter than that obtained with balloon dilatation.

## Gastroesophageal reflux disorder

Gastroesophageal reflux disorder (GERD) is characterized by retrograde regurgitation of acid through the LES into the esophagus. This causes a burning sensation in the chest, and often results in an acid taste or acid fluid contents regurgitating into the mouth. Occasional reflux is common, as questionnaires have indicated that at least 30% of the general population complain of acid reflux once per month. Frequent reflux of acid for a prolonged period can result in esophagitis, ulceration and eventual esophageal strictures. Overall, approximately 2–5% of patients with chronic GERD develop serious complications such as ulceration. However, the incidence of ulceration can be as high as 10% in patients over age 65. Older patients may present with atypical symptoms of reflux, such as hoarseness and pneumonia from aspiration, and are less likely to present with painful swallowing (odynophagia) than younger patients. Aggravating factors that predispose to reflux are similar to those in younger patients. These include obesity and exposure to agents that lower LES pressure (chocolate, peppermint, fat, alcohol, tobacco, caffeine). Women may be more prone to GERD early in menopause, owing to fluctuations in hormone release from the ovaries. Women who have a prior history of reflux during pregnancy may also be at increased risk for GERD in the geripause.

In addition to ulceration, bleeding and stricturing, chronic esophagitis is also a risk factor for development of intestinal metaplasia of the esophageal mucosa. This condition, termed Barrett's esophagus, has been implicated in the subsequent development of esophageal adenocarcinoma in some studies; however, the exact relationship is still controversial. Geriatric patients appear to be at greater risk of developing Barrett's esophagus, primarily owing to the longer duration of reflux.

Because of the increased incidence of severe esophagitis and ulceration in older patients, if GERD is suspected, diagnosis should be made using esophagogastroduodenoscopy (EGD), as this allows visualization of the mucosa and biopsy of suspicious lesions. Treatment should include lifestyle modifications similar to those recommended in younger patients. These include weight loss, avoidance of alcohol and tobacco, and elevation of the head of the bed on blocks to minimize exposure to acid at night, when most reflux episodes occur. Pharmacological treatment of mild-to-moderate esophagitis with antacids can be cost-effective, but these require frequent administration (5–6 times per day) and may have side-effects such as diarrhea. Histamine-2 ($H_2$) receptor antagonists can be used to treat mild- to-severe esophagitis and ulceration, but should be given at twice the dosage used for peptic ulcer treatment (i.e. 300 mg of ranitidine twice a day for at least 8 weeks). Cimetidine should be avoided, owing to the higher incidence of confusion and central nervous system (CNS) side-effects reported in older patients using this medication. The most efficacious treatment of severe ulceration, stricturing esophagitis, and Barrett's esophagus, is the administration of proton pump inhibitors (PPIs), such as omeprazole or lansoprazole, at twice the peptic ulcer dosage for at least 6–8 weeks. As with most medications, it is prudent to begin at a lower dose for the first 24–48 hours in patients over the age of 65, as adverse effects of drugs are more common in this age group. Dilatation of strictures with bougies or a pneumatic balloon may be necessary, and a small percentage of patients (2%) may require surgery for severe strictures. The role of endoscopic screening of Barrett's esophagus is controversial, and recent trials of PPI treatment have not demonstrated a significant decrease in the risk of development of high-grade dysplasia or adenocarcinoma. Based on current evidence, patients with high-grade dysplasia on two subsequent endoscopies should be referred for esophageal resection, as the risk of co-existing esophageal carcinoma is > 35%.

## Peptic ulcer disease

Peptic ulcers are an important problem in older patients, although the pathogenesis may differ from that in younger individuals[4]. The use of non-steroidal anti-inflammatory drugs (NSAIDs) increases with age, primarily owing to the development of chronic painful conditions such as osteoarthritis that require analgesia. An increased incidence of autoimmune disease, particularly in women, also accounts for widespread use of NSAIDs in older individuals. Although most patients using NSAIDs do not develop significant complications, the risk of complications increases with age. Twenty per cent of deaths due to ulcers occur in patients over the age of 65, primarily due to bleeding and perforation. As in younger patients, presentation is two-to-three times more likely to be duodenal ulceration rather than gastric. Unlike younger patients, older individuals may have minimal rebound or guarding with perforation, resulting in significant delay in diagnosis. In North America, women have a higher complication rate at ages over 70; however, the increased percentage of women in the older age groups probably contributes to this. Therefore, it is important to document the use of over-the-counter medications that contain NSAIDs or aspirin in geriatric patients, as these can cause significant gastrointestinal and renal disease in this age range.

The role of *Helicobacter pylori* in the pathogenesis of peptic ulcer disease in older patients is unclear[5]. *H. pylori* is clearly implicated in causing peptic ulcer disease in younger patients, as treatment with three-to-four drug regimens decreases recurrence rates from 90% to less than 10% in that population. Acquisition of *H. pylori* appears to be correlated with poor sanitation, and is endemic in many developing countries. Antibiotic treatment is less efficacious in older patients (85% clearance vs. 95% in younger patients), and relapses may be more likely. Serum antibodies may remain positive for a prolonged period despite effective clearance, and are unreliable indicators of successful treatment. There is a large cohort of aging patients with *H. pylori* serum antibodies, particularly in developing countries, in whom it is unclear whether treatment is warranted.

At present, screening for *H. pylori* in asymptomatic individuals of any age is not recommended. Asymptomatic older patients found to be positive for *H. pylori* on serum antibody screening should probably not be investigated or treated, as patients are much more likely to experience side-effects from treatment with triple antibiotic therapy than to benefit from treatment. The role of *H. pylori* in the pathogenesis of malignancy is still highly controversial. The strongest evidence indicates that it may contribute to development of gastric lymphoma; however, this is a rare condition and the causal relationship is unclear. Antibiotic treatment decreases the risk of progression of *in-situ* gastric lymphoma, and is indicated in older patients with this disease. There is no clear evidence that *H. pylori* is a pathogenic factor for the more common lesion of gastric adenocarcinoma. Therefore, investigation should be reserved for symptomatic patients, and should include endoscopy to detect both benign peptic ulcer disease and malignant ulceration (primarily gastric). Acidification of gastric contents using oral citric acid ingestion prior to endoscopy increases the sensitivity of several tests for *H. pylori*, and should be performed in patients taking acid-reducing drugs such as $H_2$ antagonists and PPIs. If ulcers are documented, then a rapid urease test of biopsy specimens is the most accurate method to document active infection.

Malignant ulceration increases dramatically with aging, therefore all gastric ulcers in geriatric patients should be biopsied. Treatment regimens recommended are based on either PPIs or bismuth preparations, and should also include at least two antibiotics. Older patients are at increased risk of side-effects from antibiotics used in these regimens, particularly nausea and sensory neuropathy due to metronidazole, and antibiotic-induced colitis from clindamycin. In addition, response rates are lower in patients over 70, probably as a result of diminished immunity. Therefore, treatment should not be undertaken lightly, and should be reserved for patients documented to have active infection in the setting of endoscopically proven gastritis or ulceration.

## Nausea and vomiting

Aging is associated with decreased ability to regulate fluid and food intake accurately. This is due to a variety of factors, including decreased sensation of thirst and hunger, impaired mobility, impaired cognition, and an increased incidence of depression. When older individuals develop nausea and vomiting, significant morbidity and mortality can result. This is likely to be of particular importance in countries that have higher rates of gastrointestinal infection due to poor sanitation. Assessment of fluid status is imperative in patients complaining of nausea and/or vomiting, and should include documentation of skin turgor and orthostatic blood pressure, preferably with the patient lying and standing. Initial assessment should also include a decision as to whether the patient can safely be managed as an out-patient, or whether further investigation should be performed in the hospital. Monitoring and social support from family or other individuals, and the ability to take in adequate fluids are helpful indications of successful out-patient management of nausea and vomiting.

Older patients are at risk for gastrointestinal infections seen in younger patients, but the consequences of 2–3 days of nausea, vomiting, and diarrhea may be much more severe in geriatric patients. If gastrointestinal infection is unlikely, then other sources of infection, including urinary and pulmonary sources, should be sought. Occult urinary tract infection is a common cause of nausea, malaise, and fatigue, particularly in older women, and can be easily detected by use of a urinalysis stick in the office or emergency room. Men with prostatic hypertrophy are also at increased risk for post-obstructive urinary infection, due to inadequate bladder emptying. Pneumonia often presents without productive cough or fever, particularly in dehydrated older patients, and requires a chest X-ray for definitive diagnosis.

Other important causes of nausea in older patients include CNS causes such as stroke, tumors, and CNS side-effects of drugs. Drugs are a notorious cause of nausea in older patients, and obtaining an accurate drug history is an important step in the diagnosis of nausea and vomiting. Almost every class of medication has been implicated; however, drugs with anticholinergic side-effects, psycho-active drugs and cardiac anti-arrhythmic medications are notorious for causing gastrointestinal side-effects. The classic example of the latter is digoxin, a medication with a narrow therapeutic window and high potential to induce nausea. Diagnosis should include questions and maneuvers to elicit nystagmus. The latter can be seen in viral infection, benign positional vertigo (spontaneous or induced by head trauma), eighth cranial nerve lesions, pontine stroke, and as a side-effect of medications such as dilantin.

## Constipation

Constipation, defined as infrequent, hard, and/or painful defecation, is very common in Western countries[6]. This is probably due in part to a decrease in fiber intake, but an additional major contribution is the slowing of colonic motility caused by age-related impairment in enteric neuromuscular function. Other regions of the gastrointestinal tract at risk for similar impairment include the oropharynx, esophagus and stomach. Small bowel motility, in contrast, is relatively unaffected by aging. Decreased neuronal conduction in extrinsic autonomic pathways, and in enteric neurons within the myenteric and submucous plexus, have been documented in animal models of aging. Diminished calcium release from intracellular storage pools leads to impaired contractile responses to chemical and neuronal stimulation in animal models of aging. Similar findings are observed in normal colonic tissue obtained from aged individuals undergoing surgery for colon cancer. Women may have additional problems due to pelvic laxity

**Table 1**  Medications that cause constipation (the 'antis')

Aluminum: antacids (Amphojel®), sucralfate
Anticonvulsants: phenytoin, carbamazepine, phenobarbital
Antidepressants: amitriptyline, nortriptyline, venlafaxine
Antihistamines: diphenhydramine (Dramamine®), chlorpheniramine
Antihypertensives: acebutolol, prazosin, amilodipine
Antilipemics: cholestyramine, colestipol
Anti-Parkinsonian: bromocriptine, L-dopa/carbidopa (Sinamet®), amantadine
Antipsychotics: haloperidol, resperidone
And opiates: codeine, morphine, hydrocodone

occurring after a lifetime of childbearing and diminished postmenopausal hormone secretion. Bulging of the rectal tissue into a rectocele can result in excessive straining and incomplete rectal emptying.

These physiological changes also predispose older individuals to experience significant complications from other superimposed conditions that impair cholinergic transmission. Medications are a particularly common cause of new-onset constipation in older patients. Culprits include drugs with anticholinergic side-effects, such as neuroleptics, antihistamines, anti-Parkinsonian medications, and tricyclic antidepressants (Table 1). Drugs that impair calcium signalling, such as calcium channel antagonists used to treat hypertension, can also result in significant constipation. Aged patients are sensitive to the inhibitory effects of opiates on motility, and this problem should be anticipated when opiates need to be prescribed. Diminished activity due to arthritis and impaired mobility also makes a significant contribution in many patients. Most bedridden patients are constipated, and need aggressive monitoring and management to avoid developing impaction.

An additional concern in older patients is the issue of colon cancer. The incidence of colonic polyps and subsequent development of colon cancer increases 5–10-fold in patients over the age of 65 according to studies performed in Western countries. Endoscopic surveillance using either flexible sigmoidoscopy or colonoscopy to remove polyps has been shown to diminish significantly the

subsequent risk of colon cancer[7]. Therefore, colonoscopy is now recommended as an integral component of colon cancer surveillance screening, in addition to fecal occult blood testing of stool specimens. However, colonoscopy is an expensive procedure, and requires special expertise to perform. Flexible sigmoidoscopy is a safer, cheaper and less difficult procedure, which can survey the distal 60 cm of colon and remove premalignant lesions such as polyps. A cost-effective strategy in a previously unscreened population might be to introduce fecal occult blood testing every 1–2 years at a cost of a few dollars/patient, and at least one flexible sigmoidoscopy or colonoscopy in previously unscreened patients[7,8]. Barium enema is a reasonable strategy to survey the entire colon, but is less sensitive at detecting polyps of < 1 cm in diameter. As most colon cancers appear to arise by mutation of tissue within colonic polyps, identifying patients at risk of forming polyps narrows the population needing repeated surveillance to those at highest risk.

Given the increased prevalence of constipation and malignancy in older patients, recommendations are primarily based on the duration of symptoms, the age of the patient and whether surveillance endoscopy has been performed. Precipitating factors for constipation, such as immobility (surgery), medication use (particularly those with anticholinergic effects) and neurodegenerative disease (Parkinson's disease), should be sought. Adequate fluid intake is necessary to prevent stool from becoming excessively hard. Stool softeners are unlikely to reverse established constipation, and should be reserved to maintain regular bowel function in patients who are defecating normally. Many older patients may require a stimulant laxative, such as milk of magnesia or senna-containing products, to initiate regular movements. If constipation is severe, then initial efforts should be directed to clean out from below using a stepwise approach of suppositories and enemas if necessary. Tap water enemas are usually effective; soapsuds or other irritant enemas such as mineral oil should not be used, owing to the risk of colitis. When bowel movements are occurring, then oral laxatives can be used. In refractory cases of recurrent constipation, endoscopy preparation solutions containing polyethylene glycol (PEG) can be very effective when used every 2–3 days. If weight loss, bleeding and anemia are present, then malignancy should be suspected, and efforts made to examine the entire colon. As polyps are usually asymptomatic, patients who have not been previously screened for colon cancer should have fecal occult blood testing and flexible sigmoidoscopy when possible. Resolution of constipation is a separate issue, and should not preclude screening within a reasonable time. It is usually worthwhile performing screening blood chemistries, as metabolic conditions such as unsuspected hypercalcemia and hypothyroidism can also cause chronic refractory constipation.

## Diarrhea

Diarrhea can be a particularly serious problem in older patients. Aged patients are at increased risk for development of infectious diarrhea due to a variety of causes, including viral, bacterial and parasitic[9]. This is primarily due to diminished cellular and humoral immunity with aging, and may be linked to decreased intestinal IgA secretion. Older patients are also at increased risk of developing dehydration and electrolyte imbalances when afflicted with diarrhea. This is due to several factors, including decreased sensation of thirst, impaired mobility and inability to obtain fluids, and use of medications, such as diuretics, that affect fluid balance.

Acute diarrhea should be treated aggressively by determining the hydration status of the patient. Older patients are less able to tolerate prolonged dehydration, particularly those with underlying cardiac or respiratory disease. Documentation of diminished skin turgor, mucous membrane dehydration and presence of orthostatic drop in blood pressure are important indications of dehydration. If fluids cannot be taken orally, administration of intravenous fluids may be necessary, and may precipitate in-patient admission. In addition to bacterial pathogens, such as *Shigella*, *Campylobacter* and *Salmonella*, that cause diarrhea in younger patients, others including *Listeria* and enteropathogenic *Escherichia coli* should be considered. Older patients are also at increased risk of developing serious diarrhea from *Vibrio*, *Giardia* and other parasites such as intestinal helminths. Classic signs of dysentery, such as fever, may not be present in older patients, and serious transmural inflammation of the bowel and even frank perforation can be missed, due to the lack of peritoneal signs in geriatric-aged individuals. Therefore, early and frequent examination, aggressive rehydration and a high index of suspicion for complications such as perforation may be life-saving in this patient population.

One cause of acute diarrhea that should be considered, particularly in demented patients, is underlying urinary tract infection. Patients may be unaware of urinary symptoms, or unable to communicate symptoms if they have cognitive impairment. Urinalysis is often rewarding in patients with new symptoms of diarrhea, nausea, fatigue, and general malaise, and should be considered whenever a previously functioning patient, with or without dementia, suddenly becomes confused. Diarrhea in a bed-bound patient should raise the possibility of fecal impaction with overflow. This is a common cause of diarrhea in patients with impaired mobility, or those at risk of anticholinergic side-effects (medications and Parkinson's disease).

Diverticulitis can cause acute diarrhea, usually associated with pain and often with bleeding. A prior history of diverticulosis, left pelvic pain and mild fever or leukocytosis are often present. Recurrent episodes can be managed with prompt use of antibiotics, but new onset should prompt investigation to check for colon cancer or other causes of inflammation, including ischemic colitis.

Chronic diarrhea is less common than constipation, but can be a difficult problem to manage. In addition to syndromes of malabsorbtion and chronic infection that may affect patients of any age, older patients are at increased risk for specific conditions that cause diarrhea. Collagenous colitis and microscopic/lymphocytic colitis affect women five times more often than men. Peak prevalence of these conditions is in patients aged 70–80. No specific etiology has been identified; however, patients do respond to prednisone and 5ASA products used to treat inflammatory bowel disease. This suggests that inflammation and/or immunological mechanisms play a role in these conditions. Inflammatory bowel diseases such as ulcerative colitis and Crohn's disease are rare, but a small increase in incidence occurs in patients aged 65–80. Lactose intolerance can develop with age, although most patients are already aware of severe problems in younger adulthood. Transient lactose intolerance following gastroenteritis is common, and simple avoidance of milk for a week or two may be helpful.

A common problem in older patients, particularly women, is a pattern of diarrhea, or diarrhea alternating with constipation. This pattern is similar to that described in irritable bowel syndrome. As in younger patients, no serious underlying condition can be documented to explain the symptoms, and treatment consists of symptomatic control. At least 60% of patients with this problem develop it in later life, suggesting that it is not simply a life-long carryover of irritable bowel disease in younger patients. It is important initially to rule out malignancy in this group, and a search should be made not only for gastrointestinal neoplasms, but also for hematological (particularly intestinal lymphoma), lung, breast, and other cancers that produce immunoglobulins or neuroendocrine products. Occult thyroid disease (both hyper- and hypothyroidism), diabetes,

electrolyte abnormalities, and hypoalbuminemia can also cause chronic diarrhea in aged patients. If initial investigation proves unrewarding, symptomatic treatment with anti-diarrheal medications such as Imodium® can improve social function by reducing urgency and soiling. Most older patients can tolerate 1–3 mg of Imodium daily. Other treatments that may work include the use of soluble fiber to increase stool bulk and cautious use of other opiates such as codeine to slow motility. Many other anti-spasmodic agents, particularly the recently released and recently withdrawn serotonin receptor antagonists, are not recommended in older patients, owing to their potential for inducing vasospasm. Use of these agents has resulted in significant rates of severe colitis in geriatric patients, some episodes of which were fatal.

## Hepatic and biliary tract disease

In Western countries, alcohol consumption is probably the most common cause of hepatitis and subsequent complications such as cirrhosis. The incidence and prevalence of alcoholism in the geriatric age group is greatly underestimated. Surveys of physicians and patients indicate that less than 20% of patients who drink heavily are identified as alcohol users/abusers by their physicians. Aging is associated with a mild decrease in the ability to metabolize alcohol, together with an increase in the relative proportion of body fat. Both processes tend to increase the resultant blood alcohol level per drink. When added to the increased likelihood of pre-existing cognitive impairment in older patients, the net result is a significant increase in confusion, balance instability, and other metabolic sequelae of drinking in geriatric patients, compared with younger individuals. The best way to diagnose alcohol abuse is to ask. Many physicians forget to ask, or are uncomfortable with the process. Direct questions about the amount, type, and pattern of drinking are usually rewarding, and can be introduced in a sympathetic and considerate manner. Unfortunately, a life time of drinking also increases the risk of developing complications such as cirrhosis or hepatoma. Patients in the geripause are much more likely to present with end-stage liver disease at the time of initial contact. Unexplained edema and new onset of heart failure may be the first overt indications of cirrhosis. Liver enzymes may not be elevated if hepatic inflammation is not present. Imaging the liver with abdominal ultrasound or computer-assisted tomographic (CAT) scan is usually helpful. The major focus of treatment should be to avoid further use of alcohol, and to assess remaining synthetic hepatic function using assays of coagulation factors, transferrin, and albumin. Abstinence can dramatically improve life span in patients with mild-to-moderate cirrhosis, and should be aggressively promoted in all age groups.

Infection with viral hepatitis is becoming increasingly common, particularly in younger age groups indulging in high-risk behaviors such as intravenous drug use. Viral hepatitis is less common in older patients; however, an increasing number of geriatric patients who emigrated from countries in which viral hepatitis was endemic are presenting with chronic hepatitis and/or cirrhosis due to hepatitis B or C. Hepatitis D occurs only in patients with pre-existing hepatitis B (usually drug addicts), and is rare in geriatric populations. Hepatitis E is a rare cause of viral hepatitis seen in patients from India.

It is unusual for older patients to acquire viral hepatitis without recent blood/body fluid exposure, therefore the majority of patients presenting with hepatitis B and C have probably been infected for years, if not decades. This has major implications for treatment, as it is highly unlikely that such individuals will respond to interferon, or other treatments to eradicate the virus. As yet there are few data available on the utility of treating older patients with anti-viral medications for hepatitis, and some indication that such treatment is more toxic in geriatric patients. Therefore, treatment should be aimed at maintaining hepatic function (including avoidance of alcohol) and managing complications. Older patients tolerate spironolactone diuretic treatment fairly well, and aggressive attempts should be made to keep salt intake low to avoid ascitic fluid accumulation. Older patients with ascites are at increased risk of developing spontaneous bacterial peritonitis, which can present with a subtle failure to thrive, rather than peritoneal pain. Encephalopathy is more common in older patients, probably as a result of underlying mild cognitive impairment, and should stimulate a search for new infection (including urinary tract). Hepatoma is a complication that is becoming increasingly common, as a larger cohort of patients survives for decades with chronic active inflammation. Resection of solitary tumors has been performed in older patients with moderate success, and should be considered in patients with stable hepatic function.

Other primary liver diseases such as primary biliary cirrhosis, autoimmune liver disease and primary sclerosing cholangitis have also been documented in increasing numbers as longevity increases. Autoimmune liver disease should be considered in patients with 'cryptogenic' cirrhosis without markers of viral hepatitis. Treatment with steroids has been shown to be beneficial in patients up to the age of 75, and immunoglobulin levels and specific markers should be tested in patients with chronic hepatitis and early cirrhosis who do not have evidence of viral hepatitis. Use of ursodeoxycholic acid in treatment of primary biliary cirrhosis and sclerosing cholangitis is suggested, but there is little evidence that it is efficacious in geriatric patients.

While gallstones are an important cause of biliary tract disease in both Western countries and developing countries, particular mention should be made of chronic sequelae of parasitic diseases affecting the biliary tract. The latter have been observed much more frequently with increasing immigration from the Middle and Far East. Clonorchis infection from cutaneous contact with infected snails can result in biliary strictures and sclerosis that often presents in late life. Cholangitis, obstruction due to pigment stones in the biliary tree and cholangiocarcinoma are recognized complications of biliary parasitic infection that increases in incidence with age.

A sudden onset of jaundice should precipitate a search for obstruction due to gallstones and/or biliary tract stones in the common bile duct. Frank cholangitis is often associated with fever, and weight loss can be seen with both cholangitis and malignancy. Pancreatic tumors are a less common cause of jaundice, and usually present with insidious onset of jaundice and/or pain. Unfortunately, the latter are usually diagnosed at a late stage, as there is no effective screening technique at present. A strong family history of pancreatic cancer is the most useful indicator at present of the need for surveillance.

# References

1. Williams ME. *The American Geriatric Society's Complete Guide to Aging and Health*. New York: Harmony Books, Crown Publishers, 1995:492

2. Blechman MB, Gelb AM. Aging and gastrointestinal physiology. *Clin Geriatr Med* 1999;15:429–38

3. Gelb AM. *Clinical Gastroenterology in the Elderly*. New York: Marcel Dekker, 1996:305

4. Pound SE, Heading RC. Diagnosis and management of dyspepsia in the elderly. *Drugs Aging* 1995;7:347–54

5. Delaney B, Moayyedi P, Forman D. *Helicobacter pylori* infection. In: Barton S, ed. Clinical Evidence 5. London: BMJ Publishing Group, 2001:324–7

6. Edwards WF. Constipation. In: Forciea MA, Lavizzo-Mourey R, eds. *Geriatric Secrets*. Philadelphia: Hanley & Belfus, 1996:25–33

7. American Gastroenterological Association. Detection and surveillance of colorectal cancer. *J Am Med Assoc* 1989;261:580–5

8. Rockey DC, Koch J, Cello JP, *et al*. Relative frequency of upper gastrointestinal and colonic lesions in patients with positive fecal occult-blood tests. *N Engl J Med* 1998;339:153–9

9. National Institute of Cholera and Enteric Diseases. *J Postgrad Med* 2000;46:231–2

# Part III
# Conclusions and Commentary

# 17

# Ethical and end-of-life issues

*Melissa M. Bottrell and Christine Cassel*

End-of-life care for the older woman is complicated by diverse factors related as much to biology as to sociological, policy and ethical issues. While many older women are living longer, healthier lives free of disability, older women also face chronic illnesses for which treatments are costly or risky, have uncertain outcomes, or lack meaningful disease modification or prolongation of life[1]. The ambiguity over beneficial outcomes colors decisions about end-of-life care and often creates difficult trade-offs between treatments that may offer potentially significant reductions in quality of life versus treatments that may not extend life but may increase comfort and thus quality of life. Decisions to move from curative interventions to more palliative care can produce anxiety for patients and/or family members. Some medical conditions limit communication and cognition. The result is often uncertainty about who should make health-care decisions, what constitutes informed consent and how to ascertain what decision should be made. Women represent 60% of Medicare recipients and all elders account for a significant proportion of health-care spending, half of which comes from public programs[2]. As such, care for older women, particularly those with chronic illnesses, leads to questions about the relative value of health care compared with other goods available in the market, and the value of marginally effective or futile treatments when survival is not likely to be long. Such issues pose ethical questions about intergenerational resource transfers, gender biases in resource allocation and ultimately issues related to rationing of medical resources.

A variety of sources are available for comprehensive analysis of these issues and many of the particular issues are discussed elsewhere in this book. In this chapter, we try to note the range of issues related to end-of-life care with particular attention to the difficulties faced by older women under the current health-care system. We also identify some issues and ideas likely to be on the horizon as medical technology continues to advance.

## Aging, ageism, and gender bias

Recognition of the particular circumstances of women is essential to understanding the context surrounding ethical issues in the elderly. Older women are more likely than men to have chronic conditions that lead to illness and disability, and they often have fewer financial and social resources to cope with these problems[3]. Women represent 60% of Social Security recipients at age 65, and by age 85, they represent 71% of recipients[2]. Social Security provides 90% of income for 41% of all older women; 25% have no other source of income. Two-thirds of home-care consumers (10 million persons) and three-quarters of all nursing home residents 65 years or older are women[2]. Hence, while considerations of aging and ageism are essential for understanding issues in end-of-life care, the particular concerns of women as the majority of the geriatric population further color those issues.

For example, cost containment efforts resulting in incentives for shorter lengths of hospital stay have pushed patients home 'quicker and sicker'. As older women tend to outlive their spouses, such cost containment policies tend to affect aging women disproportionately. The emotional and physical burden of caring for an ailing spouse can significantly impact the health of the caregiver, and thus complicate the clinical management of illnesses for which the older woman is already being treated[4].

Studies continue to find differential access to treatment between men and women, with women receiving inadequate attention to research, diagnosis and treatment of their health problems[5-8]. Efforts to refocus the health-care system so as to enhance the use of effective preventive interventions, new therapeutic interventions to manage chronic illnesses, and more cost-effective models of disease management could extend the active life expectancy of older women. Nevertheless, traditional fee-for-service Medicare has gaps in the coverage of care for chronic illness and disability that disproportionately affect women[3].

Further, debates regarding the allocation of resources, particularly cost effectiveness evaluations and tort valuation analyses, often hinge on assumptions about quality of life, particularly the number of healthy, disability-free years. Given the statistically fewer number of disability-free years typically available to an older person, such analyses tend to discriminate against elders[9]. Institutional decisions to fund or de-fund certain clinical departments, to focus on enhancing certain acute service areas at the expense of chronic care service areas, while seeming to be management and/or 'bottom line' decisions, can disproportionately affect women – given their higher rates of chronic illnesses. Even if the demographics of aging are considered simply, the clinical reality or examples of ageist policy and social circumstances may be inconsequential to clinical management of the older woman. However, such issues certainly influence the ethical context in which care is provided to older women, particularly at the end of life.

## Ageism and end-of-life care

Decisions to forego life-sustaining treatment occur under a multitude of conditions. They can be provoked when it is decided not to resuscitate a patient with advanced dementia, to maintain a resident in a nursing home rather than transfer her to the hospital for diagnostic or treatment interventions, to replace chemotherapeutic treatments focused on curing cancer with palliative radiation, or not to administer antibiotics to a bed-bound elder with severe chronic obstructive pulmonary disease (COPD). In each case, the decision-making process must use a benefit–burden analysis comparing the benefits of treatment options against potential burdens of the treatment and potential side-effects. These decisions take place within a larger social context such that benefit–burden analyses may differ for an older patient compared with a younger patient, because of personal fears about aging and disability or stereotypes of aging[10]. Some work has shown that families and physicians may be less likely to withhold or withdraw clinical care for older women than for older men. Such gender differentials may indicate continued paternalistic attitudes towards elders, particularly older women, which may inhibit older women's autonomous decision making. Some authors claim that advanced age may give persons a different perspective on what remains of life and the so-called 'closing biography' – suggesting greater acceptance of mortality. Yet providers cannot assume this stance simply because of patient age, and must approach each patient individually. Within that analysis, the decision-making team of patient, family and clinical professionals must consider how to respect the patient's autonomy within her cultural context, support the family, and to the extent possible relieve burden while also recognizing that some treatment courses may be futile.

## Respecting patient autonomy

Mechanisms to respect patient autonomy run throughout the health-care endeavor – from patient education materials regarding particular treatments or diseases, to physician training in how to communicate with patients, to forms for informed consent and advanced directives. These tools aim to create an environment in which it is possible for the clinician to ascertain the beliefs, perspectives, and concerns of the patient so as to focus health-care decisions in a manner that enhances patient autonomy. Patient choices around end-of-life decisions will vary with their personal preferences – a patient may choose to maximize quality of life or quantity of life. Concern for patient autonomy may conflict with efforts to do what is best for the patient (also known as beneficence) as, for example, when a patient refuses a proposed treatment despite the physician's best recommendation. Further, depending on their cultural or ethnic background, patients and families may express their autonomy over medical decisions in ways not typically expected in legal contexts, especially when making the emotionally and technically fraught decisions at the end of life.

## Advance directives

The practical considerations and ethical dilemmas surrounding patient autonomy can be most obviously seen through examination of advance directives. In the USA, estimates of the percentage of persons who have executed advance directives range anywhere from 4 to 20%. Highly educated Caucasians are generally more receptive than other groups to advance directives and tend to forgo life-sustaining treatment at a higher rate. Those who are poor and non-Caucasion, particularly Hispanics and African-American, may feel apprehensive about treatment limitation because they already feel that they have restricted access to care, and thus are hesitant to give the health-care system an additional reason to withhold care[11]. Further, elders commonly do not complete an advance directive because they feel they can rely on others, in particular their families, to make decisions for them, and, in fact, expect family members to help make complex health-care decisions. Thus, for some elders, the view of autonomy that stems from the individual and is expressed through a legal document does not reflect how they prefer to make health-care decisions. For these elders, decision making may require a broader family perspective that includes considerations of family burdens of care or expectations that a particular family

member (for example, a son or daughter) is the appropriate decision maker[12]. When an elder is cared for by family at home or is a long-time nursing home resident, family members and clinicians who know the patient can ensure that the patient's vision of autonomy is supported. However, modern medical practice often involves transitions between settings, through which neither the knowledge of the patient nor explicit information about the patient's end-of-life care preferences in advance directives are transferred.

Inconsistencies in care between settings often result from the patient's inability to communicate, lack of uniformity in advance directives or advance directive policies, fear of liability on the part of the institution, physician, and other health-care providers, and absence of an advance directive. Even when advance directives exist and are accessible, limitations due to ambiguous language or the lack of specific directions to apply to the situation at hand can restrict their applicability. In situations of unclear patient preferences, nursing home staff may transfer residents to hospitals or emergency medical technicians, and may administer cardiopulmonary resuscitation (CPR), although this may be contrary to the patient's wishes. A number of strategies are available to combat the lack of continuity of care and breaches of support for patient aunonomy. Primary care physicians should encourage patients to designate a specific health-care proxy or surrogate who, depending on state law, can be empowered to speak for the patient when the patient is unable to do so. Further, improved communication between health-care professionals and institutions is necessary. For example, primary care clinicians can work with local hospitals to create mechanisms to ensure that advance directives completed in outpatient settings can be easily transferred to the in-patient setting when necessary.

## Withholding or withdrawing life-sustaining treatment

While patient preferences expressed in advance directives may outline an approach to a patient's care, at some point decisions about treatment plans must consider withholding or withdrawing life-sustaining interventions. Patients have a right to refuse treatment even if it is life-sustaining[13]. Clinicians often distinguish between withholding and withdrawing. It may seem morally and conceptually easier to withhold a procedure, such as mechanical ventilation, when the outcome of procedure initiation is less certain, than to withdraw treatment; while a treatment may not provide meaningful outcomes, treatment withdrawal may clearly result in death. The timing of decisions may make distictions between withdrawal and withholding seem relevant. Withholding can occur relatively suddenly if the patient goes into cardiac arrest. Withdrawing may be a gradual process and involve the administration of analgesics or sedatives while removing treatments. In practice, withdrawing is documented more frequently than withholding[14,15]. Physicians can become morally, legally and even psychologically committed to a treatment's completion, once started[14], particularly when an intervention has been used for a long time. Thus, intervention withdrawal tends to occur more commonly for treatments that are invasive, expensive, or scarce, or lead to a quick death once withdrawn, and tends to occur less often when treatments have been in place for a period of time or for the management of iatrogenic complications[16]. For example, physicians may feel 'committed' to ventilation or dialysis support, even though the treatment fails clearly to benefit the patient. Treatment continuation may even cause patients to receive unwanted treatments despite their ethical and legal rights or that of their surrogates to refuse life-prolonging interventions. Health-care professionals, including physicians and nurses, often lack training with regard to the clinical aspects of withdrawing intensive life-sustaining treatment, such as palliation of dyspnea. Such skills are necessary to provide effective end-of-life care.

Despite the common use of the terms in practice, the definitional distinction between withholding and withdrawing lacks logical validity and moral relevance. All treatment decisions contain some of the elements of withholding or withdrawal. The morally and legally relevant fact is that the outcome is the patient's death, irrespective of whether a life-sustaining treatment was withheld or withdrawn – a right that is supported by legal precedent[17].

## Artificial nutrition and hydration

Within the context of decisions to withdraw or withhold care, decisions about artificial nutrition and hydration often raise special concerns. Legally, lines and tubes are medical procedures subject to the same benefit–burden analysis as other technical interventions such as dialysis or mechanical ventilation; surrogates and patients have the right to refuse them as with any medical treatment[18]. At the same time, providing food and water is felt by some to be a moral duty and an essential form of supportive care[19]. The idea of food and water is emotionally comforting to a family in their caring for a dying patient[13]. Decisions to forego nutrition and hydration commonly concern patients with moderate-to-severe loss of cognitive function due to Alzheimer's disease or dementia, strokes resulting in loss of ability to swallow, end-stage diseases (such as metastatic cancer), or end-stage organ failure and treatment complications (such as infection, aspiration pneumonia)[13]. Such situations, in which a family already carries a heavy emotional burden, are made worse by the emotional feelings often connected to food and water.

In the clinical setting, the eating process is a human contact quite different from intravenous gastrostomy or jejunostomy feedings. Continued intervention may result in fluid overload and significant discomfort, whereas death after withdrawal may be more comfortable. Understanding and evaluating the reasons offered to forego artificial hydration and nutrition, and thus withhold or withdraw life-sustaining treatment, are essential to providing effective end-of-life care. Clinicians, patients and family members must consider when artificial nutrition and hydration may prolong dying and patient suffering, acknowledge that these treatments may lead to poor quality of life, and thus make the more humane choice to allow the patient to die.

## Do-not-resuscitate orders

Do-not-resuscitate (DNR) orders are recommended for most terminally ill patients[20] and so require consideration in end-of-life care. People of very advanced age or with multiple advanced chronic illnesses who suffer an unwitnessed, out-of-hospital cardiac arrest, have restorative success approaching zero. Even for witnessed arrests, a return to earlier functioning is unlikely, making the success rate of CPR administered in nursing homes 0–5%[21].

A DNR order does not exclude or prohibit use of other medically suitable interventions and patients and families must be counselled as to what a DNR actually means for the patient's care. CPR success depends on how quickly it is administered after cardiac arrest, the skill of the resuscitation providers, access to a cardiac monitor, the patient's general health and well-being and the underlying medical conditions. Although CPR may restore life with effective circulation after a cardiac arrest in some patients, CPR is often unsuccessful in patients with advanced disease, and contravenes the concept of a gentle or dignified death. Elders often have mistaken perceptions of the effectiveness of CPR and poor understanding of the procedure based on television or popular media. Some studies have shown that, when elders are fully informed about the low probability of restorative success and the actual steps that occur in CPR, such as chest compression and the potential for cracked ribs in frail elders, they opt for DNR status over CPR[22]. Nevertheless, clinicians often fail to discuss CPR comprehensively[22]. Fully informed communication about end-of-life care options must include comprehensive discussion of CPR, other medical interventions and palliative care options.

Unlike most medical treatments, a presumption in favor of sustaining life exists legally, ethically and medically, making CPR the correct course of treatment unless a DNR order is in place, or unless the treatment is refused or deemed medically futile. Therefore, recommendations about CPR should be clear and definitive so the patient or surrogate, their families and other health-care providers (such as nursing home nurse aides) understand the decision and have the opportunity to ask questions. To the extent possible, a DNR decision should be made with the support and assistance of members of the care team and family to stave off potential conflicts at the last moment. The DNR order must reflect the patient's preferences, values, and beliefs, and be careful not to impose the physician's value judgments or the surrogate's wishes. Finally, consulting with social workers, spiritual guidance counselors, or ethics committees, supports sound and just decisions and ensures that the patient's wishes are respected[23].

## Futility

Decisions to withhold or withdraw care may be prompted not only by desires to focus on quality of life but also by recognition that some treatments may be futile. Consideration of treatment futility may be more common in geriatrics, because older people have limited life expectancies[24]. In terms of justice, ethicists argue that physicians have a responsibility to avoid harm to patients that may result from providing futile treatment as well as larger social concerns that wasting futile treatments limits the availability of scarce resources for use by others for whom treatments would be effective. If futility were a straightforward empirical assessment, many end-of-life decisions potentially could be easier. Unfortunately, while some futility judgements are justified, applying the concept in practice may not be an appropriate tactic, bacause futility judgments are often fraught with 'confusion, inconsistency and controversy'[1]. Nevertheless, the concept is worthy of discussion because the term and the concerns about futile treatments often inform considerations about end-of-life care in the elderly.

### Strict and loose definitions of futility

Lo has offered definitions of futility[1] that could be applied to end-of-life care for elders. These definitions include:

(1) *A small probability of success exists with the treatment*. The difficulty is in determining an appropriate cut-off point (for example, 1 vs. 5%) for futility in this probabilistic approach. Even if a quantitative threshold is stated, disagreement between patients and their surrogates may result, because no single probability can be applied to define an unacceptable risk in every potential set of circumstances. In addition, although a probability may be small, it still may be considered worthwhile. The concern then becomes how to measure a small probability of survival, especially as data regarding effectiveness of clinical interventions in elders and especially the oldest old are often unavailable.

(2) *Physicians do not believe the treatment will succeed in achieving any desired goals*. This determination raises controversial value judgements. Patients or family members may desire treatment to achieve non-medical, short-term goals, such as allowing family from far distances to see the patient prior to death. In such circumstances, physicians may have a moral duty to act with compassion and sustain life despite the lack of a legal duty to do so. Experts generally agree that patients should be informed in a comforting matter if even a small chance of success exists, because of the need to support fully autonomous decision making on the part of patients or health-care proxies. This definition of futility, however, can be used to guide treatment choices for patients when palliative care becomes the most humane treatment approach[10].

(3) *The patient's quality of life is not acceptable*. Treatments may be termed futile when patients, family members, or clinicians judge the patient's quality of life unacceptable, as when the patient is permanently unconscious and will never regain cognitive functioning. However, use of this definition by physicians exclusively to guide end-of-life decision making runs the risk of paternalistically imposing the physician's values upon patients. Advocates for the disabled and other vulnerable populations, such as the elderly, oppose the quality of life criterion as being discriminatory and disguising value judgements about the value of the lives of those less able-bodied. Moreover, competent elderly patients, having learned to cope with chronic illness and having found ways to enjoy life, tend to regard their own quality of life more highly than their family does. Patients with Alzheimer's disease who are incompetent and cannot communicate, but who do not appear to be suffering, create complex quality-of-life judgements for their family and physician[1].

(4) *The expected efforts and resources required outweigh prospective benefits*. The issue is whether the benefits to the patient are worth the costs to society as a whole. This consideration recognizes arguments about rationing, in which cost rather than benefit becomes the deciding factor and in which treating patients with poor prognoses of survival may deny other patients with better prognoses form receiving treatments[25]. Use of this criterion may appear to have an objective basis, but most implications implicit in the definition make it a poor definition to use for final determination of when treatments should or should not be applied for particular patients.

Concerns about applications of futility of patient care make futility only one of many points to consider in making decisions for patients at the end of life. The principle of beneficence speaks to the physician's obligation to do what is best for the patient. Beneficent care requires attention to both technical expertise as well as compassionate care, and allows for greater leniency in the physicians' response to patient or surrogate requests for interventions decided as futile, especially when death is imminent. Adequate knowledge of clinical medicine and biomedical science is as important as a caring approach to the patient.

In practice, physicians who are concerned that they are being asked to support futile treatment should focus on ongoing communication, consultation with ethics committees and second opinions from colleagues to help minimize potential mistakes in futility judgements, keep value judgments in check and simultaneously protect the professional and moral integrity of physician and patient autonomy. Keeping the patient informed and discussing the intervention's futility with the patient or surrogate is an important ethical and legal obligation and the best approach. Such discussions are usually beneficial to patients or surrogates and reinforce the principles of care, including respect for patients. Most patients or surrogates will eventually support the physicians' judgement[1] and appreciate unambiguous and compassionate communications and recommendations.

## Euthanasia and physician-assisted suicide

In the broadest sense, euthanasia, physician-assisted suicide, and decisions to withhold or withdraw life-sustaining treatment share common objectives such as relief of pain and suffering and respect for patient autonomy. The importance of these issues in end-of-life care for elders is highlighted by ethical, legal, political, and societal trends that frame the debate along with religious and philosophical beliefs[26,27].

Active euthanasia, also called mercy killing, causes death and ends suffering by intentionally administering medication directly to end the patient's life[20]. Euthanasia is generally categorized in three ways: voluntary, when a patient requests it; involuntary, when a patient expresses opposition; and non-voluntary, when a patient has lost capacity and cannot make decisions or express his or her wishes[1,27]. Involuntary euthanasia, while practiced in the form of lethal injections for death-row inmates, is always immoral if considered as part of a health-care plan. As respect for patient autonomy is potentially the only acceptable justification for active assistance in dying, non-voluntary euthanasia is not an acceptable practice[1].

The distinction between euthanasia and physician-assisted suicide involves the physician providing to the patient a lethal dose of medication, upon the patient's request, with the intent to allow the patient to end his or her own life[20]. The patient independently must perform the final act. Physician assistance in dying may range from providing the patient with information about committing suicide to prescribing medication. Because the patient must carry out the deed, concerns about compelling a patient against his or her wishes and abusing the powers associated with being a physician and the physician's role are lessened, although still a potential consideration. Still, being relieved of the moral responsibility for the suicidal act does not relieve the physician of further moral responsibility in physician-assisted suicide. Each situation necessitates careful consideration of the intent, motivation, justification, and results of the decision. Again, as with most end-of-life decisions, discussion with the patient and his or her family is critical and allows for more effective and meaningful palliative care practices[1].

In practice, a physician is not, however, assisting with suicide if the physician provides treatment to relieve pain and suffering even if the patient's death might be hastened[20]. In such circumstances, the underlying illness, not the treatment provided or withheld, is the cause of the patient's death. The distinction is useful in practice between 'killing', in the sense of euthanasia or physician-assisted suicide; versus 'allowing to die', in the sense of withholding or withdrawing care or providing high doses of narcotics or sedatives to relieve pain, even if they may also result in patient death. However, many philosophers consider the distinction problematic. These authors find the distinction between 'killing' and 'allowing to die' not to be a sound basis for moral judgement. Second, the idea that the disease, rather than the withholding/withdrawing of treatment, causes the patient's death may not be tenable, since death may not have occurred in the absence of this factor. Third, assisted suicide and allowing death cannot be distinguished by the intent of the patient. A patient who is refusing treatments and who has provided adequate informed consent also recognizes death as an outcome and thus the distinction lacks moral weight. Conversely, the United States Supreme Court has held that there is a rational distinction between killing and allowing to die[28,29], and that those who ask their doctors to commit assisted suicide and those who forego treatment are not similarly situated[30].

Concerns about active euthanasia and assisted suicide should not make physicians reluctant to relieve distressful symptoms in terminally ill patients. Indeed, fears that terminal distress will not be adequately relieved impel some people to seek active euthanasia and assisted suicide. Physicians should continue to partner with patients and families to ensure that patients are fully informed of consequences and feel more assured that they will not be abandoned when the plan of care moves from curative to palliative.

## Justifying physician-assisted suicide

Arguments in favor of physician-assisted suicide focus on showing respect for individual autonomy[1], recognizing the right of competent people to choose the course of their life and death, the importance of comfort and relief of suffering, and a justice argument for treating 'like cases alike'. If competent, terminally ill patients can refuse treatment and thus hasten death, suicide becomes the only option for patients where treatment refusal will not suffice to hasten death. Physician-assisted suicide then serves as a compassionate alternative to unbearable suffering since physical and emotional suffering cannot always be relieved[1]. Although society has a strong interest in preserving life, that interest may diminish when a person is terminally ill and has reached his or her 'closing biography', has said goodbye to family and wishes to exit 'on his or her own terms', usually described as death with dignity. Personal liberty is limited when there is a complete prohibition on assisted death, warranting the allowing of physician-assisted suicide in certain cases. In circumstances where suicide would occur with or without assistance,

physician-assisted suicide allows a more humane and controlled method of end-of-life decision-making[1]. Religious tolerance requires respect for personal objections to all killing, but religious tolerance also requires us to respect those whose beliefs support a right to end their own lives, especially in the context of intractable suffering and ultimately terminal illness. The political debates in numerous States and in the US Congress demonstrate the depth of feeling on both sides.

## Physician-assisted suicide and the elderly

As life expectancy grows, many older people face years of isolation and decline. Some may want to assert a right to a dignified death on their own terms, making physician-assisted suicide an option. This phenomenon may be responsible for the increase in suicide rates among elderly men in the USA. On the other hand, abuses could occur in this vulnerable population. Pressure could result, including influencing elderly people to choose physician-assisted suicide rather than more expensive palliative care options. Families may choose physician-assisted suicide to relieve caregiving burdens, and even encourage physicians to impose value judgements in quality of life on the patient or surrogate.

In one study comparing attitudes of elderly out-patients and their families towards physician-assisted suicide, family members held more favorable attitudes toward physician-assisted suicide than patients in cases of terminal illness (59.3 vs. 39.9%), chronic illness (25.3 vs. 18.2%), and mental incompetence (55.6 vs. 34%)[31]. Moreover, family members poorly predicted patient attitudes towards physician assisted suicide. Therefore, focusing on patient's interests rather than family preferences or physician moral judgements becomes an important direction and goal for end-of-life care decisions.

## Future considerations

Future technological advances may further heighten the ethical issues related to ongoing and end-of-life care for older women. Overall, rates of disability amongst the elderly seem to be declining at an increasingly rapid pace. In 1982, the US disabled older population totalled 7.1 million, but by 1999, an acceleration in the reduction in the rates of disability resulted in a lower overall number of people with disability (7 million) than there had been in 1982[32]. Numbers of individuals residing in nursing homes have also dropped significantly in the past 10 years. Reasons for the reductions in disability rates might include: improvements in maternal nutrition and public health early in the last century; better control of childhood infectious diseases; increases in the education and finances of succeeding generations reaching old age; health-related behavioral changes such as smoking cessation; improved control

and treatment of such diseases as hypertension and heart disease; development and use of new surgical interventions; and the impact of newly developed drugs[32]. Whether these rates of declining disability ease conflicts over intergenerational resource transfers but reduce the expected costs of care, or whether the resources necessary to enable further reductions in disability rates increase conflicts, has yet to be seen. In either case, the difficulties inherent in making end-of-life decisions for the young old (aged 65–84) and the old old (85+) will continue. It is up to the physician to assist patients, family and other members of the clinical care team to prepare them for these emotionally fraught decisions in order to achieve whatever the older women defines as 'the good death'.

# References

1. Lo B. *Resolving Ethical Dilemmas: A Guide for Clinicians*. Baltimore, MD: Williams and Wilkins, 1995

2. OWL-National: Older Women's League Older Women and Poverty [Web Page]. 2001; Available at http://www.owl-national.org/poverty.html. (Accessed 4 October 2001)

3. Bierman AS, Clancy CM. Making capitated Medicare work for women: policy and research challenges. *Womens Health Issues* 2000;10: 59–69

4. Fulton Picot S, Powell LL. Caregiver burden. In Mezey MD, Berkman BJ, Callahan CM, *et al.*, eds. *The Encyclopedia of Elder Care*. New York: Springer, 2001:112–14

5. Menon SC, Pandey DK, Morgenstern LB. Critical factors determining access to acute stroke care. *Neurology* 1998:51:427–32

6. Yancik R, Wesley MN, Ries LA, *et al.* Effect of age and comorbidity in postmenopausal breast cancer patients aged 55 years and older. *J Am Med Assoc* 2001;285:885–92

7. McMahon LF Jr, Wolfe RA, Huang S, *et al.* Racial and gender variation in use of diagnostic colonic procedures in the Michigan Medicare population. *Med Care* 1999;37: 712–17

8. Garg PP, Furth SL, Fivush BA, Powe NR. Impact of gender on access to the renal transplant waiting list for pediatric and adult patients. *J Am Soc Nephrol* 2000;11:958–64

9. Beauchamp TL, Childress JF. *Principles of Biomedical Ethics*. New York: Oxford University Press, 1994

10. Cassel CK. Philosophical and ethical issues in geriatrics. In Kelly WN, ed. *Textbook of Internal Medicine*, 4th edn. Philadelphia: Lippincott-Williams and Wilkins, 2000:3127–31

11. Culigari AM, Miller T, Sobol J. Race and health care: an American dilemma? *N Engl J Med* 1996;155:1893–8

12. Wolf SM, ed. *Feminism and Bioethics: Beyond Reproduction*. New York: Oxford University Press, 1996

13. Ackerman RJ. Withholding and withdrawing life-sustaining treatment. *Am Fam Physician* 2000;62:1555–60

14. Ahronheim JC, Moreno, J, Zuckerman C. *Ethics in Clinical Practice*, 1st edn. Boston: Little, Brown, 1994

15. Luce JM. Withholding and withdrawal of life support: ethical, legal, and clinical aspects. *New Horizon* 1997;5:30–7

16. Brody H, Campbell ML, Faber-Langendon J, Ogle KS. Withdrawing intensive life-sustaining treatment – recommendations for compassionate clinical management. *N Engl J Med* 1997;336:652–7

17. Gostin LO. Deciding life and death in the courtroom. From Quinlan to Cruzan, Glucksberg, and Vacco – a brief history and analysis of constitutional protection of the

'right to die'. *J Am Med Assoc* 1997;278: 1523–8

18. Annas GJ, Law SA, Rosenblatt RE, Wing KR. *American Health Law*. Boston: Little, Brown, 1990

19. Pearlman RA, Back AL. Ethical issues in geriatric care. In Hazzard WR, Blass JP, eds. *Principles of Geriatric Medicine and Gerontology*, 4th edn, vol 40. New York: MCGraw-Hill, 1999:557–70

20. Basta LL. A graceful exit life and death on your own terms. New York: Plenum Press, 1996

21. Tolle S, Tilden VP, Nelson CA, Dunn PM. A prospective study of the efficacy of the physician order form for life-sustaining treatment. *J Am Geriatr Soc* 1998;46:1097–102

22. Levin JR, Wenger NS, Ouslander JG, *et al*. Life-sustaining treatment decisions for nursing home residents: who discusses, who decides and what is decided? *J Am Geriatr Soc* 1999; 47:82–7

23. Agich GJ, Arroliga AC. Appropriate use of DNR orders: a practical approach. *Cleveland Clin J Med* 2000;67:392–400

24. van der Steen JT, Muller MT, Ooms ME, van der Wal G, Ribbe MW. Decisions to treat or not to treat pneumonia in demented psychogeriatric nursing home patients: development of a guideline. *J Med Ethics* 2000;26: 114–20

25. Schneiderman LJ, Jecker JS, Jonsen AR. Medical futility: its meaning and ethical implications. *Ann Intern Med* 1990;112:949–54

26. Scanlon C. Assisted suicide: the wrong answer. *Home Care Provider* 1997;2:159–61

27. Yong EWD. Physician-assisted suicide: where to draw the line. *Cambridge Q Healthcare Ethics* 2000;9:407–10

28. Burt RA. The Supreme Court speaks – not assisted suicide but a constitutional right to palliative care. *N Engl J Med* 1997;337:1234–6

29. Annas GJ. The bell tolls for a constitutional right to physician-assisted suicide. *N Engl J Med* 1997;337:1098–103

30. Sulmasy DP, Ury WA, Ahronheim JC, *et al*. Publication of papers on assisted suicide and terminal sedation. *Ann Intern Med* 2000;133: 564–6

31. Koenig HG, Wildman-Hanlon D, Schmader K. Attitudes of elderly patients and their families toward physician assisted suicide. *Arch Intern Med* 1996;156:2240–8

32. Manton KG, Gu X. Changes in the prevalence of chronic disability in the United States black and nonblack population above age 65 from 1982 to 1999. *Proc Natl Acad Sci USA* 2001; 98:6354–9

# Epilogue

This textbook defines and focuses upon the geripause, which is the life-phase for women that follows the postmenopause. The collaboration of both gerontologists and gynecologists has presented us with the unique opportunity to describe the results of both aging and estrogen depletion, and to distinguish between the two when approaching the care of the older patient. Using data extracted from the populations in several monitored countries, major health eras for a woman can be characterized (see Figure 2, Chapter 3). Following the reproductive period, premenopause has been defined as spanning from the age of 42 until approximately 51.4 years; perimenopause occurs from premenopause until 1 year after the menopause; and postomenopause begins thereafter.

Geripause, a term introduced by one of the authors (B.A.E), begins at about the age of 65 and can be divided into an early phase (65–85 years) and a late phase (85 years and older). The start of the early phase was defined endocrinologically as the time when elevated gonadrotropins, follicle stimulating hormone, and luteinizing hormone, begin to decline. It appears that clinical and basic biochemical changes and important clinical events in a woman's health also begin to occur.

Beyond the therapeutic interventions outlined in this textbook, the postmenopausal woman should maintain a healthy life style. The basic rules are:

(1) normalization of weight;

(2) dietary care;

(3) regular exercise;

(4) smoking cessation;

(5) control of alcohol or drug consumption; and

(6) dental care.

The chapters in this textbook include a selection of topics that deals with many of the very important issues that numerous health care providers will increasingly see in their practices. While not necessarily comprehensive, we believe that the areas covered bestow a solid foundation that will allow providers to improve and enhance their care of the elderly. We also hope that, by defining the geripause, this textbook will impart a perspective that will facilitate new advances in the care of the postmenopausal and geripausal woman that ultimately add to the quality and quantity of their remaining years.

Bernard A. Eskin, MS, MD
Bruce R. Troen, MD

# Index